CONCEPTION,
PREGNANCY
AND BIRTH

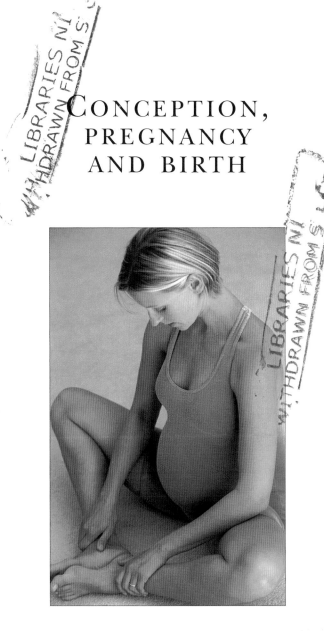

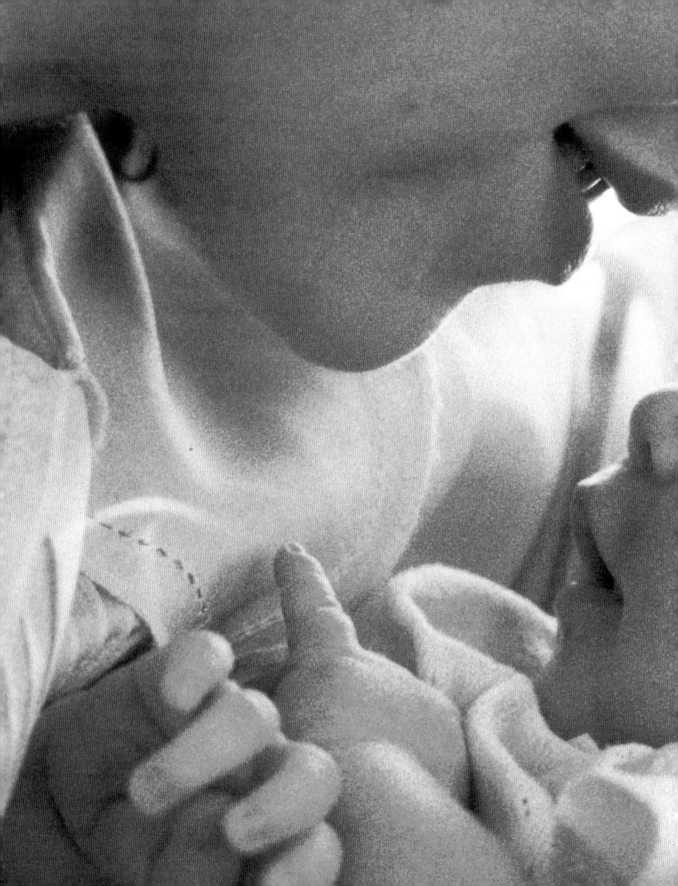

CONCEPTION, PREGNANCY AND BIRTH

Dr. Miriam Stoppard

DORLING KINDERSLEY
London • New York • Sydney
www.dk.com

For my girlfriends

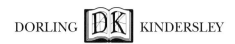

DORLING KINDERSLEY

LONDON, NEW YORK, SYDNEY, DELHI, PARIS
MUNICH AND JOHANNESBURG

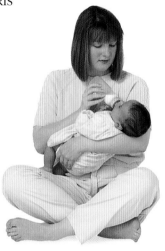

ORIGINAL EDITION
Created and Produced by
CARROLL & BROWN LIMITED

REVISED EDITION

Senior Managing Editor	Corinne Roberts
Senior Managing Art Editor	Lynne Brown
Senior Editor	Nicola Adamson
Senior Art editor	Karen Ward
Project editor	Claire Cross
DTP Designer	Rajen Shah
Production	Martin Crowshaw

First published by Dorling Kindersley in 1993

This revised edition published in Great Britain in 2000
by Dorling Kindersley Limited
9 Henrietta Street, London WC2E 8PS
Reprinted 2001

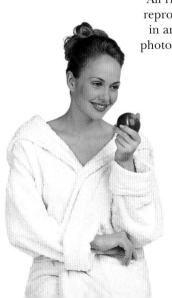

A CIP catalogue record of this book is
available from the British Library

ISBN 0 7513 3608 4

Reproduced by Colourscan, Singapore
Printed and bound in China
by L.Rex

see our complete catalogue at
www.dk.com

PREFACE

This revised edition of *Conception, Pregnancy and Birth* feels like a completely new book. It's had, so to speak, a thorough spring clean. Every page has been examined and brought bang up to date. New topics have been inserted so that the content includes the latest medical advances and newest theories. Just as important, I've re-written many passages to reflect the concerns of today's parents. In the light of these changes it seemed right to give the book a new look and we've worked hard on design and presentation to achieve a contemporary feel. The book was always big but it's bigger. This edition has two new chapters and several new sections, which any modern enquiring reader would rightly expect to find in a book on pregnancy and birth.

New fertility section

Childlessness is something fewer couples have to accept. The field of assisted conception becomes ever more sophisticated, offering undreamt of possibilities to couples who find it hard to conceive. But inevitably, the increasing sophistication of assisted reproductive technology (ART) means increasing complexity which is difficult even for the average doctor to get her mind around. I hope this large new section will lay out for the couple with fertility problems a clear road map of the successive stages of investigation and treatment they will be called on to undergo in their desire to have a baby by ART. It's never easy and the commitment of both partners will go a long way towards mitigating the emotional burden of so intimate and extended an enquiry.

New chapter for fathers

From the outset this book catered for fathers, to some extent at least, but not as much as I'd have wished. There were passages on most topics putting Dad's point of view and giving information which I hoped would be especially useful to expectant fathers. I've gone further in this edition and gathered together a whole chapter that any man, expectant or not, might be interested to dip into.

New chapter on special deliveries

Most labours are straightforward, but a few are not and require some kind of medical intervention to help the baby out. Forewarned is forearmed if only not to be taken by surprise. So I've written, reassuringly I hope, a new chapter on special deliveries outlining what you might expect to happen if your labour started to veer away from your birth plan – something everyone has to be prepared for in any event.

Notwithstanding all this updating my overall aim in this book remains the same. That you should have the birth you both want, in the circumstances you both want, helped by carers who have your needs and the needs of your new baby uppermost.

CONTENTS

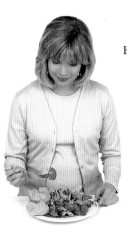

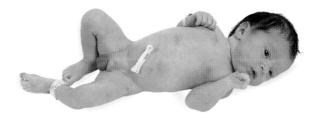

INTRODUCTION

PREPARING FOR PREGNANCY

As we find out more about what can damage ova and sperm, it seems sensible to prepare for pregnancy by changing to a more healthy lifestyle. Giving up smoking and alcohol at least three months prior to conception is a good idea for everyone. A healthy and fit body is the best possible place to conceive and carry a fetus to term. Not everything, of course, is straightforward: genes and chromosomes may be imperfect and fertilization may be difficult, but many of these problems have now been identified and some of them can be successfully treated.

One in six couples has difficulty conceiving but that doesn't necessarily mean you'll never have a baby. Most couples who think they're infertile are only subfertile and with help can conceive successfully. At least half of all problems with conception are due to male fertility problems, a fact some men have difficulty coming to terms with, but that simple fact means that infertility can only be investigated as a couple. And the first test to be done is semen analysis. Couples embarking on fertility treatment deserve and should get counselling support right from the start – their own doctor can refer them to a counsellor specialized in dealing with the stress of infertility. There is a bewildering number of treatments available to treat all kinds of infertility which is why I've greatly augmented the chapter dealing with fertility testing and treatment from simple drugs therapies to the latest complex assisted reproductive technologies (ART).

YOUR DEVELOPING BABY

For convenience, the sequence of developmental stages can be roughly divided into three phases, the first, second, and third trimesters. These are so divided because certain physiological changes occur to mother and baby in each of the three stages. In the first trimester your baby's organs form, in the second these organs become complex, and in the third they grow in size. For you, the first trimester is when your body becomes primed for pregnancy: the breasts grow, your internal organs adapt, and the muscles and ligaments start to slacken in preparation for labour. High levels of pregnancy hormones bring on pregnancy sickness, the desire to go to the lavatory more often, and tenderness of the breasts. During the second trimester the body goes into a phase of consolidation. The third trimester sees your body preparing for delivery and making sure that your baby is growing healthily.

PREPARING FOR FATHERHOOD

Many traditional stereotypes of fatherhood are outdated. Nowadays even the most hardworking Dad is considered an incomplete man if he hasn't the time and inclination to share childcare and be there for his kids. On the other hand, there are doubts – among more laddish elements at least – that greater involvement in child rearing would somehow be feminizing, and that sits uneasily with many men. The result is that some men are becoming disillusioned and anxious. Men feel they're on the horns of a dilemma; society, especially mothers, seem to know what sort of chap they want New Dad to be, but often men feel driven into a corner by being pressured into a hitherto unfamiliar role. Long ago it was established that children can do perfectly well, indeed can thrive, with only one parent of either gender. So even though some children do very well without a father, perhaps we need to encourage New Dads by offering fathers a proper New Deal. For this reason I've included a whole new chapter in this edition covering all aspects of fatherhood and fathering in the hope that, after reading it men will feel free to liberate their fathering instincts.

THE BIRTH OF YOUR CHOICE

Labour and birth can be managed in the way you choose. There are many decisions for you to make and you should be aware of all your options. In theory, it's possible to have exactly the kind of birth that you want, but this involves extensive reading, soul searching, and discussion with your partner. You'll also have to talk things over with your nursing and medical attendants so that any difficulties that might arise later on can be dealt with. Home birth is becoming more widely accepted and is something to which you can now give serious consideration. Alternatively you can choose a hospital and a team of midwives that provide the facilities, the atmosphere, and the cooperative approach that you prefer. It is extremely useful to make a birth plan outlining the kind of birth you want and, by discussing it with your attendants, you can achieve your aims. It's up to women and their partners to take a more assertive role in the way the delivery and birth of their baby will be handled.

FOOD IN PREGNANCY

Eating healthily in pregnancy is mainly a question of eating a wide variety of foods rich in essential nutrients. Emphasize fresh fruit and vegetables, whole grains, and raw food in your diet and ensure that you have a healthy intake of protein by eating fish, poultry, and low-fat dairy products, with red meat and eggs now and then. Fish is also a good source of vitamin B12 and vitamin A, which is also found in green and yellow vegetables. And if you bear in mind that your baby uses iron up so fast that it needs fresh supplies every day, you will remember to eat plenty of iron-rich foods, such as kidneys, apricots, raisins, prunes, red meat, and fish. Ideally a woman should start taking daily folic acid supplements three months ahead of getting pregnant and then all the way through pregnancy to avoid neural tube defects like spina bifida. So it makes sense to add folic acid-rich foods to your diet at all times – green leafy vegetables, nuts, and cereals.

A HEALTHY PREGNANCY

Regular exercise keeps you mentally and physically in good shape because exercise causes the body to release tranquillizing chemicals, helping you to relax, and soothing away tension. The fast circulation of the blood during exercise means that your body and your baby are well oxygenated. It is probable that labour will be easier and more comfortable if your muscles are in tone, and many of the exercises taught in antenatal classes, combined with relaxation and breathing techniques, will help to enable you to be more in touch with what is happening to you during labour and delivery. Learn to conserve energy, sleep as much as you can, and catnap whenever possible.

YOUR ANTENATAL CARE

Good antenatal care is usually rewarded with healthy mothers and babies. At the antenatal clinic, routine tests are done to spot potential problems, avoid them where possible, and enable treatment to be performed promptly. Special tests such as ultrasound scanning and amniocentesis are carried out for mothers and babies with special needs. The social and personal aspects of antenatal care are as important as the medical ones. Reassurance gained by talking to other mothers, doctors, and midwives helps you feel confident about labour and birth. The clinic provides an opportunity to ask questions, explore the different circumstances in which you can have your baby, and plan ahead for the kind of birth that you and your partner want.

CARING FOR YOUR UNBORN BABY

By being observant and aware, you can be in touch with your unborn baby throughout pregnancy. The first time that your baby communicates with you is when you feel fetal movements. Respond by talking to your unborn child. Babies have very sensitive hearing and at birth can recognize both their mother's and father's voice from simply having heard them as they were growing and developing in the uterus. It's not silly to talk and sing to your child, nor to massage it gently through your abdominal wall. Not all babies develop normally, but modern techniques are so advanced that we can even care for the developing fetus while still in utero. Advanced surgery can be undertaken while the baby is still inside you so that he has every chance of being born normal and healthy. Not all babies enjoy the perfect conditions for development but, even so, diabetic mothers and mothers with Rhesus incompatibility, for example, can, with careful monitoring and treatment, progress through pregnancy to a healthy and successful outcome.

COMMON COMPLAINTS

Very few women go through pregnancy without suffering minor complaints. In the main these are uncomfortable rather than serious. There is a group of complaints which are particular to pregnancy. Being prepared for them is half the battle in dealing with them, particularly if you are aware of the treatments that are available. The majority are easily dealt with and, for the most part, disappear within a specific length of time having no long-term effects.

MEDICAL EMERGENCIES

The risk of medical emergencies tends to be concentrated in the first and third trimesters of pregnancy. Nearly all of the classic emergencies are accompanied by classic symptoms, and should you experience any of them, you must call your doctor immediately. These symptoms would include severe abdominal pain, vaginal bleeding, a fever in excess of 100°F (37.8°C), severe nausea or vomiting, unremitting headache, blurred vision, swelling of the ankles, fingers and face, absence of fetal movement for more than 24 hours, and rupture of the membranes. In the first trimester most emergencies are associated with loss of the fetus due to haemorrhage or miscarriage, or to the blastocyst being misplaced, as in an ectopic pregnancy. Later on, an emergency might be precipitated by very high blood pressure leading to pre-eclamptic toxaemia, by recurrent late abortion, by Rhesus incompatibility, and by abnormalities of the placenta, such as placenta praevia. Nonetheless, the vast majority of babies are delivered safely.

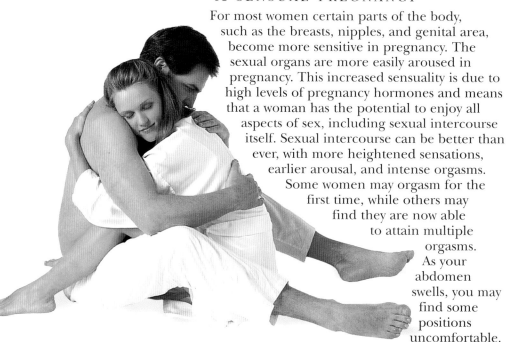

A SENSUAL PREGNANCY

For most women certain parts of the body, such as the breasts, nipples, and genital area, become more sensitive in pregnancy. The sexual organs are more easily aroused in pregnancy. This increased sensuality is due to high levels of pregnancy hormones and means that a woman has the potential to enjoy all aspects of sex, including sexual intercourse itself. Sexual intercourse can be better than ever, with more heightened sensations, earlier arousal, and intense orgasms. Some women may orgasm for the first time, while others may find they are now able to attain multiple orgasms. As your abdomen swells, you may find some positions uncomfortable.

GETTING READY FOR YOUR BABY

From the 36th week, nesting begins in earnest. There is much to do in terms of preparing the baby's room, choosing nursery equipment, buying the essential baby clothing, finalizing your baby's names, working out how long you're going to take off work, and what kind of care you will seek for your child, and for your other children. Opting to have your baby at home means that you must prepare a room for the birth and have all your equipment carefully chosen and organized. Draw up check lists, go to the hospital and make yourselves familiar with admission procedures so that you feel in control and free of anxiety.

MANAGING YOUR LABOUR

Labour is the culmination of your pregnancy and it can be divided into well-defined stages. Pre-labour is a time before labour during which you may experience dull backache or pass a "show". Your membranes may also rupture painlessly before true labour begins. The first stage of labour is entirely taken up with dilatation of the cervix to a size which will allow your baby to exit from the uterine cavity into the birth canal. This stage is usually straightforward, particularly if you remain mobile and, by maintaining an upright position, use the force of gravity to help the cervix to dilate. Very few labours are pain-free, but there are many methods and types of pain relief from which to choose. And some labours aren't straightforward so I'm devoting a whole chapter to "Special deliveries" in this new edition.

GETTING TO KNOW YOUR NEWBORN BABY

Establishing a relationship with your baby begins the second she is born and you and your partner should be left in private with a minimum of interruption. Parents who bond closely with their children are more constructive, more sympathetic parents. The importance of paternal bonding cannot be over-emphasized and your partner should be given the opportunity to hold his baby immediately after her birth. The first few days will be harder than you think. Feeding can take longer than you expect, as can your baby's daily care.

A routine is not always easy to set up but the guiding and unbreakable rule is that you take your lead from the baby. Parents of special-care babies who need to be nursed in hospital intensive care units, have no need to worry about being unable to bond with their babies. As long as parents, under the guidance of the nursing staff, become intimately involved in the day-to-day care of their baby, they should not suffer any disadvantages.

ADJUSTING TO PARENTHOOD

Getting to know your newborn baby is a thrilling experience, but don't be surprised if you feel a slight letdown at times. There are many adjustments to make and few of them are easy. Somehow you have to coax your baby to fit in with your established family routine, maintain the loving relationship with your partner, and attend to your baby's needs and constant demands for attention. Many women get bouts of sadness, and not just the "baby blues" which are so common in the first week after delivery. Much more serious is postnatal depression, which needs immediate attention from your doctor. The responsibilities of parenthood may weigh heavily upon you, but watching your baby grow and develop should bring more than enough joy to counteract the negative feelings which may occasionally creep in. Having time just for yourself will enable you to recharge your batteries, while time alone with your partner will help you to keep your relationship alive.

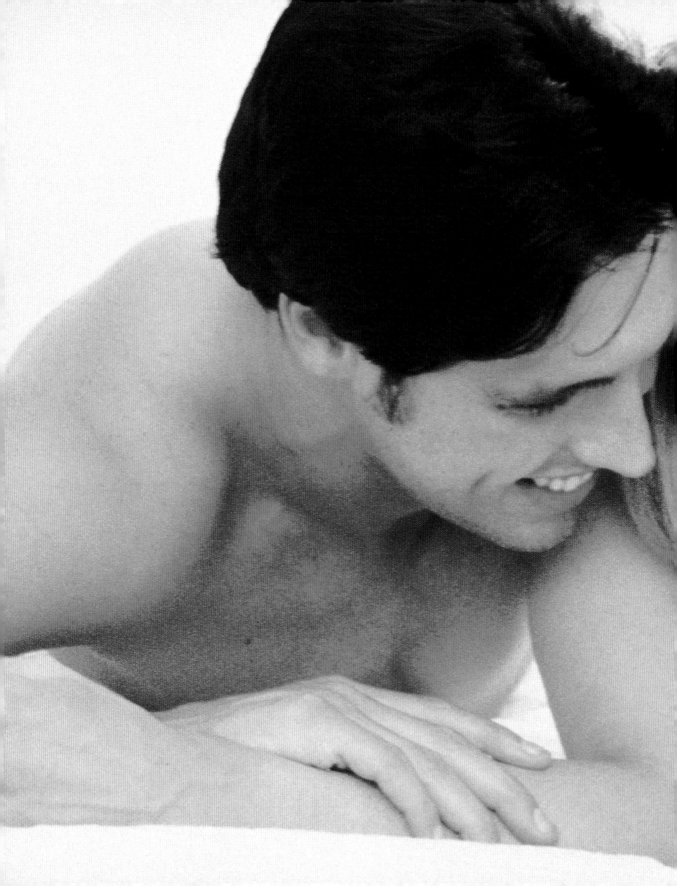

CHAPTER I

Preparing for PREGNANCY

As we find out more and more about ova and sperm and what makes them healthy, it seems common sense to prepare for pregnancy by changing to a healthy lifestyle. Not everything, of course, is always straightforward, but many of the problems surrounding conception have been identified and some can be treated.

Fit for parenthood

BELFAST PUBLIC LIBRARIES

A successful pregnancy and labour, and the birth of a healthy baby, are the responsibilities of both parents to an equal degree. A baby's health depends to a large extent on the health of her parents at the moment of conception, yet many couples do not plan for pregnancy with the same care as other important life events. Starting a family is a time of reassessment because becoming a parent will fundamentally change your life.

LIFESTYLE CONSIDERATIONS

Many things that we take for granted – who we are and what we do – will affect or be affected by a baby.

Time   Most people's lives are extremely busy and many new parents assume that their new baby will somehow fit in. They don't. Babies and children need a lot of time and attention, and parents will always have less time than they did before – for themselves, for each other, and for other people.

Costs The average experience is that you will spend 15–25 percent of your income, regardless of how much you earn or the size of your family, on child-related expenses such as clothing and equipment. But there are also hidden costs such as heating, transportation, and what you may give up for your children – meals out, holidays, and, perhaps, some of your ambitions.

Relationships It is not only your relationship with your partner that changes when you have a baby. Your relationship with your parents will alter, and you may find that you grow away from your childless friends and seek new friendships with other parents who are going through the same experiences as you.

Smoking This is one of the most damaging factors to the health of your unborn baby and the major cause of avoidable health problems. The associated risks include miscarriage and stillbirth, placental damage, a low birthweight baby that fails to thrive, and a higher risk of fetal abnormalities. Smoking can contribute to a low sperm count; a man who smokes while his partner is pregnant may also damage his unborn baby's health via passive smoking. Children of heavy smokers, whose development was tested at five, seven, and eleven years of age, were found to suffer from impaired growth and learning difficulties.

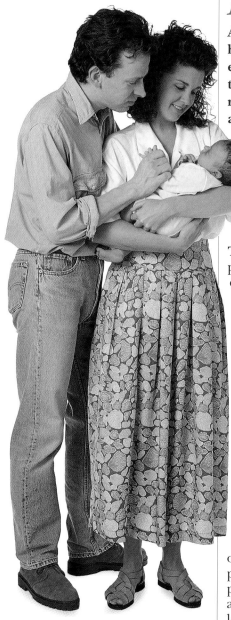

Prepared parents
Happy, healthy parents make happy, healthy children, so make sure you are fit for parenthood before you start trying for a baby.

Alcohol This is a poison that may damage the sperm and ovum before conception, as well as the developing embryo. The main risks to the unborn baby are mental retardation, retarded growth, and damage to the brain and nervous system – well documented as fetal alcohol syndrome. Alcohol can also cause stillbirth.

Research suggests that the effect of alcohol is variable: some heavy drinkers seem to get away with it, while some women who drink only a small amount don't. The only certainty is that there will be no effect if alcohol is avoided. Women tend to have a lower tolerance than men, and have a higher proportion of fat to water, so alcohol can become very highly concentrated in the blood that nourishes your developing baby.

Drugs Over-the-counter medicines should only be taken when necessary, and social drugs should definitely be cut out before you conceive. Marijuana interferes with the normal production of male sperm, and the effects take three to nine months to wear off. Hard drugs such as cocaine, heroin, and morphine can damage the chromosomes in the sperm and ovum, leading to abnormalities.

When syringes are shared, there is a high risk of contracting HIV, the virus that leads to AIDS. A mother can pass the HIV virus to her baby during pregnancy, which may lead to the baby being HIV positive in his own right (see p.19).

Diet and exercise Both are vital to your health and the health of your baby. Try to maintain a balanced diet that is low in animal fat, and to eat five portions of fresh fruit and vegetables daily. It's very important to make sure you have enough folic acid in your diet. This vitamin is known to be important in lowering the risk of neural tube defects, such as spina bifida, if taken at least three months before conception and for three months after. It's present in green leafy vegetables, cereals, and bread, and can also be taken in supplement form. Good eating habits should be coupled with regular exercise. Pregnancy puts a strain on the body, so the fitter you are beforehand, the better you'll cope.

Age Many women are delaying pregnancy until their 30s, and even 40s, and this is no more hazardous than being in your 20s as long as you are fit and healthy. Whatever your age, you are likely to have a normal pregnancy and birth, although some problems such as infertility and chromosomal defects, for example, Down's syndrome (see p.24), do become more frequent with the increasing age of both parents. Tests for chromosomal abnormalities are always offered to older women and to younger women who fall into a high risk group.

Hazards Be aware of your environment, both in and out of the home, and avoid anything that is potentially hazardous. What we eat, where we work, the places we travel to, and sometimes even the people we meet may be risky for a pregnant woman (see p.169).

STOPPING CONTRACEPTION

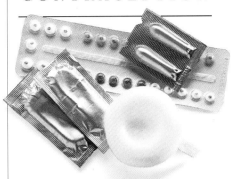

Barrier methods, such as the diaphragm and sheath, can be dispensed with immediately. However, if you are on the pill or are using an IUCD, a bit more forethought is required.

The pill It is probably advisable to stop taking the pill a month before trying to conceive, so that you have at least one normal menstrual period before becoming pregnant. However, there is some evidence to suggest that women are more fertile immediately after stopping the pill, so this could be the ideal time to try if you have previously suffered from low fertility or had a miscarriage.

If you think that you are pregnant while you are still taking the pill, consult your doctor immediately. Some forms of the pill contain a high dose of synthetic progesterone (called progestogen) that may interfere with development in the first weeks of life.

The intrauterine contraceptive device The IUCD, or coil, works by irritating the lining of the uterus so that the fertilized egg cannot implant. A very small number of women do become pregnant with the IUCD. In this case the IUCD is usually left in place as the risk of miscarriage is higher if removal is attempted. It usually comes out with the placenta after the birth.

TESTING YOUR URINE

If sugar is found in your urine it may mean you have diabetes or, as is more likely, that some sugar has leaked through your kidneys, whose threshold to sugar is lowered by your pregnant state. Further tests will need to be performed to make sure that this is indeed the case.

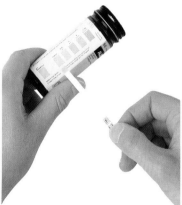

Testing urine
A chemically impregnated strip is dipped into a sample of your urine. It changes colour if sugar is present and the amount can be compared to a chart that shows glucose levels.

HEALTH CONSIDERATIONS

If you're a woman with a chronic long-term condition, such as diabetes mellitus, heart disease, or epilepsy, you should not be discouraged from having children. However, you must talk things over with your doctor before you become pregnant, so your pregnancy can be managed effectively.

Asthma The most common respiratory problem in mothers-to-be, this is usually controlled by inhalation of bronchodilator drugs and inhaled steroids. There seems to be little risk to the growing fetus from the medication, although thrush (see p.212), a condition which is often aggravated by pregnancy, can be a side-effect for the mother, and sometimes labour may be brought on prematurely.

If you are asthmatic, you need to take care of your lifestyle throughout pregnancy because stress and tension, as well as dust, pollen, and pollution, can cause breathlessness, which may put a further strain on your already hardworking heart.

Epilepsy From the momentary loss of consciousness to grand mal fits, epilepsy affects one in every 200 people. Research has found that pregnancy has a variable effect on the frequency and intensity of fits, with 50 percent of epileptic mothers unaffected, 40 percent slightly improved, and 10 percent worse.

During pregnancy, drug treatment will be continued but you will need to be seen frequently by a neurologist who can adjust your drug dosage. The drug phenytoin, often prescribed to control epilepsy, prevents absorption of folic acid. It is therefore very important to take high doses of folic acid supplements before you conceive as well as after to help lower the risk of birth defects (see p.17). However, most pregnant women can be changed over to sodium valproate which does not carry the same hazards. During labour, drugs may not be absorbed and medication should be carefully supervised to prevent fits recurring. If you suffer from epilepsy, discuss your situation with your doctor well before you hope to conceive.

Diabetes mellitus When the pancreas produces insufficient insulin to cope with glucose (sugar) levels in the body, diabetes results. Pregnancy hormones have an anti-insulin effect, which increases the severity of established diabetes, and can lead to the development of gestational diabetes in those with an underlying tendency. The urine of all mothers-to-be is routinely screened for sugar and ketones (the usual indicator of diabetes); a woman with a family background of diabetes should have a urine test before trying to conceive, and regular urine tests throughout pregnancy.

Diabetes can cause fetal heart and respiratory abnormalities, the baby to be very large, and complications for the mother ranging from chronic thrush to pre-eclampsia (see p.224). So it is important that insulin-dependent diabetic women have good control of their condition before conception, and their blood-sugar levels monitored closely with blood tests and urine tests.

Heart disease Women with a diagnosed condition will be given specialized advice according to its nature. However, as a general rule, it is advisable to avoid over-activity – try and rest each afternoon for at least two hours, and spend ten hours in bed at night. The majority of women with heart disease have easy spontaneous labours. During labour the additional strain on the heart is intermittent and, in total, is less than that imposed upon the heart in the third trimester. There is usually no reason to anticipate premature induction of labour or Caesarean section.

Kidney disease This does not necessarily preclude having children, but a pregnant woman with kidney disease must be carefully monitored. The commonest problem is recurrent urinary tract infection, but as long as the kidneys remove waste effectively, pregnancy will be allowed to continue, but if there is poor fetal growth, early induction of labour will be recommended. (Renal dialysis does pose a risk as the mother's kidneys are unlikely to be able to cope with the additional waste from the fetus.)

Sexually transmitted disease Herpes presents the highest risk of infection to your baby if you have a primary infection at the time your membranes rupture or at labour. Herpes simplex II virus infection may lead to growth retardation in your baby, and about half of infants born under these conditions will develop some form of herpetic infection after birth, possibly involving the eyes, mouth, and skin. If you have no symptoms, and are not shedding the virus from your cervix or vagina, the risk that your baby will become infected is less than one per thousand.

If you have a history of genital herpes you can expect a normal vaginal delivery even with an active secondary infection. However, if herpes ulcers are present in a primary infection just before labour commences, you will probably be advised to have a Caesarean section to reduce the risk of your baby catching herpes as he descends the birth canal.

If genital herpes occurs or recurs in pregnancy after the 34th week, your doctor will test for the presence of the virus and will probably advise a Caesarean.

HIV/AIDS The outlook for babies of mothers who are HIV positive is more optimistic than it was a few years ago. The use of oral AZT may protect the fetus from infection, and the baby will be regularly scanned to check growth. Doctors may recommend a Caesarean to protect the baby and will aim for minimal fetal trauma during labour (no use of scalp electrodes or fetal blood sampling) to minimize the risk of maternal blood contamination.

Although it is not inevitable that the baby of a HIV mother will be HIV positive and develop AIDS, there is a risk that the baby will be born with HIV antibodies; these are usually maternal antibodies and may disappear within 18 months. Because of the risks, an HIV mother will be given counselling and may be offered the opportunity to terminate her pregnancy.

GERMAN MEASLES

Before conceiving, check with your doctor to see if you have antibodies to the German measles (rubella) virus.

Don't assume you are immune to the disease if you have been vaccinated in the past – the antibodies lose their efficiency after a period of time, so check. If you are not immune, you should be vaccinated. After a successful vaccination, you should wait at least three months before you try to conceive, as the vaccine is live.

If you come into contact with someone who has, or is suspected of having, German measles, tell your doctor immediately. They will arrange for a blood sample to be taken and sent to a laboratory for antibody testing.

Depending on the result, the test may be repeated 10 days later. Should this test result in a suggestion that you have German measles, you and your partner will have to face the decision of whether to abort the pregnancy. Some doctors may recommend the administration of antibodies in the form of gamma globulin to help avoid any damage to the fetus.

TAKE CARE

German measles (rubella), particularly if caught in the first three months of pregnancy, can cause malformations in your baby. These may include deafness, blindness, and heart disease.

The importance of folic acid

Cressida has been discussing with her sister Oona and her mother the possibility of getting pregnant again. Her mother has read about the connection between folic acid deficiency and neural tube defects (spina bifida and hydrocephalus) and has been encouraging Cressida to start folic acid supplements in case she becomes pregnant.

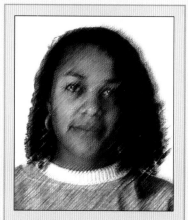

Name **Cressida King**

Age **31 years**

Past medical history
Nothing abnormal

Obstetric history
This is Cressida's second pregnancy

Cressida's first baby, a boy, was born 18 months ago and now she's planning to have a second. Her son Henry went to term and was a normal delivery. He was a normal baby apart from a brown hairy birthmark at the base of his spine. As was explained to Cressida, this is the mildest form of spina bifida, affecting only the skin. Henry is symptomless and a robust, loving little boy. Cressida, however, is worried that her second child might be severely affected by spina bifida or even hydrocephalus in the light of this past tendency.

BEING INFORMED

Cressida dislikes taking tablets even vitamin supplements. Oona has suggested that Cressida seeks medical advice to help her decide about taking folic acid now, in preparation for conception. Here are a few of the things that Cressida should consider.

SPINA BIFIDA AND HYDROCEPHALUS

The medical definition of spina bifida is a defect in which part of one or more vertebrae fails to develop completely leaving a portion of the spinal cord exposed. Spina bifida can occur anywhere in the spine but is most common on the lower back and the severity of the condition depends on how much nervous tissue is exposed.

There are different degrees of spina bifida. In one type the only defect is the failure of the fusion of the bony arches behind the spinal cord. When the bone defect is more extensive there may be neural tube defects such as a meningocele with protrusion of the meninges, the membranes surrounding the spinal cord, or more serious still a myelocele with deformity of the spinal cord.

In the developing embryo the skin, brain, the spinal cord, and nerves all arise from the same primitive layer of cells. This is why a birthmark overlying the end of the embryonic neural tube may be the only sign of late closure of the fetal neural tube.

Spina bifida symptoms depend on the severity of the spinal cord exposure; there may be paralysis, incontinence, or hydrocephalus – swelling of the brain.

REDUCING THE RISKS

The spine and the vertebral column develop from a flat layer of cells whose edges come together to form a tube which is the hollow cavity inside the spinal cord. This closure of the cord and the bones which surround it, the vertebrae, occurs very early in the development of an embryo usually within four weeks of conception.

Research in the last 10 years has proven that sufficiently high levels of folic acid in the mother's blood are necessary for normal closure of the neural tube. Mothers with low blood levels of folic acid have a higher risk of having a spina bifida baby.

There's another important factor: in normal circumstances folic acid is removed from the blood quite quickly but in pregnancy the kidneys filter it off from the blood at four times the normal rate. This means that if a mother doesn't eat folic acid-rich foods or doesn't take folic acid supplements regularly she can become relatively deficient in folic acid and the levels may drop low enough to put her baby at risk.

It's therefore crucial for all pregnant women to take daily supplements of folic acid in order to keep the blood levels high.

TAKING FOLIC ACID

1. I pointed out to Cressida that it's not enough to start folic acid when pregnancy is confirmed. Cressida's mother is right, it's essential that Cressida's folic acid levels are topped up at the very moment she conceives whenever that may be. It's therefore essential that she takes folic acid before conception. Experts recommend that all women contemplating pregnancy start folic acid supplements three months before trying for a baby.
2. It's also essential to take enough and experts agree on a daily dose of 400 micrograms.
3. Folic acid is available in several different forms:
• in foods such as liver (only about once a week);
• in green leafy vegetables – the darker green the better, mushrooms, lima beans, kidney beans, wholewheat bread, nuts, particularly walnuts, peas, and beans – so all pregnant women should enrich their diets with these foods months before they become pregnant;
• as folic acid capsules in 400 microgram doses, available from all pharmacies – one a day should be taken from three months prior to pregnancy through to term;
• in a nutritious folic acid milk drink available from pharmacies,

one carton of which (about a glass full) contains the daily folic acid requirements – this is ideal for women who don't like taking tablets or capsules.

WOMEN AT RISK

Parents who've had one child with spina bifida are more at risk than parents who've had completely normal children. And while Henry is developing normally, he does have a birthmark which means Cressida's future children could be at risk of a more severe form of spina bifida. She and all women like her must therefore embark on a rigorous regime of folic acid supplements well before pregnancy and through to term.

NUTRITIONALLY VULNERABLE WOMEN

I told Cressida that potentially all babies are at some risk of spina bifida and other neural tube defects like hydrocephalus whatever the mother's age whether she's a first-time mother or

already has healthy children – even if she's in the best of health herself. But some women should be especially rigorous about taking folic acid supplements. So I asked Cressida if she'd experienced any of the following:
• allergy to certain key foods, such as cows' milk or wheat;
• being generally run down, underweight, or eating a poor, unbalanced diet;
• a period of overzealous dieting or worse anorexia nervosa;
• a recent miscarriage or stillbirth;
• drinking or smoking heavily;
• working particularly hard or being subject to a lot of stress.

Women who have babies close together or a multiple birth may be nutritionally compromised as a result and will be in particular need of folic acid before falling pregnant again.

Cressida was persuaded by these arguments and decided to start on folic acid immediately in the form of the milk drink each morning with breakfast.

FOLIC ACID IN FOOD

Foods high in folic acid (50mcg per serving and above)
Cooked black-eyed beans, brussels sprouts, beef extract, yeast extract, cooked kidney, kale, spinach, granary bread, spring greens, broccoli, and green beans.

Foods with medium folic acid content (15–50mcg per serving)
Cooked soya beans, cauliflower, cooked chick peas, potatoes, iceberg lettuce, oranges, peas, orange juice, parsnips, baked beans, wholemeal bread, cabbage,

yoghurt, white bread, eggs, brown rice, wholegrain pasta.

Foods fortified with folic acid
Bread: most supermarket chains stock one own-label soft grain bread which is fortified with folic acid. A two-slice serving of one of these will provide approximately 90mcg of folic acid. A few leading brands of bread are also fortified.

Cereals: many cereals are fortified but to widely different levels so it is important to always check the label. Some have over 100mcg per 30g serving.

INHERITING GENES

Half of a baby's genes come from his mother, via the ovum, and half come from his father, via the sperm.

Each ovum and sperm contains a different "mix" of the parents' genes, so each child inherits a different and unique selection of genetic information than that inherited by his siblings.

Most of our individual mix of genes blends together but some genes are dominant to their counterparts. In those cases, the dominant gene, say for brown eye colour, will prevail over a recessive, such as the gene for blue eyes.

The genetic mix
Your baby will be a unique combination of his parents' genes.

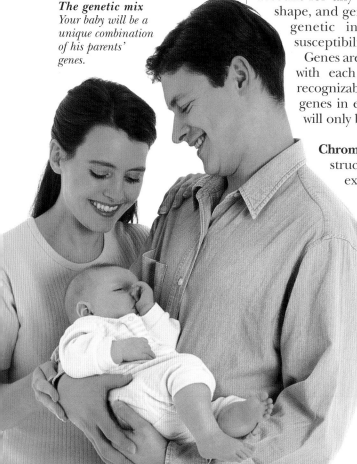

What is a gene?

A gene is a minute unit of DNA (deoxyribonucleic acid) carried on a chromosome, which also consists of DNA. In the nucleus of every body cell, there are at least 50,000 unique genes divided among 23 pairs of chromosomes.

THE "BLUEPRINT" OF THE BODY

Genes influence and direct the development and functioning of all the organs and body systems. They determine the pattern for growth, survival, reproduction, and possibly ageing and death for each individual. Because all cells (except for egg and sperm cells) derive from the single fertilized egg, the same genetic material is duplicated in every cell in your body. However, not all the genes contained within a cell are active; it is the site and function of the cell that determines which genes are active. For example, different sets of genes are active in bone cells and blood cells.

Except for identical twins, individuals differ greatly in the composition of their genes, and it is their genes that entirely account for any variation in height, hair and eye colour, body shape, and gender, for example, among them. An individual's genetic inheritance will also determine his or her susceptibility to certain diseases and disorders.

Genes are held in pairs along a chromosome (see opposite) with each gene being either dominant or recessive. A recognizable effect is the result of the dominant gene or genes in each individual pair; the effect of recessive genes will only be noticeable when there are two recessive genes.

Chromosomes Twenty-three pairs of these threadlike structures are found in the nucleus of every cell, except for egg and sperm cells. These cells contain only 22 chromosomes plus an X or Y chromosome. Each chromosome contains thousands of genes arranged in single file along its length. Chromosomes are made up of two chains of DNA, which are arranged together to form a ladder-like structure, the sides of which are sugar-phosphate molecules. This spirals around upon itself and is known as a double helix. DNA has four bases – adenine, cytosine, guanine, and thymine, which are arranged in different combinations according to the functions of the genes on the different parts of the chromosome. Each combination of bases provides coded instructions that regulate the various activities of the body.

CHROMOSOMES, GENES, AND DNA

Chromosomes
There are 23 pairs – 22 general plus the gender chromosomes (see left) – of these thread-like structures in the nucleus of every body cell. But the egg and sperm cells carry only half this amount – these cells contain the information that controls the body's functioning and growth.

Chromosome

The double helix
The 2 chains of DNA, which make up each of the 46 chromosomes, are arranged to make a long spiralling ladder.

Each of the 4 DNA bases – adenine, cytosine, guanine, and thymine – is represented here by a different colour

Sugar-phosphate molecules form the sides of the DNA ladder

DNA replication
When a new cell is about to be formed, the DNA in each of the chromosomes "unzips" along the centre of the rungs of the ladder, and each half of DNA then duplicates itself. The new DNA chains that are created are genetically identical to the original chromosomes.

Gene

MUTANT GENES

Sometimes when a cell divides and duplicates its genetic material, the copying process is not perfect, and a fault occurs. This leads to a small change, or mutation, in the structure of the genetic material.

Carrying a mutant gene normally has a neutral or harmless effect – most, if not all, of us have a mutant gene as part of our genetic make-up. Occasionally, however, it can have a disadvantageous effect and, more rarely, a beneficial one.

The effects of a mutant gene depend largely upon whether it is carried within the fused ovum and the sperm, or whether it is a fault in the later copying process of the cells (somatic or body cells).

A mutation in the ovum or sperm will reproduce itself in all of the body's cells, resulting in genetic disease such as cystic fibrosis (see p.24). A mutated somatic cell, at worst, will multiply to form a group of abnormal cells in a specific area. These may have only a minor local effect, or they could cause deformity or disease. This type of mutation is usually triggered by an outside influence, such as radiation or exposure to carcinogens.

DOWN'S SYNDROME

This chromosomal disorder (see column, right) occurs when a fertilized egg has 47 chromosomes instead of the usual 46.

In most cases, the egg itself is defective, being formed with the extra chromosome; the sperm may be similarly affected. This type of Down's syndrome is known as trisomy. Less commonly, one parent may have a chromosomal abnormality that results in his or her child inheriting faulty chromosomal material. This is known as translocation. Down's syndrome may be diagnosed by chorionic villus sampling or amniocentesis (see p.185). Maternal blood alphafetoprotein levels (see p.184) are generally lower if a mother has a fetus with Down's syndrome.

In women, the risk of having a Down's syndrome baby increases with age (see p.185). The risk increases dramatically over age 35.

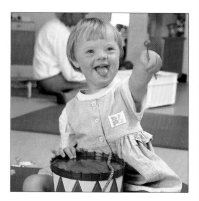

Down's syndrome child
One baby in every 1,000 will be born with this disorder. Most cases of Down's syndrome occur randomly and are non-recurrent. However, one cause – translocation – is inherited, so it is important to explore any family history of Down's syndrome.

GENETIC CONSIDERATIONS

Within the nucleus of each cell are genes and chromosomes that contain DNA, which determines the growth and functioning of the body (see also p.22). Genetic disorders occur when genes and chromosomes are abnormal. Genetic diseases can occur because a single gene may be defective, there may be a fault in the number or shape of chromosomes, or several genes may be faulty. There may also be complicating environmental factors. A single defective gene that results in a genetic disorder can be either dominant or recessive, a mutation, or attached to the X chromosome (see below). Abnormal chromosomes that result in genetic disorders are usually new mutations, but may be inherited (see column, left).

Where more than one gene or environmental factor is involved in producing a disorder, there is as yet no straightforward method of determining why it has happened.

If either partner has a history of a genetic disease in their extended family, counselling (see p.26) should be sought. The number of tests for genetic diseases that can be performed is increasing yearly, although they cannot predict the severity of the condition. The ultimate decision about whether to attempt to conceive, to go ahead with an existing pregnancy, or to request a termination will always rest with you, the parents. Bear in mind, however, that although a handicapped child will need special care, many such children are both affectionate and responsive, and can lead happy, fulfilled lives.

DOMINANT GENETIC DISEASES

Fatal diseases due to dominant genes are rare because affected individuals normally die before they can pass on the genes. However, some diseases, such as familial hypercholesterolaemia (see below), present a manageable risk to health.

Familial hypercholesterolaemia FH is the most common dominant genetic disease. In it, blood cholesterol levels are so high that there is a risk of heart attacks and other complications caused by narrowing of the arteries. The condition affects one in 500 people and can be detected by a blood test at birth.

RECESSIVE GENETIC DISEASES

A defective recessive gene is usually masked by a normal dominant one. However, if both parents carry a defective recessive gene, each of their children has a one in four chance of inheriting both recessive genes (and therefore one of several disorders) or neither, and a two in four chance of being a carrier. Thus there are always more carriers than sufferers.

Cystic fibrosis CF is the most common recessive gene disorder. One in 20 of the white population carries the CF gene, and one in 2,000 white babies born is affected by the disease. In non-whites, the incidence is about one in 90,000. This disease mainly affects the lungs and the digestive system. The mucus within the lungs becomes thick and sticky, and accumulates, causing chest infections. The mucus also blocks the ducts of various organs, particularly the pancreas, preventing the normal flow of digestive enzymes. If not treated promptly, CF results in malnutrition. Rapid and accurate carrier testing involving analysis of blood or mouth cells is possible. Over 60 percent of sufferers survive into adulthood; some have been helped by heart transplant surgery.

Sickle-cell anaemia This is the most common genetic disease among black people (one in 400). It is so called because the red cells are sickle-shaped from defective haemoglobin; this causes them to break down and the small blood vessels to clog, which may result in a stroke. It is usually diagnosed by a blood test, and the mother will be offered CVS if both parents are sufferers. Sufferers are susceptible to meningitis and other serious infections but can, with care, live a productive life despite some ill health. Carrier status protects against malaria.

Thalassaemia This is common among Asians, blacks, and people of Mediterranean descent. The gene may be dominant or recessive. It produces anaemia and chronic ill health, and blood transfusions may be necessary. Blood tests will reveal the disease and can indicate if the haemoglobin level is reduced. Not all cases are severe, and some sufferers may survive for many years.

Tay–Sachs disease Common among Ashkenazic Jews, this is a fatal condition resulting in deterioration of the brain caused by a deficiency in enzymes. Few children with the disease live beyond three years, and no adequate treatment is known. Tay–Sachs is diagnosed by testing blood for enzyme deficiency.

GENDER-LINKED DISEASES

These are conditions caused by defects on the X chromosome. If a second normal X chromosome is present, as in a healthy female, the defect won't show because it is masked. Women therefore carry the disease. However, in males, who have a Y chromosome instead of a second X chromosome, the disease will express itself. Therefore men are affected.

Haemophilia This results when the crucial clotting factor VIII is missing and causes profuse bleeding from any injury, external or internal. Effective treatment with factor VIII derived from normal blood is now available, and haemophiliacs can lead relatively normal lives. Diagnosis can be made from a sample of fetal blood at 18–20 weeks of pregnancy.

Duchenne muscular dystrophy This is the most common type, affecting one boy in 5,000. In childhood, sufferers lose the ability to walk and are usually confined to a wheelchair for their comparatively short lives. It can be detected before birth.

CHROMOSOMAL DISORDERS

These are usually due to some fault in the process of the chromosome division in the formation of the egg or sperm, or during the initial divisions of the fertilized ovum. More rarely, one parent has an abnormal arrangement of chromosomes.

The severity and the type of abnormality depends on whether one or both sex chromosomes, or one of the other 44 chromosomes (autosomes) are affected. The latter are slightly less common than sex chromosomal abnormalities, but tend to produce more serious, widespread effects. An extra autosome means that one of the 22 pairs of autosomes occurs in triplicate, known as a trisomy (see p.198). The most common trisomy is Down's syndrome (see column, left).

In a trisomy, part of a chromosome is missing or an extra bit is joined to a chromosome. Trisomy can cause mental and physical defects.

Occasionally the problem can be caused by translocation. This happens if there is a normal number of chromosomes but they are not arranged correctly (part of one is joined to another). The parent carrier is normal but the child may have an abnormality if he or she inherits the translocated chromosomes.

Abnormalities of the sex chromosomes result in defects in sexual development, infertility, and occasionally mental retardation. Boys may suffer from Klinefelter's syndrome, girls from Turner's.

Abnormalities can be diagnosed by chromosome analysis, which may be offered during genetic counselling (see p.26).

CAN YOU BENEFIT?

It is important to seek expert advice if you fall into any of the following groups:

• if a previous child was born with a genetic disorder such as cystic fibrosis, or a chromosomal disorder such as Down's syndrome

• if a previous child was born with a congenital defect, for example, a club foot (see p.199)

• if there is a family history of mental handicap, or abnormal development

• if there is a blood relationship between you and your partner

• if you have a history of repeated miscarriages (see pp. 218 & 222).

Genetic counselling

Genetic counselling is aimed at determining the risk you run of passing on an inheritable disease to your child. The second goal is to help you to decide whether or not to go ahead to conceive in the light of that assessment. You may be concerned because you have a blood relative (including, perhaps, a previous child) who has suffered from an inheritable disorder.

HOW GENETIC COUNSELLING WORKS

When you are referred for genetic counselling, the counsellor will ask both of you about your health, and discuss your family background. Virtually every case dealt with by a genetic counsellor is unique. The advice depends on a precise diagnosis of the disease (what it is and why it occurred), and on the creation of a comprehensive family tree, which details all blood relationships and any diseases suffered. Birth or death certificates may be used if necessary and it is important that you take along as much information as you can. Be prepared for the whole project to take some time as it can be a long and involved process of investigation. Genetic counsellors are trained in genetics and psychology: they will assess the degree of risk and help you make an informed decision. If there is a small risk, you may decide to go ahead and try for a baby. If, however, the risks are very great, you may prefer not to take that chance.

For many genetic disorders, such as sickle-cell anaemia or Tay–Sachs (see p.25), it is possible to establish whether the parents are carriers. This can be done by seeing the disease itself, such as sickle-shaped cells on a blood sample; by looking for the product of the disease, such as the proteins that are present in Tay–Sachs; or by flagging a gene or chromosome. Flagging is a sophisticated technique that is used to find out if a fragment of DNA will attach itself to the patient's chromosome. If it does, the gene, and therefore the disease, is present; if not, it is absent. However, in most diseases, more than one gene is involved, so it can be difficult to check all the elements that are involved. This is true of cystic fibrosis, for example, although at present the diagnosis can be over 90 percent certain.

If a couple has already had an affected child, the counsellor will first rule out a cause which is not inherited, for example, German measles (rubella – see p.19). Possible causes such as exposure to radiation, drugs, or injury will also be considered. The counsellor will examine the child and will arrange for genetic testing to be done on blood or cells washed from the mouth with water.

Sometimes it can be difficult to pinpoint the exact cause, but you will be given as thorough a diagnosis as possible, and your chances of having another affected child outlined. It is worth bearing in mind that many disabilities do not have a genetic origin and cannot be predicted; genetic evaluation can only reassure you that there is no evidence of an inheritable disease.

The importance of your family history

By examining the medical history of your family network, a counsellor will be able to detect the pattern of a disease over several generations. For example, James, a six year-old boy, was suffering with painful, swollen joints. During a conversation with James' parents, the counsellor learned that a cousin, and probably a great-uncle, suffered from the genetic bleeding disorder known as haemophilia (see family tree, below). This information pointed almost immediately to the probable diagnosis – James, too, suffered from haemophilia. The pain and the swelling that he was experiencing was caused by the blood that was leaking into his joints.

How genes are inherited

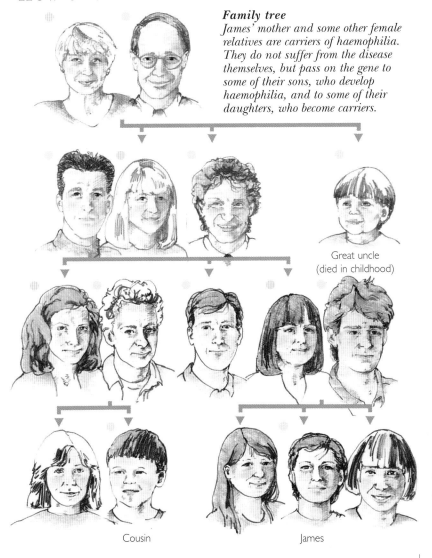

Family tree
James' mother and some other female relatives are carriers of haemophilia. They do not suffer from the disease themselves, but pass on the gene to some of their sons, who develop haemophilia, and to some of their daughters, who become carriers.

Great uncle
(died in childhood)

Cousin

James

Males with haemophilia

Unaffected males

Probable female carriers of haemophilia gene

Possible female carriers of haemophilia gene

YOUR HORMONES

The ovarian cycle is mostly controlled by the hormones oestrogen, progesterone, follicle-stimulating hormone (FSH), and luteinizing hormone (LH).

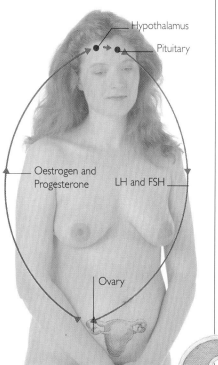

Hypothalamus

Pituitary

Oestrogen and Progesterone

LH and FSH

Ovary

Hormonal control
Ovarian follicle development is triggered by FSH from the pituitary gland. The follicles produce oestrogen, which causes the pituitary to release a burst of LH that cuts FSH production. The LH triggers the release of the egg from the most mature follicle and the corpus luteum, which forms from the follicle after the egg has been released, then produces progesterone.

Conceiving a baby

The miracle of birth begins when a sperm from the father fuses with an egg from the mother to form a single cell with its own unique genetic blueprint. This single cell then divides and redivides until eventually a new human being is created. The vast majority of normally fertile couples achieve a pregnancy within the first two years of trying.

A woman's entire stock of ova, or eggs, are formed in her two ovaries before her birth. By the fifth month of pregnancy, a baby girl's ovaries contain around seven million eggs. Many of these eggs will die before she is born leaving her with approximately two million eggs at birth. This process of degeneration continues until puberty, by which time between 200,000 and 500,000 eggs survive. Of these, only 400–500 mature and are released by the ovaries during a woman's fertile years – roughly one per lunar month. The ovaries are located in the pelvis, close to the trumpet-like endings (fimbriae) of the fallopian tubes. The germ cells that ultimately develop into a woman's ova are formed in the yolk sac that sustains the embryo in the first weeks of life. If the embryo is

THE FEMALE REPRODUCTIVE TRACT

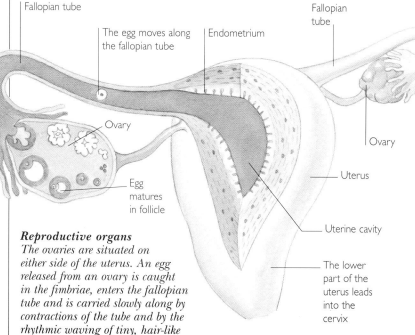

Fallopian tube

The egg moves along the fallopian tube

Endometrium

Fallopian tube

Ovary

Egg matures in follicle

Ovary

Uterus

Uterine cavity

The lower part of the uterus leads into the cervix

Reproductive organs
The ovaries are situated on either side of the uterus. An egg released from an ovary is caught in the fimbriae, enters the fallopian tube and is carried slowly along by contractions of the tube and by the rhythmic waving of tiny, hair-like projections (cilia) in its lining.

male, these cells are reabsorbed as the placenta develops. When the embryo is female, however, about 100 germ cells actually move from the yolk sac, along the umbilical tissue, and into the minute female embryo. Once inside the embryo, they migrate to the tissues that will later develop into the ovaries, and there they begin to multiply.

THE OVARIAN CYCLE

During a woman's reproductive life, her ovaries release ova in cycles. Each of these ovarian cycles lasts about 28 days, and the development and release of an ovum ready for fertilization by a sperm is called ovulation. Ovaries usually ovulate alternately. In the first half of each ovarian cycle, about 20 ova begin to ripen, and occupy fluid-filled sacs (follicles). One of these follicles, outgrowing the others, matures and ruptures, thus releasing its ovum. This happens on or around 14 days before the end of the cycle, regardless of the total length of the cycle. The other follicles that had started to ripen then shrivel up and their eggs die.

The ruptured follicle becomes a yellow-coloured structure, called the corpus luteum, that grows for some days and produces the hormone progesterone, which is essential for the development of an embryo. In the absence of pregnancy, however, the follicle withers away, and a new cycle begins when the lining of the uterus is shed at the beginning of the woman's next period.

FERTILITY FACTS

Fertility varies from person to person and at different stages of our lives. The following facts are true for most people:

• the fertility of both men and women reaches its peak at about the age of 24

• among couples having intercourse regularly without contraception, 25 percent of women will conceive in the first month, 60 percent within six months, 75 percent within nine months, 80 percent within a year, and 90 percent within 18 months

• after ovulation, an egg can only be fertilized for approximately 12–24 hours.

THE MONTHLY CYCLE

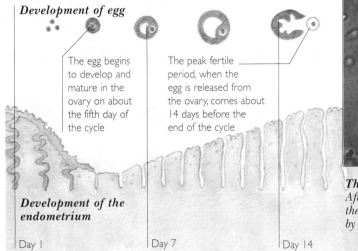

Development of egg

The egg begins to develop and mature in the ovary on about the fifth day of the cycle

The peak fertile period, when the egg is released from the ovary, comes about 14 days before the end of the cycle

Development of the endometrium

Day 1   Day 7   Day 14   Day 21   Day 28

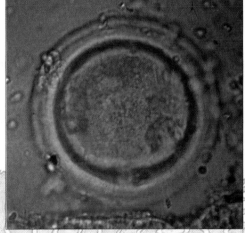

The mature egg
After leaving the ovary, the egg is drawn into the fallopian tube, where it awaits fertilization by a sperm.

The cycle begins
Menstruation, the shedding of the endometrium, heralds the start of the ovarian cycle. Under the influence of oestrogen the endometrium is then rebuilt.

Fertile period
After ovulation, under the influence of oestrogen and progesterone, the endometrium becomes thicker and spongy to receive a fertilized egg.

The cycle ends
If the egg is not fertilized, the corpus luteum dies and, because oestrogen and progesterone levels fall, the endometrium is shed.

The role of a man

The process of sperm production takes place within a man's testes and is known as spermatogenesis. Sperm production is continuous and the whole process, from the initial generation of a sperm to its maturation and ejaculation, takes about seven weeks.

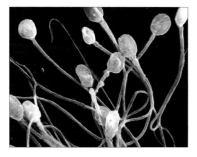

Sperm
Each sperm has a head that contains its genetic material, and a tail for propulsion. A complex network of microscopically tiny tubes within the testes produces spermatids, the forerunners of sperm.

The testes
A cross-sectional view of a testis shows the network of minute tubes that contain the spermatogonia, the cells from which spermatids are created. These tubes connect with about eight larger tubes; these are the efferent ducts that convey the developing sperm into the epididymis where they mature and grow their tails. The testes also produce hormones, the most important being the male sex hormone testosterone, which is the most powerful of the androgens – the hormones that are responsible for male secondary sexual characteristics such as facial hair and deepening of the voice, and male and female sex drives.

Sperm, a man's contribution to the conception of his child, are formed in his testes (testicles). Sperm formation begins at puberty under the influence of testosterone from the testes, and luteinizing hormone (LH) and follicle-stimulating hormone (FSH), which are produced by the pituitary gland and act on the testes as they do on the ovaries. Production continues throughout a man's fertile life and, although the numbers and quality of sperm produced diminish from the age of 40, men in their nineties have fathered children. Sperm production speeds up at times of sexual activity, but if ejaculation is very frequent, sperm numbers decrease, lowering a man's fertility.

The mature sperm Each individual sperm is tadpole-shaped and, because it is only about a twentieth of a millimetre long, it cannot be seen by the naked eye. It has a head that is dark in colour owing to the concentration of genetic material within it, and a strong, lashing tail five to six times longer than the head, with which it "swims". The tail is attached to the head by a short middle section or body. This contains special cell components called mitochondria, which are its energy-producing apparatus.

The newly formed sperm pass into the epididymis at the rear of each testis, where they mature. From the epididymis, matured sperm travel up a tube, the vas deferens, to a small, sac-like structure called the seminal vesicle. When a man ejaculates, the sperm is mixed with fluid produced by the seminal vesicle and this, together with fluids secreted by the prostate and other glands, makes up the seminal fluid (semen) that is discharged from the penis via the urethra.

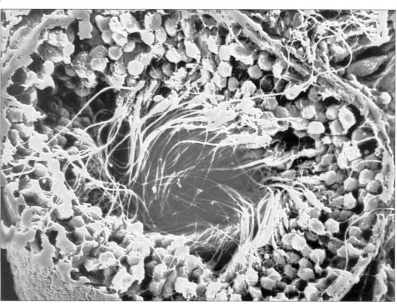

THE MALE REPRODUCTIVE TRACT

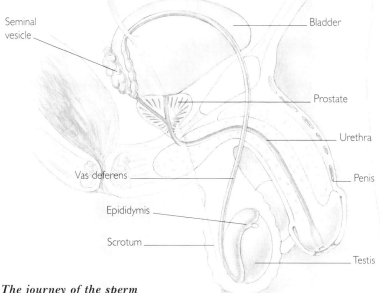

- Seminal vesicle
- Bladder
- Prostate
- Urethra
- Vas deferens
- Penis
- Epididymis
- Scrotum
- Testis

The journey of the sperm
The sperm leave the epididymis via a tube called the vas deferens. Each vas deferens, which is about 4 mm (⅙ in) in diameter, runs up the spermatic cord, from which the testis is suspended. From there, each vas deferens loops up around the bladder, down past the seminal vesicle and into the prostate gland. From the seminal vesicle

onwards, the vas deferens is known as the ejaculatory duct. At the prostate each ejaculatory duct joins the urethra, which is the hollow tube within the penis through which the semen is ejaculated.

EJACULATION

The average amount of seminal fluid ejaculated is three and a half millilitres (about two-thirds of a teaspoonful), the normal range being from two to six millilitres. Each millilitre contains 60–150 million sperm, of which nearly a quarter are abnormal. Only about three-quarters are motile (able to wriggle).

Reaching the egg Although sperm can move two to three millimetres per minute, their actual speed varies with the acidity of their environment – the higher the acidity, the slower their movement. The vaginal secretions are slightly acidic; thus sperm ejaculated into the vagina probably move quite slowly until they reach the more friendly alkaline environment of the uterine cavity. After withstanding the hostile acidic vaginal conditions, they then face a longer and more dangerous journey before they reach the egg way down a fallopian tube. Of a total sperm count of 300 million per ejaculation, only a few hundred will actually reach the egg. A large quantity of the remainder may trickle out of the vagina, or be destroyed by vaginal acidity. Others may be swallowed up by cleansing cells within the uterus, enter the wrong fallopian tube, or enter the correct tube but miss the egg altogether.

YOUR BABY'S SEX

The gender of a child is determined by whether the fertilizing sperm is an X sperm (female) or a Y sperm (male), as the woman's ovum is always female, X.

The X and the Y sperm have different properties, the X sperm (female) being larger, slower, and longer-lived than the Y sperm (male). The X sperm also appears to be favoured by the slightly acidic conditions in the vagina.

Bearing in mind that there is very little scientific evidence to support them, the following ideas may be of interest if you are trying to choose the gender of your baby.

When For a female baby, make love up to two or three days before ovulation as only female sperm survive this long; for a male baby, make love on the day of, or just after, ovulation, as the faster male sperm will reach the ovum before the female sperm.

Frequency For a female baby, make love fairly frequently, as this lowers the proportion of male sperm in the semen; for a male baby, make love infrequently, as this will increase the proportion of male sperm.

PENETRATION

This sequence of pictures, taken with an electron microscope, shows fertilization taking place – a sperm penetrating the tough outer membrane of an egg and then entering the egg itself.

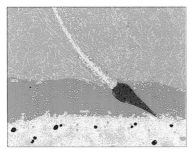

Membrane penetration
The sperm penetrates the membrane of the egg by releasing enzymes that create a hole in it.

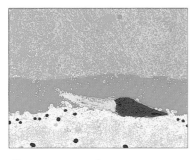

Oocyte penetration
The sperm prepares to penetrate the oocyte, the innermost part of the egg.

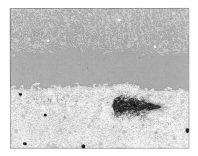

Chromosome transfer
Prior to joining its chromosomes with those of the egg, the sperm sheds its body and tail.

Fertilization

Fertilization occurs when a sperm meets and penetrates an ovum. All human cells contain 46 chromosomes, thread-like structures that carry their genetic information.

The exception to the rule are sperm and ova, which have only 23 chromosomes, so that when they meet, the single fertilized cell that results has the full 46 chromosomes. The new cell (zygote) splits first into two identical cells, each with 46 chromosomes, and then continues to divide slowly as it travels down the fallopian tube, until it reaches the uterus. By the time it reaches the uterus it is called a blastocyst or blastula, and is a hollow clump of about 100 cells.

CONCEPTION

Egg meets sperm
The egg is released from its follicle. It travels one-third of the way along the fallopian tube, where it is fertilized.

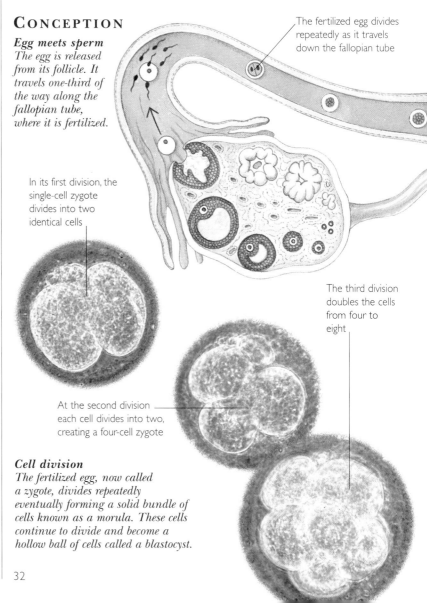

The fertilized egg divides repeatedly as it travels down the fallopian tube

In its first division, the single-cell zygote divides into two identical cells

The third division doubles the cells from four to eight

At the second division each cell divides into two, creating a four-cell zygote

Cell division
The fertilized egg, now called a zygote, divides repeatedly eventually forming a solid bundle of cells known as a morula. These cells continue to divide and become a hollow ball of cells called a blastocyst.

Implantation A week after fertilization the blastocyst secretes a hormone which helps it to burrow its way into the endometrium. Implantation is usually in the upper one-third of the uterus. The pregnancy is now established and the placenta will start to form.

Twins When a woman produces more than one egg at a time, non-identical (fraternal) twins may develop from two separate eggs, fertilized by two separate sperm. Each has its own placenta within the uterus. Identical twins come from a single egg, fertilized by a single sperm. This egg divides into two, and each develops independently into a genetically identical twin sharing a single placenta. Other multiple pregnancies, such as triplets, originate in the same ways as twins and, similarly, the siblings may be identical or fraternal.

BOY OR GIRL?

Of the 46 chromosomes that carry the complete human genetic blueprint, the sex of a child is determined by just two, the X and the Y.

The sex chromosomes
A woman's eggs each contain a single X chromosome, while a man's individual sperm have either an X or a Y chromosome. If an egg is fertilized by an X chromosome sperm, the baby that is created will be a girl (XX). If the sperm has a Y chromosome, the resulting child will be a boy (XY).

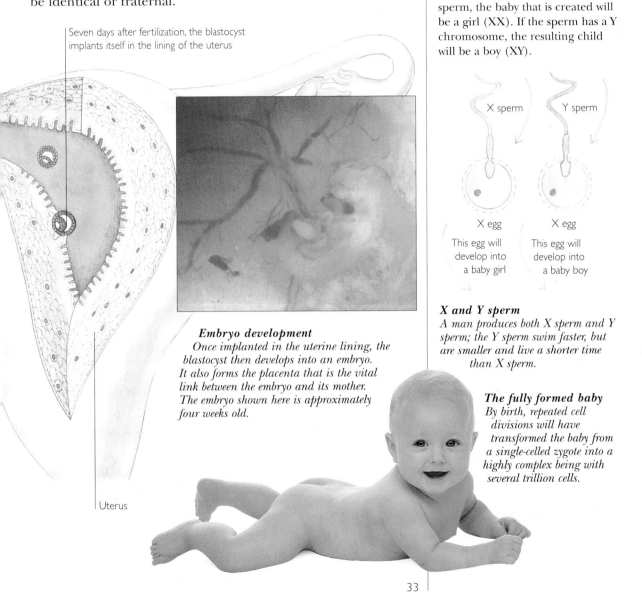

Seven days after fertilization, the blastocyst implants itself in the lining of the uterus

Uterus

X sperm   Y sperm

X egg   X egg
This egg will   This egg will
develop into   develop into
a baby girl   a baby boy

Embryo development
Once implanted in the uterine lining, the blastocyst then develops into an embryo. It also forms the placenta that is the vital link between the embryo and its mother. The embryo shown here is approximately four weeks old.

X and Y sperm
A man produces both X sperm and Y sperm; the Y sperm swim faster, but are smaller and live a shorter time than X sperm.

The fully formed baby
By birth, repeated cell divisions will have transformed the baby from a single-celled zygote into a highly complex being with several trillion cells.

THE AGE FACTOR

The older you get the longer it takes to conceive so take your age into account when assessing whether you are having problems and should consult a doctor. Then again, the older you are the less time you have so you should seek advice early.

• The number of infertile women increases with age: between the ages of 20 and 24, one in ten women are infertile, but by 40–44 years, this increases to nearly 30 percent.

• All treatments for infertility are significantly more successful in couples under 30.

• The overall quality of women's ova diminishes with age as does the number of healthy ova produced at any one time.

• The receptivity of the uterine environment to implantation of a fertilized ovum decreases with age.

THE HORMONE FACTOR

In women, incorrect amounts of luteinizing hormone (LH) and follicle-stimulating hormone (FSH) can affect ovulation (see p.28). In men, these same two hormones, LH and FSH, stimulate the testes to produce sperm so if a man's pituitary gland does not release enough FSH and LH, his ability to produce sperm will be impaired. In men and women, incorrect functioning of the thyroid and adrenal glands will affect sperm production and ovulation respectively.

Problems in conceiving

Having problems conceiving doesn't always mean you are infertile. Infertility means different things to different people; it certainly means something different to doctors and to couples. Most couples who think they are infertile are only subfertile and with help can conceive successfully.

WHAT IS INFERTILITY?

To most people infertility means the inability to have children but it's more complex than that. A couple may have no difficulty in conceiving their first child but find they cannot have a second; this means that they are suffering from secondary infertility. Another couple, who have both had children by their previous partners, may now find that they cannot conceive together. This is known as subfertility and happens because the fertility of a couple is the sum of their individual fertilities.

If both partners' fertilities are marginal conception may not occur. But if one partner's fertility is strong, it still may be possible for the couple to conceive. The majority of couples achieve conception within four to six months of trying; if a couple hasn't conceived within six months and then approaches their doctor for advice, he or she is most likely to send them away with encouraging words but advising them to come back if nothing has happened after a year. However, age is undoubtedly a factor for women (see sidebar, left) who produce lower quality eggs as they get older. Statistics show that around 90 percent of women in their twenties will become pregnant within a year of trying, and the remainder still have a high statistical chance of becoming pregnant naturally within a further year or so. However, women in their thirties have a much lower statistical probability of becoming pregnant after a year of trying, so should seek help after that time has elapsed.

There are now many ways in which a couple can be helped to conceive a child – they range from simple advice on sexual technique to drug treatment, surgery and ultimately to the new assisted reproductive technologies (ART) (see p.48). However, the emotional costs can be exceedingly high – and not just for you and your partner – but for other family members including the child or children you may conceive.

THE EMOTIONAL IMPACT

Most couples dealing with problems in conceiving have to cope with difficult psychological, family, and social factors too. The investigation or treatment of infertility may pose additional psychological trauma, interfere intolerably with sex life, and even erode the love a couple feel for each other. Then, of course, there can be an onerous financial burden on the couple due to the cost of investigation and treatment, which can add to the overall stress of the situation.

Most couples see children as an extension of themselves, as bearers and perpetuators of the family name as well as an expansion of their hopes, aims, and ambitions. The inability to have children is therefore often perceived as a denial of basic human rights; worse, as an injustice, a disappointment, sometimes bordering on grief.

THE IMPORTANCE OF COUNSELLING

Given the tensions that surround the treatment of infertility, couples deserve and should get psychological support. When you decide to embark on investigation and treatment, ask your doctor to refer you to a counsellor trained in dealing with the stress of infertility at all stages of its management. You shouldn't have to wait until you find yourselves well on into secondary referral; you both need help and advice at the start. The unfulfilled wish for children represents a major life crisis for some couples and, without support, has sadly been known to cause disenchantment with life, personal suffering, and guilt. One or both partners may become introspective and antisocial, leading to depression and the irretrievable breakdown of the relationship.

Some procedures require deep self-questioning and a couple will need a great deal of support because of the lengthy and invasive nature of the treatment, and especially the ethical issues surrounding assisted reproductive technologies, insemination, and any technique involving donors.

Psychological factors affecting fertility The way you feel can in itself affect your fertility by causing a hormone disturbance or impotence. So, without proper support, fertility treatment may make matters worse. On the other hand, doctors have plenty of anecdotal evidence that couples suddenly conceive very soon after making the decision to have their infertility investigated, as if taking the plunge releases the psychological tensions that may have been affecting fertility.

UNEXPLAINED INFERTILITY

In the UK, 12 percent of couples investigated for fertility problems, will, in the end have to face the fact that their infertility cannot be explained. In those couples it's tempting to consider radical treatments, but the agreed approach is to wait for up to three years depending on the woman's age. After this there are treatments that have been successful like GIFT (see p.49) and intrauterine insemination (see p.48) as well as ovarian stimulation by FSH (follicle-stimulating hormone). Drug treatments with clomiphene, danazol, and bromocriptine are not effective. Investigation for immunological factors may be fruitful (see p. 39).

ISSUES TO CONSIDER

Even before you have professional counselling, it's worth asking yourselves some searching questions, so that some of the issues are out in the open from the very beginning.

• Would you tell friends and family, or would you attempt to keep your fertility treatment a complete secret?

• If you intend to keep it a secret, can you be sure that the truth won't come out, perhaps destructively, at a time of crisis?

• Could you cope with a multiple pregnancy?

• What if one, some, or all of the babies died?

• Having committed so much time and money to having a baby, how easy will you find it to let her go once she grows up?

• How long would you persist with infertility treatment?

• Would you consider donor eggs or sperm?

• Is adoption an option?

To optimize your chances of conceiving each of you may have to make some basic lifestyle changes. You are both equally involved in your infertility and you must both take joint responsibility.

• Both partners must stop smoking.

• Both partners should drink relatively little (women not more than two units per week, men not more than seven units per week).

• Overweight women should try to lose weight. Obesity compromises ovulation and losing weight helps. In one study, 12 out of 13 women who lost 6.0 kg or more began to ovulate and 11 out of 12 conceived.

• Men should wear loose fitting underpants to allow circulation of air around their testes and avoid situations where overheating is a possible hazard.

• Don't use temperature charts to find ovulation days (fertile days) and don't confine intercourse to fertile days; couples used to be advised to time intercourse for these days, but the stress involved was found to be counterproductive.

• Have penetrative intercourse two to three times a week.

• Although very frequent sex can diminish the number of sperm in each ejaculate, don't abstain for longer than 10 days or the sperm count will start to fall.

• Women should start taking 0.4 mg of folic acid supplements daily.

• Recreational drugs are disallowed; many affect fertility.

• Both should eat a healthy diet and take regular exercise.

Seeking advice

The first step is to chat with your family doctor together to air your concerns and ask questions. Many doctors find that it is the woman who seeks advice first, but it really is important for you both to accept that whatever the reasons for your problems turn out to be, you are both going to need investigation. So if at all possible make the first visit a joint one.

A crowded appointment book doesn't permit the kind of detailed, relaxed conversation you need with your doctor, so it's a good idea to request a full half hour's appointment, perhaps at a more relaxed time of day when your doctor is less pressured. A good alternative is to explore seeking advice from the sexual health clinic in your local hospital which you can attend without a referral from your doctor, or from your family planning clinic. At either of these, you'll find a team of sympathetic experts who'll focus on your problem.

HOW YOUR TREATMENT WILL BE MANAGED

At your initial discussion with your doctor, you have a right to know how your treatment will be managed. Each stage in the investigation and treatment should be fully explained to you in the appropriate language and you should be given lists of addresses and self-help organizations to contact. Ask for these if they aren't offered.

After the initial tests are completed, either by your family doctor or at the sexual health clinic, you should be referred for all secondary tests and further management of your case to a dedicated specialist infertility clinic, which will be run by a professional, multi-skilled team. You have the right to insist on being referred to such a unit.

Given the acknowledged stress surrounding the whole process of infertility treatment, you should expect discussions with the doctors caring for you to be relaxed and friendly and to take place in a sympathetic atmosphere, where you feel your contributions will be valued and your goals and expectations explored. There should also be explanatory talks or written information on what will be involved, including the pros and cons of alternative treatments that are relevant to your own particular situation. In addition, you have a right to expect that your preferences will be given weight by the professionals and that any disagreements will be negotiated between you both. Your doctor and the fertility unit to which you're referred will want to provide the best outcome for you both – that is, a healthy baby – but the route to this goal is going to be rocky and it's as well to be prepared from the outset.

PRIMARY TESTS

Primary tests are carried out by your primary care physician – your family doctor. Initially your doctor will take notes on your fertility history as a couple, including your ages, how long you've been trying to conceive, any past illnesses and surgery or medication that might affect fertility (see column, right). The woman will also be asked about her menstrual cycle, how regular it is, the duration of menstruation and whether it's accompanied by pain. You'll also be asked about your job in case either of you, but especially the man, is exposed to occupational hazards that may affect fertility. The doctor will also want to know about any past sexually transmitted disease in either partner, including chlamydia, and he'll look at past smear test results.

Both of you will have some initial tests done by your family doctor after your initial consultation. More specialized tests are called "secondary tests" (see pp.41 & 44) and are only done in a special fertility unit.

Primary tests for the woman:
- smear test (if not done recently)
- test for chlamydia infection (see p.44), which will be treated if detected
- physical examination, including an internal examination
- a simple blood test for progesterone levels in the second half of the cycle to confirm whether ovulation is taking place.

Primary tests for the man:
- physical examination of the man's penis and testes
- two semen samples which will be analyzed by the laboratory at the fertility clinic where further investigations, secondary tests (see p.41), will be done.

Rapid referral for secondary tests Although your doctor will probably conduct the primary tests (above), there are circumstances in which you'll be referred as quickly as possible for secondary investigations at a specialist unit. These include:
- if either partner is over 35 years of age
- if the woman has a history of amenorrhoea (absence of periods), or oligomenorrhoea (sparse or infrequent periods)
- abnormal anatomy on internal examination of the woman or a varicocoele of the scrotum (see p. 39) in the man.

Seeing a counsellor
It is important to have a thorough initial discussion with your doctor, who will advise you on the treatment stages of infertility and refer you to a specialist fertility clinic where you can see a counsellor.

DRUGS TO AVOID

Many medications may have a deleterious effect on fertility, affecting sperm, eggs, or sexual activity. Your doctor will want to know if you have been treated with any of the following drugs.

Men
- Sulphasalazine: lowers sperm count
- Nitrofurantoin: lowers sperm count
- Tetracyclines: lower sperm motility
- Cimetidine: causes impotence
- Ketoconazole: causes impotence and lowers sex drive
- Colichicine: lowers fertilization power of sperm
- Antidepressants: cause impotence
- Propranolol: causes impotence
- Chemotherapy: lowers sperm count
- Recreational drugs: cannabis and alcohol cause sperm abnormalities; cocaine lowers libido as well as sperm motility and count

Women
- NSAIDS: affect egg follicles
- Chemotherapy: causes ovarian failure
- Cannabis: stops ovulation and interrupts menstruation

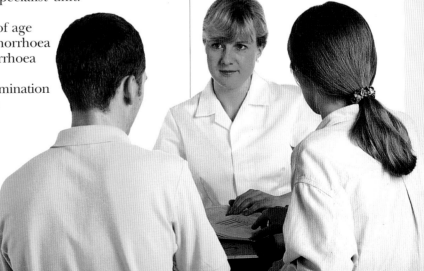

Male infertility

The most common cause of male infertility is some kind of problem with the sperm themselves, although there may be anatomical problems that prevent sperm from being released into the ejaculate. Great strides have been made in the past 15 years to increase our knowledge of male infertility and the role of sperm in particular.

PROBLEMS WITH SPERM

Sperm are extremely vulnerable cells; they take seven weeks to form and can be affected by outside influences at any point in their development. Because of this it is entirely possible for a man to give sperm samples on separate occasions that differ widely both in quality and quantity.

Testicular failure The cause is usually hard to establish, but may be due to a chromosomal problem such as Klinefelter's syndrome (when the man has two or more X chromosomes rather than one), testes that did not descend properly after birth, a blow to the testes, such as a sports injury, or mumps in adulthood.

WORKPLACE HAZARDS

Men are particularly vulnerable to hazards at work that may depress their sperm count.

Let your doctor know at the initial consultation if you work with any of the following:

• pesticides

• X-rays

• solvents used in paint products

• heavy metals such as lead, mercury, or arsenic.

ANATOMICAL PROBLEMS

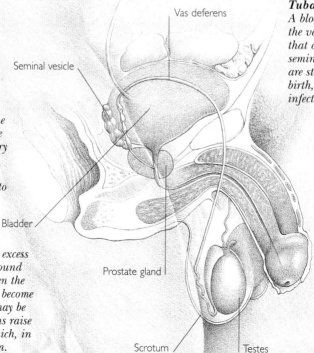

Transport of sperm
Obstruction of the vas deferens may impede the movement of sperm out of the testis.

Ejaculation problems
About one percent of men find that they do not ejaculate at the time of orgasm. This is because of retrograde ejaculation (a "dry run"), when the semen is ejaculated backwards into the bladder instead of forwards into the urethra.

Scrotum
A hydrocoele (when there is an excess of normal lubricating fluid around the testis) or a varicocoele (when the veins of the scrotum and testes become enlarged, see column, right), may be present. Both of these conditions raise the temperature of the testes which, in turn, inhibits sperm production.

Tubal blockage
A blockage of either or both of the vas deferens – the tubes that connect the testicles to the seminal vesicles where sperm are stored – may exist from birth, or be the result of an infection, such as gonnorhoea.

Testicular failure
Sperm production may be non-existent, or may be inhibited. A rare condition is testicular failure when semen contains no sperm (see opposite). Complete testicular failure, like complete ovarian failure, tends to be untreatable. It does not, however, always affect both testes

Vas deferens

Seminal vesicle

Bladder

Prostate gland

Scrotum

Testes

Low sperm counts These in themselves do not mean infertility. Many men with low sperm counts father children but conception tends to take longer. Unfortunately, however, when there are few sperm the majority tend to be abnormal or have poor motility (activity). Low sperm counts and sperm abnormalities may be caused by hormonal problems, anatomical problems, immunological problems, or even environmental factors.

IMMUNOLOGICAL PROBLEMS

Both men and women can produce antibodies to sperm which may interfere with fertilization but it's mainly a problem for men. In men the antibodies are on the surface of sperm, in the semen or in the blood. In women antibodies are found in the cervical mucus or in the blood. Antibodies are found in 5–10 percent of infertile couples. However, two out of 100 fertile men also have antibodies.

How antibodies affect fertility In terms of fertility, the most important antibodies are those that are attached to the sperm themselves: they can affect sperm motility, the ability of sperm to penetrate the cervical mucus, and the ability of sperm to fertilize the ovum. Antibodies can also affect a normal acrosome reaction (see p.41).

How fertiltiy treatments are affected Antibodies on the surface of the sperm can interfere with IVF (in vitro fertilization) and other kinds of ART (assisted reproduction technologies) (see p.48). The antibodies can immobilize the sperm, even destroy them. However, the presence of antibodies doesn't necessarily abolish the ability to conceive so many specialists recommend that antibody testing is not carried out routinely, but only in couples with "unexplained infertility" (see p.35) when all other tests are complete. This is because treatment is difficult and hazardous. The mainstay is very high dosage with steroids, which can only be justified as a research procedure in the light of serious side effects.

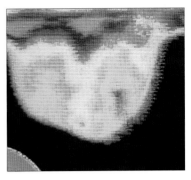

Healthy testes
This thermal photograph shows how healthy testes (blue) are at a lower temperature than the body (orange, top of picture).

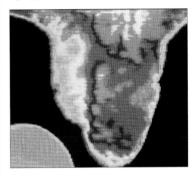

Varicocoele
The orange patches on the nearer testis are a varicocoele; the orange colour indicates a raised temperature, which can inhibit sperm production.

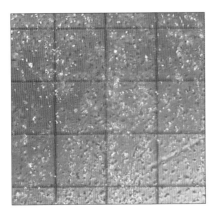

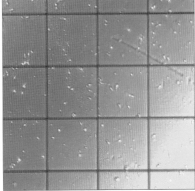

The sperm count
This basic determinant of male fertility is ascertained by two semen analyses which also check for any sperm abnormalities. Each millilitre of semen should contain at least 30 million sperm, the majority of which should be normal. The picture on the left is of a good sperm sample. If fewer than 20 million sperm are visible and there is a high proportion of abnormal sperm, the semen is described as being poor. The sperm sample shown in the picture on the right is an example of poor semen.

SEMEN ANALYSIS

Care in following instructions for collecting a sample of semen for analysis ensures that results are conclusive and the analysis won't need repeating more than twice.

Taking the sample After abstaining from sex for three days, a man produces a semen specimen by masturbating into a sterile plastic pot marked with name, date, and the time. The sample is protected from temperature extremes and delivered to the laboratory.

What's healthy? The laboratory would expect the following findings from a healthy semen sample:

Amount: 2–5 ml (half to 1 tsp)

Numbers: over 20 million sperm per ml

Motility: more than half the sperm wriggle

Normality: more than one third of the sperm are normal

White blood cells: less than 1 million per ml of sperm

Male tests

Even though a woman perhaps feels more driven to seek advice early on getting pregnant, there's no point in her doing it on her own. If a couple is having difficulty in conceiving it really doesn't make sense for the man to delay. It is important to have sperm tests done as early as possible so that treatment of both partners can proceed in tandem.

HOW MEN CAN BE HELPED

Taken overall, sperm counts in the Western world have declined in the last fifty years, and many scientists suspect that this may be due to common environmental factors (see p.38). Fertility clinics offer andrology services, which deal with male problems and diseases, as well as gynaecology services, which deal with female problems and diseases, so there is a greater chance than ever before that men who are subfertile or infertile can be helped to achieve natural fatherhood.

Male infertility can be a touchy subject because men still equate it with virility. This is a shame as the two are not linked at all. A man's sperm may be incapable of fertilizing an egg, yet he may be an excellent lover. In contrast, a man who is unable to make love to a woman may have perfectly viable, fertile sperm.

SEMEN ANALYSIS

One of the first tests for a man is semen analysis. This is organized by the doctor or clinic looking after your primary care. Two samples are usually analyzed as sperm counts can vary according to circumstances, such as how often you have sexual intercourse.

ABNORMAL SPERMATAZOA

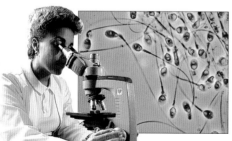

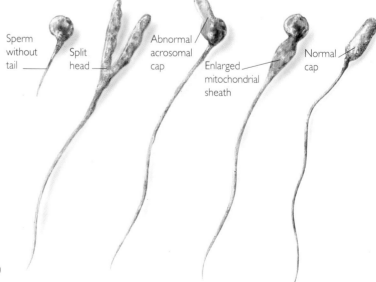

Sperm without tail — Split head — Abnormal acrosomal cap — Enlarged mitochondrial sheath — Normal cap

Examining sperm
In order for a sperm to successfully fertilize the female ovum, it needs all its essential components. The sperm's tail enables it to swim, which is vital for it to reach and fertilize the egg. The head of the sperm has a cap, the acrosome, containing enzymes that play an important role in egg penetration.

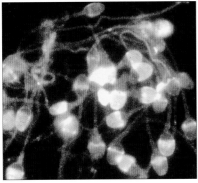

Normal sperm

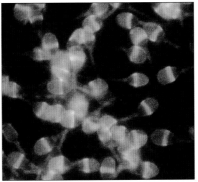

Defective sperm

Sperm acrosome test
The head of a normal sperm is surrounded by a cap, the acrosome, containing enzymes that enable the sperm to break through the outer membrane of the egg. If sperm lack this acrosomal cap, they are incapable of fertilizing an egg. Sperm are tested by using chemicals that fluoresce (glow) when they react with the acrosome. These pictures show defective sperm (on the left) and normal sperm (far left).

The analysis looks for numbers of sperm, sperm motility (how well and how much the sperm can move) and shape (known as morphology). Many specialists believe that even a relatively low sperm count may not affect fertility, but if the sample reveals a low sperm count combined with many sperm that are malformed, or have low motility, or both, or if there is a high white blood cell content, then it is likely that the man's fertility will be affected.

Low sperm counts There are several types of low sperm count. A semen analysis (see column, left) decides which of the following definitions apply to a particular sperm sample.
• Azoospermia: semen is devoid of sperm, either due to a failure to make sperm, a blockage affecting the sperm transportation, or failure to ejaculate, all of which result in sterility
• Oligospermia: there is less than 20 million sperm per ml of semen. A mild case is less then 10–20 million, a moderate case is 5–10 million, and a severe case would be less than 5 million
• Aesthenospermia: low motility (sperm are unable to wriggle) even if the count is normal
• Teratospermia: a high number of abnormal sperm. It is severe if there are more than 70 percent abnormal sperm, possibly due to a chromosomal abnormality or a harmful environmental contact. However, the cause is usually not found.

SECONDARY TESTS FOR SPERM FUNCTION

After routine semen analysis (see column, left), microscopic tests of sperm function would only be done at a specialist clinic as part of the *secondary stage* of investigation of an infertile couple. Specialist tests examine:
• the ability of sperm to penetrate mucus so that they can traverse the cervix and reach the uterus, and thence the tubes and ovum
• the ability of the sperm to recognize the ovum and latch on to it – the first step in fertilization (the acrosome test)
• the ability to fuse with and fertilize the ovum (the egg penetration or hamster test, see column, right)

These tests can be useful in predicting fertility but at present are restricted to those few centres with relevant expertise, and are not generally available.

EGG PENETRATION TEST

The potential of sperm to fertilize an egg can be tested very accurately with the egg penetration test.

Done in a laboratory, the egg penetration test involves introducing sperm to ova taken from hamsters and then measuring how well the sperm can penetrate and fuse with them.

Hamster ova are used so that your partner does not have to go through stressful hormone treatment in order to provide eggs for testing. There is no danger of an embryo resulting from the fusion of sperm and these laboratory eggs.

POLYCYSTIC OVARY SYNDROME

Many women have benign ovarian cysts that don't affect fertility. However, *polycystic ovary syndrome* (POS or PCOS) is a condition where hormone abnormalities interfere with ovulation.

True polycystic ovary syndrome is caused by excessive production of male hormone by the adrenal glands, leading to an abnormally high ratio of LH to FSH of more than 3:1. The result is that the ovary becomes filled with cysts of immature follicles which fail to generate eggs. Periods are infrequent, there's a tendency to obesity and excessive facial and body hair.

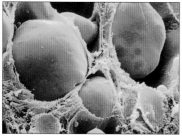

Developing eggs
Viewed through an electron microscope, this picture shows part of a normal ovary, with eggs developing in their follicles.

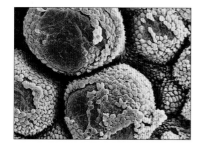

Polycystic ovary
In POS, follicles develop into cysts so eggs fail to develop or remain immature.

Female infertility

The inability of some women to conceive has been rigorously investigated over the last 30 years, and great advances in diagnosis and treatment have been pioneered. The causes of female infertility tend to fall into four main areas and all of these types can now be treated with varying degrees of success.

FAILURE TO OVULATE

The inability to release an egg is the most common cause of female infertility and is found in about a third of all infertile women. Failure to ovulate (release an egg) is usually due to hormonal problems. Occasionally, however, the ovaries are damaged or, rarely, have run out of eggs.

Hormonal problems We have already seen in the normal ovarian cycle (see p.28) that hormones from the pituitary gland and the ovary are responsible for the healthy growth and maintenance of the ovum. However, in many cases of infertility, too little of one or too much of the other hormone may be present. For example, at mid-cycle the hypothalamus should stimulate the pituitary gland to release a massive amount of FSH (follicle-stimulating hormone) and LH (luteinizing hormone) to bring about ovulation but in 20 percent of cases it fails to do so. Therefore, although there is some FSH and LH, there is not a sufficient amount for ovulation to take place. Alternatively, the pituitary gland may be damaged or malfunctioning, and either produce none or too much FSH and LH. Or, as a result of excessive LH stimulation and a relative deficiency of FSH, the ovaries may become polycystic (see column, left) and no longer capable of producing mature ova.

Problems due to abnormal levels of hormones are often treated by fertility drugs that include clomiphene, human chorionic gonadotrophin (hCG), and human menopausal gonadotrophin (hMG), in addition to female and pituitary hormones themselves. For 90 percent of women whose problems are hormonal, modern drug therapy can result in regular ovulation but, for reasons unknown, only about 65 percent of these women will achieve a pregnancy.

HORMONAL IMBALANCE

Hormones may interfere with conception in other ways than influencing ovulation. For example, a fertilized egg needs progesterone in order to survive. If too little progesterone is produced or it is produced for too short a time, the egg may not survive. Known as *inadequate luteal phase* this condition is treated with drugs.

Hyperprolactinaemia This is quite a common condition whereby there is an excessive production of the pituitary hormone responsible for milk production in women. Often, there is no apparent reason why the pituitary gland produces too much of this hormone. At other times, the condition may be due to a small benign tumour, a prolactinoma. This leads to an imbalance of FSH and LH, resulting in infrequent or absent periods in women and depressed sperm production in men.

FIBROIDS AND FERTILITY

Fibroids are benign muscle tumours that form anywhere within the uterine wall. They can sometimes be a cause of infertility, though this is rarely the case. They can cause the uterus to become misshapen and may compress either or both of the fallopian tubes.

How fertility is affected If the fibriods are very near to the surface of the uterine lining, they can interfere with the normal implantation of the embryo in the uterus, and if they occur near the junction of the uterus and the fallopian tubes, they may prevent the fertilized egg from successfully reaching the uterus to implant. Fibroids appear most frequently in women who are over the age of 35 and if they are causing problems they can be removed by surgery. The operation is called a myomectomy. It is a simple and straightforward operation that leaves the uterus and ovaries intact.

ENDOMETRIOSIS

If at your initial investigation you indicate that you suffer from very painful periods (dysmenorrhoea), your doctor may suspect endometriosis.

In this condition there are minute patches of menstruating endometrium (the uterine lining) distributed through the pelvis, ovaries, and tubes. It's not clear why it occurs but it is often associated with diminished fertility. The current theory is that the body forms antibodies to the endometrium – "autoantibodies". Not only is fertility diminished but there is excessive pregnancy wastage with sometimes repeated miscarriages. Endometriosis should always be looked for in cases of repeated miscarriage.

STRUCTURAL PROBLEMS

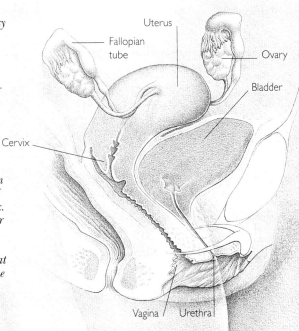

Tubal damage
A previous ectopic pregnancy (see p.225), pelvic inflammation, previous surgery, or an infection, particularly chlamydia (see p.44), may cause blocked or damaged tubes that will prevent natural conception

Problems with fertilization
In order to reach an egg to fertilize it, sperm must swim through a large quantity of mucus secreted by the cervix. If there is too little mucus or if it is thick, sperm cannot traverse the cervical canal. If it contains antibodies that attack the sperm directly, the sperm will never reach the egg and fertilization cannot occur

Damage to the ovaries
The ovaries may fail to produce mature eggs. Scarring, which is due to surgery, infection, or as a side effect of radiation treatment, can damage the ovary. Or the supply of eggs may become exhausted prematurely. This can be due to the menopause or its premature onset, surgical damage, or radiation therapy.

Uterine conditions
Problems with the uterus account for about 10 percent of infertility cases. The uterus may be congenitally abnormal in shape; contain adhesions (scars), polyps, or fibroids; or be subject to endometriosis (see above)

Uterus

Fallopian tube

Ovary

Bladder

Cervix

Vagina   Urethra

CHLAMYDIA INFECTION

Chlamydia is a sexually transmitted parasite that is so small that it is likened to a virus. Many people have unknowingly been infected with chlamydia, with a consequent impact on fertility.

It is very important for you to be tested for chlamydia infection as part of your primary investigations as this condition can cause pelvic inflammatory disease (PID). One episode of PID has a 10 percent chance of causing tubal blockage, with the risk rising to 50 percent after three episodes.

Up to 70 percent of infections in women may give rise to no symptoms and therefore go untreated. The incidence of PID can be reduced by the following:

• selective screening of high risk women for cervical chlamydia infection, which can be done with a smear test

• screening all women age 25 years or younger, plus women who have had two or more partners in the last year, who make up nearly 90 percent of infections

• any infertility test requiring the insertion of an instrument into the uterus can aggravate a cervical infection so this should not be done without first excluding chlamydia.

Testing for chlamydia infection includes a blood antibody test, cervical swabs for culture, and DNA tests. Sexual partners must be notified, assessed, and treated as chlamydia has been implicated in male infertility too.

Female tests

When primary tests indicate that you are probably ovulating, fertility clinics employ a range of more advanced tests to help them discover why you have been unable to conceive. These tests investigate the condition and functioning of your hormones, ovaries, uterus, and fallopian tubes.

HORMONE AND OVULATION TESTS

Measuring the levels of hormones in your blood or urine every day for an entire menstrual cycle can give useful information. It shows how the ovaries, brain, pituitary, and hypothalamus are interacting, and highlights any imbalance in your hormones that may be causing a problem with ovulation. Usually, your oestrogen, progesterone, and LH levels are measured and compared to normal. Other hormones that can affect ovulation are FSH, testosterone, and prolactin so blood levels will be checked.

Ultrasound scanning With a simple scan your fertility specialist can check the development of your ovarian follicles and confirm you're ovulating. This tracking of the follicle can also be of great value when ovulation is being stimulated by drugs (see p.46), as it can help avoid dangerous overstimulation. Accurate assessment of follicular growth is essential to perform complex assisted conception procedures such as IVF (in vitro fertilization) (see pp.50–1).

Endometrial biopsy The endometrium (lining of the uterus) undergoes cyclical changes under the influence of oestrogen and progesterone. There is a clear stepping-up of endometrial thickening and growth in the second half of the menstrual cycle following ovulation, due to increased progesterone production. However, if progesterone output is inadequate, development of the endometrium may not be sufficiently advanced to allow the embryo to implant successfully. In a biopsy, a tiny sample of your endometrium is taken and examined under a microscope in the second half of the menstrual cycle when any changes due to progesterone levels will be visible.

TUBAL PATENCY TESTS

The fallopian tubes are extremely delicate structures, less than four millimetres in diameter at their narrowest, and they are easily damaged. Up to a third of all of the women who attend an infertility clinic are found to have a fallopian tube problem. A number of tests exist that can demonstrate their health. This testing should always be done after the primary assessment by your family doctor. It's one of the first investigations of an infertile couple at a specialist clinic.

Hysterosalpingogram This special X-ray may be used as a screening test for tubal patency. Dye is slowly injected into the uterus and fallopian tubes through the cervix and then observed on an X-ray screen. It gives valuable information on the uterine cavity but if closer scrutiny is required you will be offered a diagnostic laparoscopy.

Laparoscopy The laparoscope (see below) uses fibreoptics to enable the surgeon to view the internal organs and evaluate the whole pelvis, giving information on adhesions, endometriosis, and ovarian disease. Laparoscopy involves hospitalization and a general anaesthetic. Any woman with pelvic disease or one who shows positive results for chlamydia antibodies would proceed straight to laparoscopy – in the latter case because the presence of antibodies are as good an indicator of tubal damage as a hysterosalpingogram.

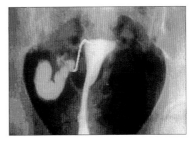

Blocked fallopian tubes
This X-ray image, produced duing a hysterosalpingogram, shows that the right fallopian tube is blocked near the uterus.

USING A LAPAROSCOPE

The surgeon uses a laparoscope – a thin viewing tube inserted through a tiny incision in the patient's abdomen. This is one of the most important and informative tests in determining whether your tubes are damaged or blocked.

Reasons for a laparoscopy
This procedure is commonly used during female infertility treatment. During this procedure, ova may be removed for use in IVF (in vitro fertilization) (see p.50).

Heathy ovary
Laparoscopy can show that organs are healthy as well as reveal any problems. This picture, taken via a laparoscope, shows a healthy ovary with a mature follicle that will soon burst to release an egg.

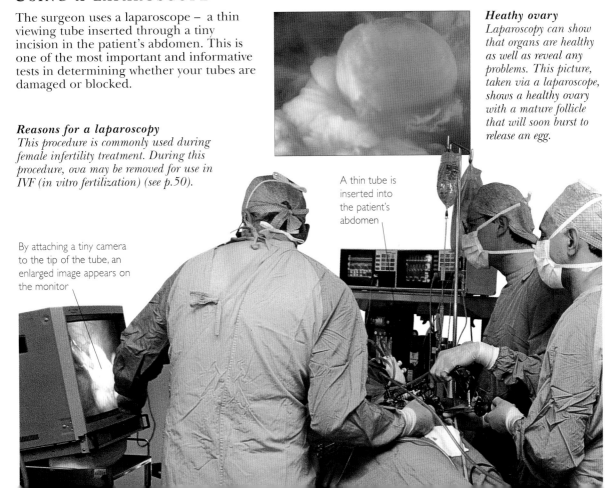

A thin tube is inserted into the patient's abdomen

By attaching a tiny camera to the tip of the tube, an enlarged image appears on the monitor

TREATING POLYCYSTIC OVARY SYNDROME

The aim of treatment is to stimulate ovulation and produce a healthy mature egg. Several methods may be tried.

Drug treatments
• Clomiphene to induce ovulation.

• FSH injection in clomiphene-resistant women.

Surgical treatments
All methods of surgery involve "damaging" the ovary in some way to bring about ovulation, either by cutting out a portion (wedge resection) or drilling holes in the surface with diathermy or laser. Surgical methods are restricted to women with clomiphene resistance.

FIMBRIOPLASTY

If a fallopain tube is blocked, it can be opened up with a microsurgical technique known as fimbrioplasty. An ovum released at ovulation can then enter the tube and so meet up with sperm one third of the way down to bring about fertilization.

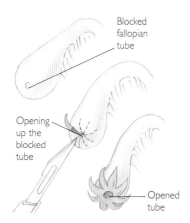

Blocked fallopian tube

Opening up the blocked tube

Opened tube

Treatments for female infertility

If you are found to be ovulating irregularly or not at all, there are extremely successful drug treatments to correct this. These treatments used to result in a large number of multiple pregnancies but doctors are now extremely sensitive to overstimulation of the ovaries, so control drug dosage very carefully and monitor you closely.

DRUG TREATMENTS

Clomiphene   In the US, clomiphene accounts for two-thirds of all fertility drugs prescribed. This is the first line treatment for amenorrhoea and oligomenorrhoea, though exactly how the drug works is still unknown. It leads to a 50 percent increase in FSH, which in turn stimulates follicles to grow and produce eggs. Ovulation usually happens around 5–10 days after the last clomiphene tablet is taken. The dose is 50–250mg and must be carefully controlled to avoid multiple pregnancies, so the formation of eggs in the ovary will be monitored closely with ultrasound. The conception rate per treatment cycle is about five percent. There is a possible association with ovarian cancer after 12 cycles so if conception isn't achieved after about six cycles, you may be advised to try ART instead (see p.48).

FSH for clomiphene-resistant POS   If you are suffering from polycystic ovarian syndrome (POS) (see p.42) but have failed to ovulate or conceive after six months' treatment with clomiphene, you'll be offered follicle-stimulating hormone (FSH) by injection. The success rates are quite high – an ovulation rate of about 95 percent per cycle and pregnancy rates of up to 25 percent after three cycles.

Pulsatile GnRH So called "hypothalamic" infertility with amenorrhoea is due to the absence of a hormone called *gonadotrophin releasing factor*, (GnRH), produced in the part of the brain called the hypothalamus. The role played by GnRH in fertility is to force another part of the brain, the pituitary gland, to release FSH and LH which in turn stimulate the ovary to ovulate. GnRH deficient women can be treated with hormone replacements usually given in intravenous "pulses" to mimic normal secretions at 60, 90, and 120 minutes, in an increasing dose per pulse. Ovulation rates as high as 75 percent and pregnancy rates up to 15 percent per cycle can be achieved after GnRH replacement treatment.

Bromocriptine High prolactin levels (hyperprolactinaemia) suppress normal GnRH pulses, which causes failure of ovulation and consequent infertility. Bromocriptine is the gold standard treatment for this condition and will suppress prolactin production and restore ovarian function. Because it is cleared from the blood quite quickly, bromocriptine usually needs to be taken around three times a day, though some newer similar drugs need only be taken once a day or even once a week. After treatment with bromocriptine, ovulation rates can be as high as 75 percent. If pregnancy occurs, treatment should stop. There are no reported cases of miscarriage, prematurity, fetal abnormalities, or multiple pregnancies as a result of this treatment.

SURGICAL PROCEDURES

Microsurgical techniques, involving laparoscopy (see p.45), have greatly improved doctors' ability to repair any damage to the fallopian tubes.

Tuboplasty (see below, right) Scarred and narrowed fallopian tubes can be unblocked by an operation known as tuboplasty. A small balloon-tipped catheter is inserted into the blocked fallopian tube and the balloon inflated to open the damaged tube and create a passage for fertilized or unfertilized eggs to pass through to reach the uterus. The balloon is then deflated and removed.

Fimbrioplasty (see left) Sometimes the frond-like ends of the fallopian tube (known as the fimbriae) fuse together, blocking the opening of the tube and thus preventing ova from entering from the ovary. Microsurgical techniques enable the blocked end of the tube to be peeled back and opened, allowing free access for ova once again.

Reversal of sterilization Known technically as "reanastomosis after sterilization", reversal of female sterilization is an increasing part of the treatment of infertility. Around three out of every 100 women who are sterilized then regret the operation later and ask for it to be reversed, very often because they have begun a new relationship and wish to have children with their new partner.

The rejoining of the severed ends of the fallopian tubes gives a good chance of achieving a normal pregnancy, rates being as high as 92 percent, but this does depend on the expertise of the surgeons at your particular centre. Unfortunately, in some centres, success rates may be less than 50 percent so it is worth checking this.

Sterilization with clips has the highest chance of being successfully reversed. However, IVF (see p.48) may be the treatment of choice for sterilized women, the pregnancy rate being about 1 in 6.

TREATING ENDOMETRIOSIS

Drug treatments do not help infertility due to endometriosis (see p.43) but it can be treated surgically quite successfully.

Laparoscopic surgery (see p.45) can be used to destroy all visible signs of endometriosis. This increases the possibility of conceiving by almost 75 percent in the first 36 weeks after treatment in women under the age of 40 with mild endometriosis.

ART (see p.48) should be considered for women who fail to conceive after laparascopic surgery whether or not they have tubal obstruction and for women with moderate to severe endometriosis.

Some US specialists believe it is better to go straight to ART, without prior surgical intervention.

TUBOPLASTY

This procedure is usually performed if the fallopian tubes have become scarred or blocked.

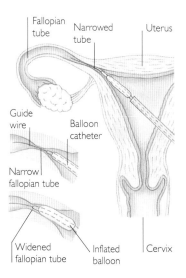

Fallopian tube — Narrowed tube — Uterus

Guide wire — Balloon catheter

Narrow fallopian tube

Widened fallopian tube — Inflated balloon — Cervix

MEDICAL RISKS OF ART

ART can bring hope and optimism for many couples and – of course – result in a healthy pregnancy and a bouncing baby. But it's as well to be aware that, even after successful conception, the pregnancy is at a higher risk than usual:

• high miscarriage rate (25 percent)

• high rate of ectopic pregnancies (4 percent)

• high rate of complications (15 percent)

• high rate of premature births (20 percent)

• high rate of Caesarean sections (15 percent)

• high rate of multiple pregnancies (15 percent).

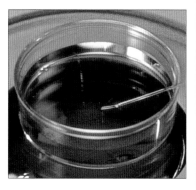

IVF
Harvested eggs are placed in liquid in a special dish and mixed with sperm. A fertilized egg(s) is then placed in the uterus for implantation.

ART
(assisted reproduction technology)

Assisted reproduction technology has helped many childless couples to become parents. What was once known as in vitro fertilization (IVF) has grown into a sometimes bewildering number of techniques which manipulate the fundamental biology of human reproduction in both men and women. Before embarking on ART treatment, couples should be aware that the emotional costs can be high and should receive the appropriate support and counselling.

WHAT IS ART?

ART is an umbrella term that describes a range of infertility treatments (see chart, right). Through drugs, laboratory techniques, and even the use of donors, the reproductive potential of both men and women can be maximized by bringing about sperm production, ovulation, fertilization, implantation, conception, and birth.

WHY YOU MAY NEED IT

If any crucial step is compromised in the chain of events resulting in a healthy baby, either of you may need ART. Possible problems include failure to produce mobile sperm, failure to ovulate, and failure of healthy sperm to penetrate and fertilize an ovum.

ETHICAL CONSIDERATIONS

The science of assisted reproduction technology raises enormous ethical questions that affect the individual, the couple, the family, the community, and society. Most of us would say that whatever enhances the moral status and dignity of everyone can be considered morally acceptable. But each situation can be complicated by experience, cultural background, the law, and religious teaching.

Discussing alternatives In becoming a family each person becomes part of a couple, but each still has a unique perspective and interest. In addition, there are the interests of the potential child to consider. I don't feel that doctors have the right to question a couple who opt for treatment for infertility. To my mind, the only option is to offer counselling to discuss alternatives like adoption and the use of donor sperm or eggs.

It's important for specialists to understand that an infertile couple is in a vulnerable position and that they bear a heavy responsibility to see that the couple receives impeccable investigation and therapy.

Contentious issues It is generally agreed that there is no moral problem with ART using the sperm and eggs of partners, the only objection being from the Roman Catholic church. However, the use of donor eggs, sperm, or even embryos is highly sensitive. Arguments against it include that it violates marriage vows and blurs a child's genetic make-up. On the other hand, all the evidence points to a reassuring track record for such children.

The view in the UK is that financial compensation for donors or surrogacy should be avoided and the anonymity of donors and surrogates is paramount. However, elsewhere in the world payment for egg donors is inevitable as there simply aren't enough donors to go round.

Cryopreservation (freezing of donor sperm or pre-embryos) is another area of concern. Despite religious opposition, cryopreservation has proved to be very useful in improving pregnancy rates while avoiding multiple pregnancies. It's worth remembering that most moral arguments object only to the fact that some pre-embryos will not survive. In principle, cryopreservation preserves individual human life.

Ethics is not an exact science. There is no absolute moral right and wrong. To impose a moral imperative unwillingly on another person is nothing less than tyranny and flies in the face of enhancing the moral dignity of a couple and their children.

PSYCHOLOGICAL IMPACT

Because we all feel that our fertility and sexuality are intimately bound together we can feel profoundly disturbed when either is questioned. So counselling is important. The biggest strains occur at key moments, for example:

• **during ovarian stimulation** – anxiety about techniques and the hormonal effects leads to fear and tension, constraining sexual needs

• **during laboratory investigation** – couples fear that embryos may get mixed-up, or be damaged

• **after embryo transfer** – there is worry about implantation problems, or complications such as ectopic pregnancy, or multiple pregnancy.

ART: WHAT THE INITIALS MEAN

IVF	*In vitro fertilization (see p.50). Fertilization takes place outside the body, in a glass dish (in vitro means "in glass"), and the fertilized embryo or embryos are replaced into the uterus. Helpful for couples where the woman's fallopian tubes are damaged, in cases of severe endometriosis, immune problems, unexplained infertility, and older women who have deteriorating egg production.*
GIFT	*Gamete intrafallopian transfer. Sperm and ovum are mixed outside the body and immediately transferred back into the fallopian tube so that fertilization can happen "naturally". GIFT is cheaper and has a higher pregnancy rate than IVF, but can only be used for women with healthy fallopian tubes.*
ZIFT	*Zygote Intra-Fallopian Transfer. As GIFT, except a very young embryo is transferred to the fallopian tube.*
SUZI	*Sub-zonal Insemination. A type of IVF in which sperm are carefully selected and injected underneath the zona pellucida (the outer layer of the egg). This helps men with low sperm counts.*
MIST	*Micro-insemination sperm transfer. See SUZI above.*
ICSI	*Intra-Cytoplasmic Sperm Injection. An amazing technique in which a single sperm is selected, specially treated and injected directly into the egg itself (see p.52). When fertilization has taken place by IVF, the embryo is transferred in the usual way.*
MESA	*Micro-Epididymal Sperm Aspiration. The surgical extraction of sperm from the epididymis is needed for men who have no sperm in their ejaculate, because of a blocked vas deferens. It precedes ICSI.*
TESE	*Testicular Sperm Extraction. As MESA, except the sperm are collected from the testis for ICSI.*

The typical pattern of an IVF treatment

Several difficult and complex steps have to be negotiated so that you can have your baby: harvesting the mother's eggs; fertilization of eggs by healthy sperm; implantation of at least one embryo into your uterus; pregnancy to term, and delivery of a healthy baby.

ENSURING A GOOD EGG SUPPLY

In order to maximize the chances of a successful pregnancy through IVF treatment, more than one egg at a time is removed for fertilization. Normally a woman will only shed one egg during each ovarian cycle. A few days after the end of your period your ovaries will be stimulated to make them produce more than one egg. You will be given ovary-stimulating drugs, such as clomiphene or hMG (human menopausal gonadotrophin), so

RETRIEVING THE MATURE EGGS

Using ultrasound to give a clear picture of the reproductive tract, a gynaecologist delicately guides a thin, hollow probe through the vagina and uterus and along a fallopian tube towards the ripened eggs. These eggs are then drawn into the probe by gentle suction.

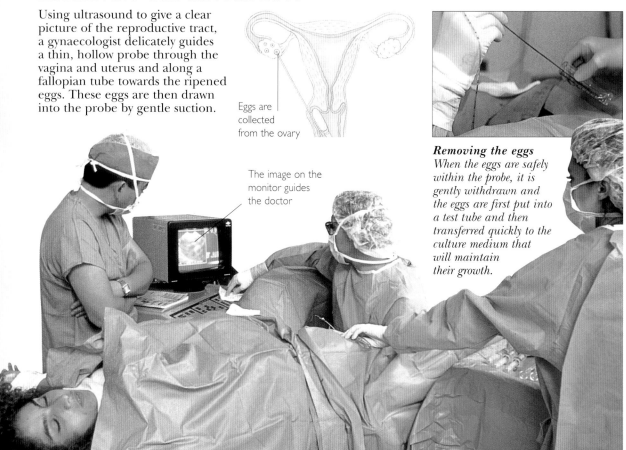

Eggs are collected from the ovary

The image on the monitor guides the doctor

Removing the eggs
When the eggs are safely within the probe, it is gently withdrawn and the eggs are first put into a test tube and then transferred quickly to the culture medium that will maintain their growth.

that your ovaries produce a number of eggs simultaneously. Over the next week or so you will make daily visits to the fertility clinic so that the development of the eggs can be carefully monitored with ultrasound scans. As the eggs mature, the follicles containing them swell and produce increasing amounts of oestrogen. A series of blood tests will detect this increase in oestrogen and the growth of follicles can be precisely measured and tracked by a daily scan.

COLLECTING THE EGGS

When ovulation is imminent, your mature eggs are collected at your clinic under ultrasonic or laparoscopic guidance ready for fertilization by your partner's sperm.

Ultrasonic guidance The use of ultrasound pictures to guide the egg retrieval probe is less invasive than using a laparoscope (see below). It's carried out under light or local anaesthetic and you will need to spend only a few hours at the fertility clinic instead of staying in overnight as you would have to do if you had a laparoscopy.

Laparoscopy (see p.45). This is key-hole surgery. A laparoscope, a small, thin telescope is passed into your pelvic cavity and a fine, hollow probe collects ripened eggs from your ovaries under direct vision. While you're anaesthetized a small amount of carbon dioxide gas is injected into your abdominal cavity to separate the organs so that they can be seen more easily. The laparoscope is inserted through a small incision made in your navel and your eggs are carefully collected with the probe.

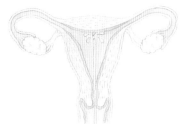

Returning eggs
Once the eggs and sperm have been mixed outside of the body, a successfully fertilized egg is then injected through the cervix via a thin tube for implantation in the uterus.

CONFIRMING CONCEPTION

18 hours after they have been mixed with your partner's semen, the eggs are inspected under a microscope to find out if any have been fertilized. It is uncommon for all the eggs to be fertilized and develop into embryos, but two or three usually do. Fertilized eggs are incubated for 48 hours or more, when they will have divided into about 2–4 cells. Providing they show no signs of abnormality, a maximum of three embryos are transferred (see p.53) to your uterus. The picture on the right shows a sperm approaching an egg.

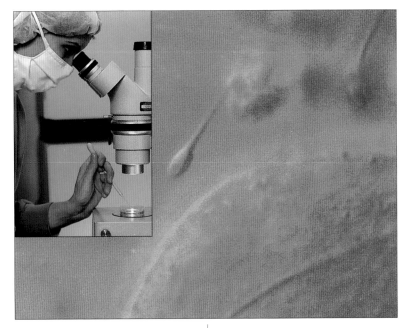

Advanced ART

A major advance in reproductive technology, the micromanipulation of sperm and eggs, has made it possible for a man with a very low sperm count and virtually no motile sperm to fertilize his partner's ovum and go on to have a healthy baby.

MICROMANIPULATION

ICSI (intra-cytoplasmic sperm injection) (see p.49) is one technique which uses micromanipulation. A prepared ovum is placed under a microscope and injected directly with an individual sperm (see below). Sperm may be collected by masturbation or from the testis itself through surgical techniques such as MESA or TESE (see p.49). Once fertilized the embryo is incubated and implanted by embryo transfer (see opposite) when it's reached 2–4 cells in size. ICSI may be offered to couples who fail to conceive by other methods. The first ICSI pregnancy was in 1988.

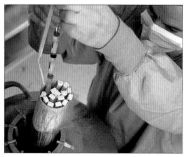

Frozen sperm
Sperm frozen in liquid nitrogen can be used during ICSI procedures. This is particularly effective for men with a low sperm count or for sperm with poor motility, as the sperm can be stored and then injected directly into the prepared egg.

ICSI (intra-cytoplasmic sperm injection)
In ICSI, an egg is placed under a microscope and then injected with an individual sperm (see right). If the egg is fertilized it is placed inside the woman's uterus ready for implantation, a process known as "embryo transfer" (see opposite).

Timetable for ICSI
Below is a timeline showing the steps in ICSI through drug treatment to embryo transfer: the principles would be the same for other forms of IVF.

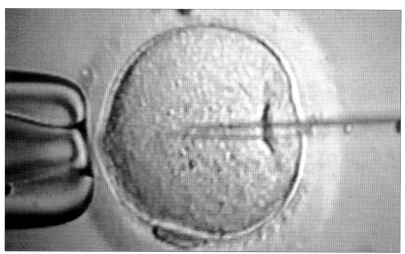

TIMETABLE FOR ICSI (INTRA-CYTOPLASMIC SPERM INJECTION)

DAY 1	2	3	4	5	6	7	8	9	10	11	12	13	14	15	16	17	18	19	20

⟵ **DRUG TREATMENT TO ENSURE GOOD EGG SUPPLY** ⟶

Days 1–10
Drugs (LH/RH agonists) to suppress menstrual cycle

Days 11–21
Daily gonadotrophin (FSH) injections to stimulate follicles

Day 1
1st day of menstrual cycle

Day 10
Blood test to confirm suppression

Day 14
1st ultrasound scan to check follicle development

Days 18–21
Daily scans to check growth of follicles. On day 21 final scan confirms one follicle is 16–18mm, others at least 14mm, then final FSH injection is given

However, there are controversial issues surrounding this technique. For example, there is concern that an ovum could be fertilized with a sub-standard, weak sperm, possibly resulting in damaged or unhealthy children. Although the pregnancy rate with ICSI is not high, the babies born so far have been normal with no chromosomal abnormalities.

EMBRYO TRANSFER

All forms of IVF (see p.49) require taking an embryo, usually between two and three days old, from the incubating dish in the laboratory and placing it inside a woman's body. Sadly, two out of three embryo transfers fail to implant. Successful implantation is dependent on the age of the mother, the quality of the embryo, and the receptivity of the uterus.

One of the problems with this treatment is that doctors still don't know when is the best time to transfer an embryo. Studies seem to suggest that delaying the transfer of an embryo to the uterus can increase the chances of implantation. However, in one study, there was no difference in pregnancy rates between embryos that were replaced 44 hours after insemination and those that were replaced 68 hours after insemination. Also, pregnancy rates increase with the numbers of embryos that are replaced: for example, one embryo gives an eight percent chance of becoming pregnant, two embryos give a 25 percent chance, and three embryos give a 33 percent chance of pregnancy. Often, therefore, doctors may be keen to transfer more than one embryo.

Cryopreserved embryos (see p.49). It's also possible to thaw out cryopreserved (frozen) embryos or eggs from liquid nitrogen (-273°C) and transfer them in the same way. The embryo is thawed slowly, at a rate of 8°C per minute. However, not all embryos survive this process in a good enough state to implant. Replacement in the womb is done at a point in the menstrual cycle, 100 hours after the LH (luteinizing hormone) peak, which is determined by serial blood tests. Pregnancy rates vary from 1 in 6 to 1 in 4.

THE FUTURE OF ART

Great progress in ART has been made in the last decade of the twentieth century. Living proof of the advanced technology are the many thousands of babies who are now alive and well.

Many doctors feel that ART has gone as far as it can, the pregnancy rate having reached the natural chance to conceive – a rate of 22 percent. However, there seems to be a lot left to learn and to do:

• superovulation of the ovaries will probably be achieved

• further studies will be made on embryos before transfer

• there is still much research to be done on the implantation of the embryo in the uterus

• male infertility will probably be studied increasingly, perhaps as the result of refinement of ICSI (see opposite) or the invention of some other method of sperm treatment

• more investigation is needed into cryopreservation techniques, to improve egg freezing methods and the low pregnancy rate with freeze-thawed embryo to open up new horizons for infertile couples

• in vitro maturation of eggs.

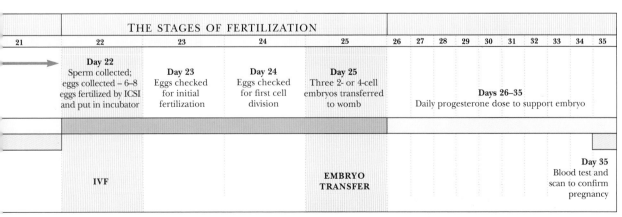

THE STAGES OF FERTILIZATION														
21	22	23	24	25	26	27	28	29	30	31	32	33	34	35

Day 22
Sperm collected; eggs collected – 6–8 eggs fertilized by ICSI and put in incubator

Day 23
Eggs checked for initial fertilization

Day 24
Eggs checked for first cell division

Day 25
Three 2- or 4-cell embryos transferred to womb

Days 26–35
Daily progesterone dose to support embryo

IVF

EMBRYO TRANSFER

Day 35
Blood test and scan to confirm pregnancy

Using donors, or a surrogate mother, is not something to embark on without careful thought and specialized counselling.

The use of donors is an area of potential conflict between partners and you need to try to be sympathetic to each other's reactions. Sometimes one partner has seen it as a corrective measure for poor sexual performance, or procreative failure, which can lead to destructive guilt or subconscious accusation or blame. You also need to think about your relationship with a child conceived this way. Ask yourself these questions:

• if you were to have a child using donor sperm, or eggs, or both, would the fact that the child wasn't "yours" prevent you from loving her as your own?

• would you feel jealous if a donor conceived a child with your partner when you couldn't?

• would you tell your child about how she was conceived, or would you try to keep it a secret?

• if your child was conceived using donor eggs, or sperm, or both, how would you cope if she wanted to trace her genetic history in later life? What if she couldn't because records were destroyed – as they often are?

Using donors

Sperm, egg, and even embryo donation have helped many childless couples become parents. Surrogacy is also a form of donation when a woman donates her uterus to bear another couple's biological child. However, emotional costs can be high, and it is essential that all the issues should be discussed openly. Counselling for couples considering assisted conception is provided by clinics and hospitals.

DONOR INSEMINATION

In cases where men are sterile or have subfertile (very low) sperm counts that do not respond to treatment donor insemination is an option. So too where there is a major blood group incompatibility between the couple (for example, where a Rhesus-negative woman has developed antibodies to the Rhesus-positive blood of her partner); when either partner carries a hereditary abnormality; or when a mature, stable, single woman wants a child but not a partner.

Donor insemination (DI) can seem an ideal solution for many couples but there are a number of points to consider carefully. Foremost are the feelings of your partner. It is not uncommon for men to feel inadequate or jealous of donors who impregnate their partners. This can rebound on your life together, and on the child after it is born. In addition, some women are repelled by the circumstances in which they conceive or by the fact that a different man's sperm is used at each visit. Others worry about what sort of man the donor was, or idealize him as a "perfect man", or wonder if their child will meet, and perhaps marry, a half sibling. Using sperm from a donor that you know, or are related to by marriage, can relieve some of these problems but can magnify others. It also raises its own problems, such as what happens if the father wants visiting rights.

It is still usual for doctors to advise secrecy (records are normally destroyed to ensure the anonymity of the donor), but that can be a heavy burden for a couple to carry. DI could also be very damaging to the child, especially if other people know and let it slip, or if it comes out at a time of crisis, such as divorce. Most couples feel hesitant about this method of conception. It is exceedingly stressful, so good counselling is essential. You can insist that there is no mention of DI in your maternity records, and you and your partner's names can be given on the birth certificate.

EGG DONATION

In cases where a woman is unable to produce an egg, those of a donor may be used during IVF treatment. Egg donation has the advantage that both of you are involved: your partner fertilizes the egg, and you will carry and give birth to the baby. However, it is more complicated than sperm donation. It relies on hormonal drugs and egg collection techniques (see p.48). Consequently, donor eggs are hard to find, the main sources being anonymous donors, IVF patients who may donate extra eggs, and relatives. Problems can arise from these sources: the eggs donated by IVF mothers have an increased risk of chromosomal disorders because IVF patients tend to be older than average, and donated eggs from relatives or friends may lead to family tensions. As with sperm donations, records of donors are often destroyed, and this secrecy may adversely affect your child later in life.

If you are not producing eggs, you probably will not be menstruating, and this means that the lining of your uterus (endometrium) will be thin and incapable of nourishing a developing embryo. Consequently, you will be given drugs to stimulate it to thicken so that the embryo can implant.

EMBRYO DONATION

This happens occasionally when couples donate unused embryos that have been frozen and stored to childless couples. This has been the focus of much debate, and raises many sensitive issues, such as the donor parents' feelings if their own child, or children, die, and the chances of the siblings meeting and perhaps having children together. However, it does mean that it is an "adopted" child for both of you.

SELECTING SEMEN AND EMBRYOS

Semen Fresh semen is usually frozen and stored and then used for donor insemination. While the semen is being stored, the clinic has time to test it and the donor for infections. The semen is put into a sterile vial and frozen by immersing it in liquid nitrogen. It is then stored for a period of months, during which time tests are carried out on the donor to ensure that he is free of infections, such as hepatitis B or HIV, that could be transmitted via his semen. When it has been established that the donor was free of infection at the time of donation, the semen is tested for harmful microorganisms, such as bacteria; if these tests prove negative, semen can then be used for insemination.

Up to 50 percent of sperm in the semen are unlikely to survive the freezing and thawing, although this fall in sperm numbers is partly offset by the fact that it is the healthiest, most robust sperm that will survive the process. Donor insemination is carried out under exactly the same conditions as artificial insemination with sperm from a partner (see p.49).

Embryos Storage by cryopreservation (CRP) (when embryos are frozen, see p.53) prevents embryo wastage when several embryos have been fertilized and avoids the necessity of transferring all the embryos to the uterus and the risk of a multiple pregnancy. Pregnancies that result from CRP embryos has raised the success rate of a cycle of IVF treatment from one to 10 percent.

SURROGATE MOTHERS

Surrogate motherhood – where a woman bears a child on behalf of another – is physically straightforward but fraught with potential emotional, legal, and moral difficulties.

Full surrogacy The simplest form of surrogacy is where a surrogate mother conceives and carries the child of an infertile woman's partner. Insemination may be indirect (the surrogate is artificially inseminated with the man's sperm) or direct (the man has sexual intercourse with the surrogate).

Partial surrogacy In this arrangement an egg from the woman who is unable to conceive is fertilized with her partner's sperm and then implanted into the surrogate mother's uterus.

Surrogacy problems After the child is born it is handed over to the couple who commissioned it. They then legally adopt it and the surrogate mother subsequently has little or no involvement with it. The surrogate may, however, find it very hard to part with the child, especially if she is its genetic mother. In some well-publicized cases couples have had to take lengthy and costly legal action in order to get custody of the baby.

Other problems can arise if the child is born handicapped or if the surrogate wants to maintain a close relationship with her child and is not allowed to do so. There is also the possibility that either or both of the commissioning parents may find it hard to accept the child fully and lovingly.

Male infertility

Such was male pride in the past that the possibility of a man being infertile was never mentioned let alone openly discussed and male doctors, in the main, connived. We now know that men are responsible for half of all infertility and it's time to come to terms with that regardless of sensitivities. After all, women have been doing it for decades.

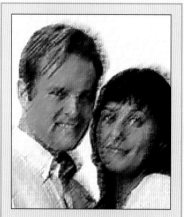

Names **Peter and Jane**

Ages **29 and 27 years**

Past medical history **Peter had NSU (non-specific urethritis) three years ago and was treated at a G.U. (genito-urinary) Clinic with no recurrence. Peter had mumps when he was 12 years of age. Jane has no relevant medical history**

Obstetric history **Peter and Jane have been trying for a baby for three years without success**

With 30 approaching fast, Jane feels her biological clock is ticking away and she doesn't want to leave conceiving to chance any longer. She would like to get some medical advice about what she and Peter should do next and asks Peter if he'll see the doctor with her. However, Peter is shifty and makes excuses about why he can't go, so in the end she visits the doctor on her own.

TAKING THE INITIATIVE

Like most women, Jane shoulders the responsibility for starting a family. Like a lot of men, Peter would rather not know when there appears to be a problem with conceiving. Women are nearly always the ones who seek advice first about infertility. Quite a lot of men write to me in confidence and independently of their wives to seek advice. Perhaps its having to face another man in the form of a male doctor that puts men off. In public men are defensive.

Joint responsibilities

Whatever the reason, many men are loath to discuss the possibility of their being infertile, which in itself is sad. Firstly, infertility should not be equated to virility and men need to understand this and separate these two things in their minds. Secondly, if a man is found to have less than perfect fertility, nowadays there is much that can be done to help him and his partner conceive successfully. Either way, men have to face up to the possibility of infertility. In half of all infertile couples the infertile partner is found to be the man. Responsibility must be shouldered jointly.

Overcoming reservations

Reticent though Peter is to become involved, I've pointed out that the failure to have a baby can never be tackled by Jane alone. Even if he turns out to be blameless, infertility investigation is only ever undertaken as a couple and if he really wants to have children he must overcome both his embarrassment and any sense of guilt and shame.

PRIMARY TESTS

Jane's doctor said more or less the same and after about a week of soul-searching, Peter agreed to a joint consultation. Poor Peter, it was only the beginning.

The doctor took very seriously Peter's past attack of NSU (non-specific urethritis) as any sexually transmitted disease can interfere with fertility. As can the mumps virus, which may cause inflammation of the testes and damage future sperm production. At the pubertal age of 12 Peter's testes were extremely vulnerable. At the end of the intial interview, prospects didn't look too bright for Peter. Nor did they improve when the doctor asked Peter to attend the fertility clinic for semen analysis on two separate occasions.

By this time, Peter felt very much the injured party. However, the doctor explained that both

Jane and he would need to have primary tests done. Jane's would be in the form of a smear test, a test for chlamydia, an internal examination, and blood tests to confirm ovulation. Peter's part of the bargain would entail a physical examination of his penis and testes *and* semen analyses.

As the doctor explained, analysis to examine the form and health of his sperm is only logical: it would be a difficult task to obtain Jane's eggs for examination but his sperm are available through the simple expedient of masturbation (see page 40).

Strains on the relationship

Things went steadily downhill from this point. Peter hated attending the fertility clinic and having to supply semen samples: it was so cold and clinical and inhuman. He felt torn. He wanted to do what was necessary, to please Jane if nothing else, but he felt isolated and persecuted. His morale fell lower and lower at the prospect of finding that it was all his fault.

Jane did her best to reassure Peter and show her love for him, but he went deeper and deeper into his shell, refused to talk about the problem, and became very uncommunicative. Jane felt increasingly estranged from Peter. Peter felt unloved and they stopped having sex altogether. Jane, feeling desperate, suggested that they should get some counselling. Peter cut short the conversation by leaving the room.

All seemed lost when the results of the semen analysis came back. Peter's sperm count was 5–10 million, and less than 30 percent of his sperm were active.

Getting support

At this point I insist that both Peter and Jane give serious consideration to seeing a counsellor if only to outline that all was not lost. It was a great struggle, but Peter finally swallowed his male pride and made an appointment to see a fertility counsellor with Jane so that they could be prepared for what was to come.

SECONDARY TESTS

The counsellor explained that, although a low sperm count with low motility is, of course, a blow, Peter does have some sperm, and some are mobile. This means that even if Peter's sperm fail the ovum penetration test, an advanced form of ART (assisted reproduction technology) called ICSI (see p.49), in which an individual sperm is injected into one of Jane's healthy ova, could lead to a successful pregnancy and a healthy baby at the end of it.

This possibility is a cause for rejoicing not for sadness, nor for Peter's feelings of worthlessness.

EMBARKING ON IVF

An IVF treatment programme (see p.50) isn't straightforward for either of them: Jane, despite her normal fertility, will need to be heavily involved too. In order to increase the chances of having several eggs on which to perform ICSI with Peter's sperm she will have to undergo drug treatments and serial tests to make sure her ovaries are goaded into producing several eggs at the same time rather than the usual one. This part of the treatment takes the best part of three weeks and both Peter and Jane must be prepared

for the effect of the fertility hormones on Jane. At the very least she could become moody, irritable, even weepy and tearful. She'll have to make daily visits to the fertility clinic for ultrasound scans during the third week, which will play havoc with her normal life and work. She will have to make special arrangements and Peter has to be prepared to help her out.

In fact the maximum impact of Peter's infertility falls on Jane. Even though Jane is desperate to have a baby it's easy for resentment to build, especially if the initial treatments aren't successful and she has to undergo several programmes. Peter's involvement, by comparison, is miniscule – all he has to do is provide two specimens of semen each treatment programme. That in itself can cause estrangement from Jane. If he's not careful it's all too easy for Peter to feel shame and guilt and begin to hate Jane (as well as himself) for putting him in this position. It could all sadly backfire.

No couple should face such a painful situation without psychological support and I think Peter is beginning to accept that. Their fertility clinic has a team of counsellors and Peter and Jane have made an appointment to see one next week. Once they've had all the different steps of the fertility programme explained to their satisfaction and all their questions have been answered (I advise them to sit down and make a list together) I strongly advise them to keep on talking about their feelings to each other and to their counsellor, every step of the way.

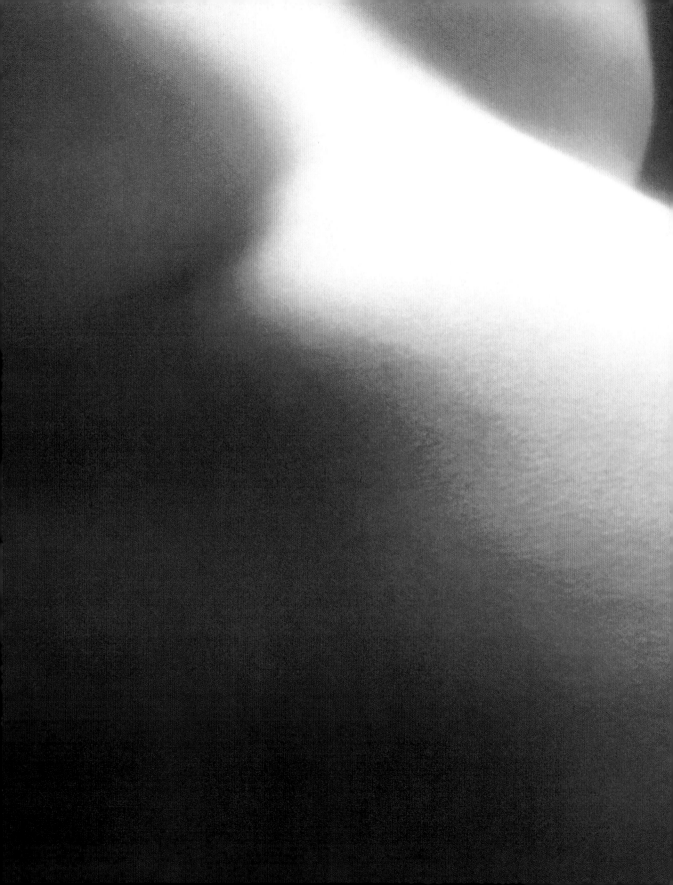

CHAPTER 2

You and your DEVELOPING BABY

There is very little as exciting as the month-by-month development of your baby. Understanding exactly how he grows will help you establish a relationship with your baby even before he is born.

Pregnant!

Many women "know" when they conceive. This special intuitive feeling is probably due to the very early outpouring of female hormones, initially prolonged high levels of progesterone (which a woman does not experience unless she is pregnant), followed by the production of human chorionic gonadotrophin (hCG) by the fetal tissues as soon as the embryo achieves implantation, about seven days after fertilization.

SUSPECTING THAT YOU ARE PREGNANT

There are certain classic signs that can make you suspect that you are pregnant before seeking confirmation.

Amenorrhoea Within two weeks of fertilization, a woman may miss a period. Although pregnancy is the most common cause of amenorrhoea, it is not the only one, so a missed period should not be taken as an absolute sign of pregnancy. Several other factors such as jet lag, severe illness, surgery, shock, bereavement, or great stress also can cause amenorrhoea. Periods, however, do not always stop in pregnancy: some women have been known to have light periods up to the sixth month, and occasionally all the way through their pregnancies.

Frequency of urination As soon as progesterone levels rise and the embryo starts to secrete hCG, the blood supply to the pelvic area increases, which leads to pelvic congestion. This is communicated to the bladder, which becomes irritable and tries to expel even the smallest quantity of urine. Most women therefore experience the desire to pass urine (micturition) more frequently than usual, although it may be in only very small quantities. This can happen as early as one week after conception.

Tiredness Fatigue is partly due to very high levels of progesterone, which has a sedative effect. During early pregnancy your metabolism speeds up in order to support your developing embryo and your vital organs, which have to cope with an enormously increased amount of work. This can lead to utter fatigue, which is sometimes so great that it is uncontrollable and you may just have to sleep. If so, you must – for your sake and for your baby's.

Odd tastes and cravings The saliva·often reflects the chemical content of the blood and, with rising hormone levels, the taste within your mouth can change, often being described as metallic. This can also make the taste of certain foods different from

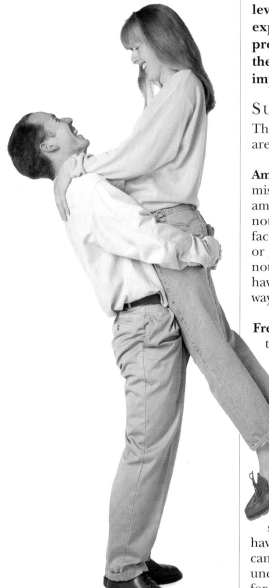

Discovering a new life
Finding out that you are pregnant is often one of the most special moments in your life.

normal, with some that you may usually enjoy (coffee is a common example) even becoming intolerable. There is no real scientific explanation for cravings, which can occasionally be for very odd things such as coal, but they are thought to be the body's response to deficiency in certain minerals and trace elements. Try to control or distract cravings for inedible substances as well as high-calorie foods that are low in nutritional value. Otherwise feel free to indulge yourself within reason.

Morning sickness   Most common in the morning, morning sickness can come on at any time of day especially when you do not eat often enough and your blood sugar is allowed to drop.

Smell   Pregnancy often heightens your sense of smell, and you may find that common odours such as cooking smells make you nauseous. Perfume can also have a similar effect, and you may notice that the way your perfume smells also changes, owing to alterations in your skin's chemistry.

Breast changes   Even at the start of pregnancy, breast changes may be quite obvious: your breasts can become quite lumpy and sore to the touch; the nipple area may become tender and sensitive, and will also deepen in colour; and veins can become enlarged over the surface of the breasts.

CONFIRMING PREGNANCY

Once you suspect that you might be pregnant you should seek confirmation as soon as possible. There are a variety of tests available that can be performed at different intervals following conception. Some are more accurate than others.

Blood test   This test has to be performed by your doctor and is becoming more widely available. It can accurately detect the pregnancy hormone hCG (human chorionic gonadotrophin) in the blood as early as two weeks after conception – about the time your next period is due.

Urine tests   HCG can also be detected in your urine. Urine tests can be conducted at home, in hospital, at your doctor's office, at family planning clinics, or chemists. These tests are over 90 percent reliable and can be performed as soon as two weeks after conception, although you will get the most reliable result if you wait four weeks longer (see also p.62).

Internal examination   The routine use of ultrasound at around 12 weeks (see p.180) means that women almost never have to suffer internal examinations during pregnancy. Once they were used to confirm the pregnancy because pregnancy hormones soften the cervix and uterus and cause more blood to be directed to the pelvis, giving the vagina and cervix a classic purplish tinge visible through a speculum. Slight uterine enlargement could also be felt.

TELLING THE WORLD

You will obviously tell your partner, and possibly your immediate family, as soon as you know yourself.

Doctor   Your pregnancy may be confirmed by your doctor, so he or she will obviously know immediately. If not, you should get in contact as soon as you can to discuss birth options and antenatal care.

Employer   You should tell your employer before you attend your first antenatal clinic (see p.174), which will probably be when you are about three months pregnant.

Friends and acquaintances   Many women delay telling friends and acquaintances that they are pregnant until after the first trimester. Although this is understandable, it is probably unnecessary once your doctor has confirmed your pregnancy.

DO YOU HAVE THE CORRECT RESULT?

A number of factors can affect whether your pregnancy test results are accurate.

• In older women, hormonal changes caused by approaching menopause can give false positives or negatives.

• Incorrectly collected or stored urine can lead to errors.

• If the test is performed too early, the concentration of hCG will be too low to detect. It is important to know when your period was due. Irregular or infrequent periods can affect an accurate indication of pregnancy.

• Antidepressant or fertility drugs containing hCG or hMG can change the results. Contraceptive pills, antibiotics, and painkillers should not have any effect.

• If the equipment used for the test is too hot, the result may be false. Urine must be room temperature at the time of the test.

HOME TESTING

Finding out whether you are pregnant in the privacy of your own home may help to ease any nervous feelings and you can be sure of complete confidentiality. There are a variety of pregnancy testing kits available from chemists, which are simple to use and offer immediate results with an accuracy of over 90 percent.

How the tests work All the urine tests check for the presence of hCG (human chorionic gonadotrophin), the hormone that is manufactured by the blastocyst. Two of the main types, the ring and the colour tests, involve mixing a chemical solution with a sample of your urine. The chemicals react according to the amount of hCG in your urine. The reaction is shown by a colour change in the tube or window strip, or coagulation is prevented, causing a dark ring to appear in the tube. A third test can be done by simply placing the absorbent part of the test in contact with the urine. From two weeks after conception, hCG may be detected in urine. Most kits advise using the test between one and four days after the first day of your missed period. However, if you do perform the test then, repeat it two weeks later when the hCG is more concentrated and the result will be more reliable. Most kits provide two tests for the purpose of confirmation.

Necessary precautions Make sure your sample of urine is the first passed that morning (it will have a higher concentration of hCG) and that it is collected in a clean, soap-free container. Do not have any liquids before the test as this will dilute the sample. Follow the kit's instructions very carefully and do not use the test if it has been damaged in any way or is past its use-by date. If you cannot perform the test immediately, store the specimen in the refrigerator, but don't keep it for more than 12 hours.

Unexpected result It is possible that a test will show a positive result that becomes negative when repeated, and your period may start a few days later. Don't worry. Half of all conceptions do not become established pregnancies, as the fertilized egg fails to implant in the lining of the uterus and there is a natural termination. The test may have been positive because it was done before the loss of the fertilized egg. To avoid this error do the test around the time of your first missed period. If there is a weak but positive result, repeat the test a few days later with a fresh sample.

EXPECTED ARRIVAL DATE

Once you have confirmed that you are pregnant, your next question almost certainly will be, "When will my baby be born?".

About 266 days or 38 weeks pass between conception and birth. This is the same as 40 weeks from the start of your last menstrual period (LMP) because ovulation, and therefore conception, is normally two weeks after the start of your LMP (see chart, right). You can work out the approximate date of your baby's arrival with calculations using the first day of your LMP. The estimated date of your baby's delivery (EDD) is therefore at 280 days (40 weeks) from the first day of your last period. The accuracy of this date is dependent on a regular 28-day cycle. If you have a shorter or longer menstrual cycle, your delivery date may be earlier or later. If you conceived immediately after coming off the pill it may be difficult for your doctor or midwife to give you a firm date and they will probably have to be guided by your baby's development.

Medical staff use the EDD when monitoring the baby's development to ensure that there are no problems with the expected rate of growth. Unnecessary intervention can occur if too much emphasis is put on this date and doctors may decide to induce labour if they believe your baby is overdue. However, risks to you and your baby do not rise much until after 42 weeks, and most doctors are prepared to let the pregnancy continue, without inducing, if tests show the baby is not at risk (see p.260).

HOW THE EDD CHART WORKS

Find the first day of your last period on the chart by looking for the month in bold type on the left-hand side, then looking along the line until you find the actual date of your LMP. Then look at the figure below it. This is your baby's estimated date of arrival.

YOUR BABY'S ARRIVAL

Don't be anxious if your baby does not show signs of arriving on the day you had planned. About 85 percent of babies born from normal pregnancies are delivered within a week before or after the date predicted.

The EDD is used to give you an approximate idea of when to expect your baby's arrival. You should be prepared to allow for flexibility and not see it as the exact day you will go into labour. A healthy pregnancy may last between 38 and 42 weeks.

YOUR ESTIMATED DATE OF DELIVERY

January	1 2 3 4 5 6 7 8 9 10 11 12 13 14 15 16 17 18 19 20 21 22 23 24 25 26 27 28 29 30 31
Oct/Nov	8 9 10 11 12 13 14 15 16 17 18 19 20 21 22 23 24 25 26 27 28 29 30 31 1 2 3 4 5 6 7
February	1 2 3 4 5 6 7 8 9 10 11 12 13 14 15 16 17 18 19 20 21 22 23 24 25 26 27 28
Nov/Dec	8 9 10 11 12 13 14 15 16 17 18 19 20 21 22 23 24 25 26 27 28 29 30 1 2 3 4 5
March	1 2 3 4 5 6 7 8 9 10 11 12 13 14 15 16 17 18 19 20 21 22 23 24 25 26 27 28 29 30 31
Dec/Jan	6 7 8 9 10 11 12 13 14 15 16 17 18 19 20 21 22 23 24 25 26 27 28 29 30 31 1 2 3 4 5
April	1 2 3 4 5 6 7 8 9 10 11 12 13 14 15 16 17 18 19 20 21 22 23 24 25 26 27 28 29 30
Jan/Feb	6 7 8 9 10 11 12 13 14 15 16 17 18 19 20 21 22 23 24 25 26 27 28 29 30 31 1 2 3 4
May	1 2 3 4 5 6 7 8 9 10 11 12 13 14 15 16 17 18 19 20 21 22 23 24 25 26 27 28 29 30 31
Feb/Mar	5 6 7 8 9 10 11 12 13 14 15 16 17 18 19 20 21 22 23 24 25 26 27 28 1 2 3 4 5 6 7
June	1 2 3 4 5 6 7 8 9 10 11 12 13 14 15 16 17 18 19 20 21 22 23 24 25 26 27 28 29 30
Mar/Apr	8 9 10 11 12 13 14 15 16 17 18 19 20 21 22 23 24 25 26 27 28 29 30 31 1 2 3 4 5 6
July	1 2 3 4 5 6 7 8 9 10 11 12 13 14 15 16 17 18 19 20 21 22 23 24 25 26 27 28 29 30 31
Apr/May	7 8 9 10 11 12 13 14 15 16 17 18 19 20 21 22 23 24 25 26 27 28 29 30 1 2 3 4 5 6 7
August	1 2 3 4 5 6 7 8 9 10 11 12 13 14 15 16 17 18 19 20 21 22 23 24 25 26 27 28 29 30 31
May/Jun	8 9 10 11 12 13 14 15 16 17 18 19 20 21 22 23 24 25 26 27 28 29 30 31 1 2 3 4 5 6 7
September	1 2 3 4 5 6 7 8 9 10 11 12 13 14 15 16 17 18 19 20 21 22 23 24 25 26 27 28 29 30
Jun/Jul	8 9 10 11 12 13 14 15 16 17 18 19 20 21 22 23 24 25 26 27 28 29 30 1 2 3 4 5 6 7
October	1 2 3 4 5 6 7 8 9 10 11 12 13 14 15 16 17 18 19 20 21 22 23 24 25 26 27 28 29 30 31
Jul/Aug	8 9 10 11 12 13 14 15 16 17 18 19 20 21 22 23 24 25 26 27 28 29 30 31 1 2 3 4 5 6 7
November	1 2 3 4 5 6 7 8 9 10 11 12 13 14 15 16 17 18 19 20 21 22 23 24 25 26 27 28 29 30
Aug/Sept	8 9 10 11 12 13 14 15 16 17 18 19 20 21 22 23 24 25 26 27 28 29 30 31 1 2 3 4 5 6
December	1 2 3 4 5 6 7 8 9 10 11 12 13 14 15 16 17 18 19 20 21 22 23 24 25 26 27 28 29 30 31
Sept/Oct	7 8 9 10 11 12 13 14 15 16 17 18 19 20 21 22 23 24 25 26 27 28 29 30 1 2 3 4 5 6 7

PATERNITY LEAVE

At present in Britain and the USA there is no provision in law for paid paternity leave, although European Union directives may change this for the UK within a few years.

In practice, most fathers take some time off around the birth of a child. This time is usually taken either as unpaid leave or as part of their paid leave entitlement.

Trade unions and enlightened employers are coming to recognize the importance of this time and are beginning to include paternity leave in their contracts.

In Scandinavian countries fathers receive pay while taking paternity leave, which means that nearly all fathers take it, to the benefit of all concerned. The family group is strengthened and bonded.

Your rights

Pregnant women are entitled to certain rights and benefits depending on their circumstances and national insurance contributions. The entitlements, particularly for those on low incomes, are complicated but any Department of Social Security, citizen's advice bureau, or legal advice centre should be able to work out what you can claim for. Any maternity leave and pay from your employer will be explained by your employer or trade union representative.

STATE BENEFITS

These include the maternity grant and the maternity allowance, a tax-free allowance payable for a maximum of 18 weeks and dependent on your national insurance contributions (the amount is the same as unemployment benefit), as well as a cash payment from the Social Fund for some women on a low income. The rules are explained in leaflets FB.8 and N1.17A which you can get from your local social security office, citizen's advice bureau, or antenatal clinic. You can also get free prescriptions and dental treatment, and you may get free milk and vitamins for yourself and any children under five if you are on a low income.

WORKING WOMEN

It is the law in Great Britain that your job be kept open for you irrespective of your length of service. The Basic Maternity Leave period is currently 18 weeks. You are entitled to Extended Maternity Leave if you have been employed for more than one year at the 11th week before your expected delivery date. This period is up to 11 weeks before the birth and 29 weeks after the birth.

In payment terms, if you have been employed for more than 26 weeks at the 15th week prior to your expected delivery date, you are entitled to six weeks' pay at 90 percent of your average weekly earnings, followed by 12 weeks' Statutory Maternity Pay (currently £59.55 per week). If you have been employed for less time, you only get the latter amount throughout your maternity leave. These monies will be paid even if you don't return to work. The government refunds 92 percent of the sum to your employer, who may have more generous maternity pay and leave entitlements than those provided by law. You are also legally entitled to time off with pay to attend antenatal clinics and you are protected against unfair dismissal when pregnant. If your job is dangerous or it would be illegal for you to continue doing it (see p.169), your employer must find you an alternative job.

The chart opposite gives you a timetable for claiming benefits and notifying your employer so that you can be sure of getting your maximum entitlement in terms of money and rights. The information is taken from leaflet FB.8 issued by the DSS.

WHEN	WHAT TO DO	WHY
As soon as you know you are pregnant	1 Ask doctor or midwife for form FW8. 2 Tell dentist if you need treatment. 3 Check leaflets MV.11, H.11, and G.11, tell social security office if getting supplementary benefit. 4 Tell employer.	1 Apply for free prescriptions. 2 Apply for free dental treatment. 3 Check right to free glasses, free milk and vitamins, help with hospital fares. 4 No loss of pay for keeping antenatal appointments.
As soon as you can	If you are unemployed or sick, check leaflet N1.17A and ask social security office about maternity allowance claim.	It can affect the amount of maternity allowance you may get.
26 weeks	Ask at antenatal clinic for forms BM4 and Mat B1. Apply BM4, and give Mat B1 to your employer.	You can apply from now for maternity grant and allowance.
3 weeks before you stop work	Tell your employer in writing: the date you stop work, the week the baby is due, and whether you intend to return to your job.	To protect your right to maternity pay, and return to work.
29 weeks	If getting supplementary benefit, claim single payments for maternity clothes and baby's needs.	Maternity grant, maternity allowance, and maternity pay are paid from now.
As soon after the birth as you can	1 If more than one baby, fill in BM4X. 2 If baby was late, fill in form BM9. 3 Register baby's birth. 4 Send off CH2 or CH11A if you are a single parent. 5 Check low income benefits.	1 Extra maternity grant for each baby. 2 To claim extra maternity allowance 3 To get the birth certificate. 4 To get child and one-parent benefit. 5 To see if you qualify for FIS, supplementary benefit, free prescriptions, dental treatment, spectacles, milk, vitamins, hospital fares, or help with rent and rates.
3 weeks after birth	Register baby (if you live in Scotland).	Latest date.
6 weeks after birth	Register baby (places other than Scotland).	Latest date.
7 weeks after the date which the baby was due	Write to your employer stating that you will be going back to work.	To protect your right to return to work.
3 months after the birth	If you haven't already, apply for maternity grant for single or multiple births.	You may lose maternity grant if not claimed by now.
3 weeks before returning to work	Write to your employer stating the date that you wish to return.	To protect your right to return to work.
When the baby is 29 weeks old	Latest time by which you have a right to go back to your job.	You may lose your right to return to work.

In the first three months you will probably gain approximately 1–2kg (2–4lb), if nausea hasn't been a problem.

Of this, only 48g (1.7oz) will be your baby. The rest is made up of the baby's support system (the placenta and amniotic fluid), your enlarged uterus and breasts, and your increased blood volume. Maternal fat stores will account for about the same weight gain as your baby.

First trimester

During pregnancy, the trimesters are the major milestones of the mother-to-be. Rather than representing three three-monthly periods, they are periods of uneven length, and are defined by the physiology of fetal growth. By convention, the trimesters date from presumed conception (two weeks after your LMP), and the first trimester represents the first twelve weeks of your baby's fetal life. The second trimester ends at 28 weeks, and the third trimester encompasses the rest of your pregnancy.

During the first trimester, your body adjusts to pregnancy. At the beginning you won't look pregnant, and you may not feel pregnant either, but the activities of your hormones will soon start to affect you in various ways. Your moods may change capriciously, your libido may decrease or increase, and you may find that your appetite changes and that you prefer simpler, blander food.

PHYSICAL CHANGES

Your pregnant body is having to work very hard to accommodate the developing embryo and the placenta. Pregnancy induces a higher metabolic rate – between 10 percent and 25 percent higher than normal – which means that the body accelerates all of its functions. Your cardiac output rises steeply, almost to the maximum level that will be maintained throughout the rest of the pregnancy. Your heart rate rises too, and will continue to do so until the middle of the second trimester. Your breathing becomes more rapid as you now send more oxygen to the fetus and exhale more carbon dioxide.

Owing to the action of oestrogen and progesterone, your breasts quickly become larger and heavier, and are usually tender to the touch from very early on. Fatty deposits are increased and new milk ducts grow. The areola around the nipple becomes darker and develops little nodules called Montgomery's tubercles. Underneath the skin, you will notice a network of bluish lines appearing as blood supply to the breasts increases.

Your uterus enlarges even in early pregnancy, but it cannot be felt through the abdominal wall until the end of the first trimester, when it begins to rise above the pelvic brim. While it is still low in the pelvis, your uterus will increasingly press upon your bladder as it enlarges, so that you will almost certainly find that you will need to urinate more often.

In addition, the muscle fibres of your uterus begin to thicken until it has become very solid indeed. However, you probably won't notice any increase in your waistline until the end of this trimester.

TAKING CARE OF YOURSELF

You have an increased need for carbohydrates and protein to supply your growing baby and the placenta, as well as your uterus and breasts, so it is imperative that you eat healthily right from the beginning of your pregnancy. You will have an increased need for fluids, so try to drink a minimum of eight glasses of fluid a day. Make sure, too, that you are getting plenty of rest. Drugs, caffeine, junk food, alcohol, and smoking should be avoided throughout the whole of pregnancy, but particularly at this time.

Clothes You should make sure that your clothes are comfortable. While there is probably no need to invest in maternity clothes just yet, there's nothing worse than having to put up with your clothes feeling tight and uncomfortable, even if it's only for a few days, so do make sure that you keep one step ahead of your increasing size. However, you will almost certainly need a larger bra from early on, and this should be a properly fitted maternity bra (see **Maternity wear**, p.163).

YOUR ANTENATAL CARE

Your doctor may be the one that confirms your pregnancy, or you may make an appointment with the antenatal clinic as soon as you have a positive test result. If this is the case, you may not be seen until your next trimester. At the first visit, you will be asked about your own and your family's medical histories and will have a thorough physical examination, which will include urine and blood tests.

MAKING PLANS

Your doctor will be able to advise you as to the childbirth options that are open to you in your area, and may offer antenatal care, whether complete or shared with your hospital. You will need to start thinking about the type of delivery you want and where you are most likely to get it. Books like this one can help you determine your choices in childbirth as well as provide in-depth information on aspects of pregnancy, birth, and baby care. Soon after pregnancy is confirmed, most women are unable to resist buying their unborn babies at least one small gift, such as a teddy bear, although many feel that to do more than this is to tempt fate. If you feel inclined to do so, this is the time to start keeping a daily journal, so that you will have a complete record of your pregnancy.

YOUR PREGNANCY

Finding out that you are pregnant, especially for the first time, is extremely exciting, and you will undoubtably long for the physical signs that will confirm the pregnancy test.

• Your breasts will grow larger, heavier, and more sensitive.

• The pigmentation of your nipples, and any moles and freckles, will increase.

• You may feel very tired.

• You will probably experience nausea, especially first thing in the morning.

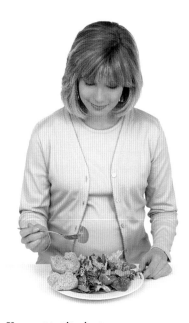

Your appetite in pregnancy
You may experience unusual food cravings or go off foods that you normally like.

Second trimester

Your weight gain

In the second three months, you will probably gain approximately 6kg (12lb).

Of this, only 1kg (2lb) will actually be your baby. The rest is made up of the baby's support system (such as the placenta and amniotic fluid), your enlarged uterus and breasts, and your increased blood and fluid volume. Maternal fat stores will usually account for approximately the same weight gain as your growing baby.

Now is the time when pregnancy is well established and many of the minor complaints associated with early pregnancy will have disappeared. It is the time when certain tests may need to be done. Amniocentesis, for example, will be offered to women over 35, those with a family history of congenital abnormalities, and those for whom other tests such as the nuchal scan indicate the need for more detailed analysis.

Physical changes

You may notice that your nipples begin to secrete colostrum. You will notice that your waistline gradually starts to disappear and you will now "look" pregnant. Pigmentation may also increase (see p.158). Your gums may become slightly spongy; this is probably owing to the action of pregnancy hormones. However, there is no evidence to suggest that women experience an increase in dental decay during pregnancy and there is absolutely no evidence to suggest that there is any truth in the saying "a tooth lost for every child".

Digestion The entire musculature of your intestinal tract is relaxed and this is the cause of many of the minor discomforts that occur during pregnancy.

Oesophageal reflux may cause heartburn because of the relaxation of the sphincter at the top of the stomach. Gastric secretion is also reduced and therefore the food remains for longer in the stomach.

The relaxed intestinal muscle also leads to fewer bowel movements and although this permits more complete absorption of foodstuffs, it can also often lead to constipation in pregnancy.

Your increasing size Once your uterus has grown above your pelvis, your waistline will begin to disappear and you will need to wear larger and looser clothing (see p.162).

On the other hand, the second trimester is a classic time for women to be told that they look small-for-dates. If this happens to you, don't worry. How big you will look will depend on many factors, including your height and particular build; whether this is your first pregnancy or not, because the uterine muscle tends to get stretched after the first child; and the size of your baby. If your doctor is satisfied with how your pregnancy is progressing, then you should be too.

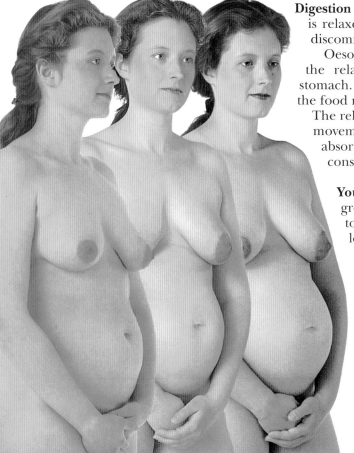

TAKING CARE OF YOURSELF

This is the trimester in which you will gain the most weight overall (approximately 6kg/12lb) and it is essential that you continue to eat well (see p.128). Your posture may also change as the muscles of the abdominal wall become increasingly stretched in order to accommodate your enlarging uterus. As your uterus enlarges it will produce an alteration in your centre of gravity because you are carrying an increasing amount of weight in front. If you find yourself leaning backwards to try and counter this, it may result in backache (see also p.160).

Backache This usually happens due to the increased blood flow to the whole of your pelvis, which causes some softening and relaxation of the ligaments of the sacroiliac joints (the sacrum), which attach your pelvic bones to your spine at the back. In addition, the ligaments and the cartilage at the front of your pelvis also loosen and so the mobility of these joints is slightly increased.

To help prevent backache, sit with a straight back and don't slouch, don't wear high-heeled shoes, and preferably sit on a hard chair or the floor. Always bend with a straight back or, if lifting, bend from the knees and lift from a crouching position. Avoid lifting if you possibly can (see also p.160).

YOUR ANTENATAL CARE

Regular checks of your urine, weight, and blood pressure may be supplemented by testing for chromosomal defects, if this is determined to be necessary. From this time, too, your doctor will concentrate on measuring the adequate growth of your fetus. He or she will palpate your abdomen to feel the size and shape of the uterus and check for the height of the fundus (see p.178), and will listen for the baby's heartbeat.

During the fourth month you will probably have an ultrasound scan, and it will give you a special thrill to see your baby for the first time. You will also be able to hear your baby's incredibly fast heartbeat (see column, p.178) and you may see your baby moving.

PREPARING FOR BABY

Towards the end of this trimester, when you are feeling better and will probably be full of energy, is the ideal time for you to make most of the preparations for your baby, such as sorting out your baby's room and shopping for the layette and baby equipment. It is better to do at least some of these things now than to wait until the third trimester, when your size will increase rapidly and you may find that you begin to feel very tired once again.

YOUR PREGNANCY

During the second trimester you will begin to feel comfortable with being pregnant. You will enjoy the sensation of your baby moving within you and will feel energetic and full of life.

• Your libido will return or increase – it is not uncommon for women to experience orgasm or multiple orgasm for the first time.

• Your abdomen will become rounded. You will lose your waistline and "look" pregnant.

• Pigmentation will continue to increase and you may notice a darker line developing down the centre of your abdomen – the linea nigra (see p.158).

• You may suffer from indigestion and rib pain.

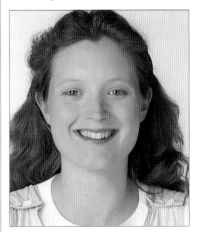

Hormonal effects
As the placenta takes over the production of pregnancy hormones, your hormone levels should begin to balance out. This means that you will feel more serene and positive than you did in the first trimester. Your appearance will also benefit, with thicker and shinier hair and a clear and glowing complexion.

Third trimester

YOUR WEIGHT GAIN

During the final months you will probably gain approximately 5kg (10lb).

Of this, approximately 3–4kg (6–8lb) will be accounted for by your baby. The rest is made up of the baby's support system (consisting of the placenta and amniotic fluid), your enlarged uterus and breasts, and your increased blood volume. Maternal fat stores will usually account for approximately the same weight gain as your baby.

You will probably feel anxious about labour and wish you could have the baby now. This doesn't mean that there is anything wrong with your baby. The sense of urgency is due to metabolic changes in the brain. Subtle shifts have gone on in each trimester, bringing about the fatigue of the first, the elation and vigour of the second, and now the anxiety of the third.

PHYSICAL CHANGES

Your size is now increasing rapidly and you are bound to feel tired. You may find that you are not sleeping as well as usual and this will increase your need for rest (see opposite). As your ligaments stretch and give way, you may find walking about rather uncomfortable. Once your baby has settled into your pelvis, you will find that your breathlessness will diminish because the pressure on your diaphragm has been relieved.

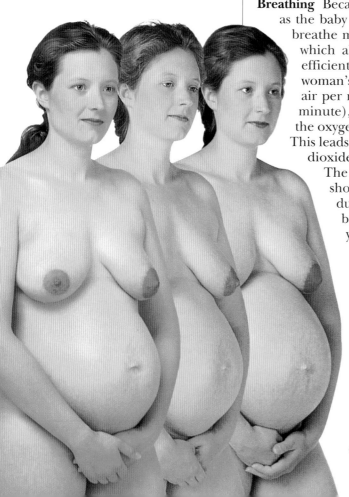

Breathing Because of the reduced movement of the diaphragm as the baby grows bigger in the abdomen, pregnant women breathe more deeply, taking more air in with each breath which allows for better mixing of gases and the more efficient consumption of oxygen. This lifts a pregnant woman's ventilation rate from the normal seven litres of air per minute to ten litres (three pints to five pints per minute), giving an increase of over 40 percent. However, the oxygen requirements are increased by only 20 percent. This leads to overbreathing, which means that more carbon dioxide is exhaled per breath than is normally the case. The low level of CO_2 in the blood gives rise to a shortness of breath, which you may find bothersome during this trimester. Relief from this shortness of breath should come when your baby engages in your pelvis and pressure on your diaphragm is eased. Meanwhile, you should sit in a semi-propped up position whenever possible and should avoid overdoing things.

Possible problems Hypertension (high blood pressure – see p.178) may be a problem in later pregnancy. The major warning signs are swollen and puffy hands, wrists, ankles, feet, and face, and your doctor or midwife will look for these during your antenatal visits. Pre-eclampsia (see p.224) may interfere with the functioning of the placenta and prevent it from transporting nutrients to your baby efficiently. You may have to be hospitalized.

CARING FOR YOURSELF

As the third trimester continues, the extra weight that you are carrying can result in further backache and may make you feel continually tired. Sleep can become a problem, as you will probably find that very few positions in bed are comfortable. Don't take sleeping pills; they will make the baby sleepy too. Take your time with everything and make certain that you get enough rest; you should catnap and set aside periods when you can relax.

As your desire for making love may either diminish or be frustrated by your increasing size, you may find that massage can help you to relax. Eat lots of fresh fruit and vegetables and drink at least eight glasses of fluid per day as you'll probably pass urine more often. You may be constipated at times.

YOUR ANTENATAL CARE

You will be checked more frequently during this time. There are many tests that your doctor may use to judge the baby's health or well-being such as ultrasound, fetal heart rate monitoring, and hormonal measurements. Your doctor will discuss at each stage what is being done and why. Unlike the special tests in the first and second trimester – chorionic villus sampling, amniocentesis, and cordocentesis (see pp.184–187) – none of the tests at this time are invasive of the uterus. Urine and blood pressure testing will be done frequently as will checks for possible swelling of your feet and hands, although such swelling may be normal if it is not accompanied by other symptoms. From the 36th week up to the onset of labour you'll be asked to visit the antenatal clinic on a more frequent basis than you did in the earlier months of your pregnancy.

PREPARING FOR BABY

By the end of this trimester you should have sorted out the nursery and purchased essential clothing and equipment. Labour may be increasingly on your mind, and some women find that they worry obsessively about it. Although no-one can predict what will happen during labour as your experience will be unique, be reassured that most births go without a hitch.

YOUR PREGNANCY

In this trimester, practical matters such as attending childbirth classes and preparing your baby's clothes and room will vie with daydreaming and fantasizing about the new arrival.

• You will probably be feeling easily tired although you may find it hard to rest.

• You will become increasingly aware of Braxton Hicks' contractions (see p.270).

• You will have visited the hospital and become familiar with it and the staff. If you are having a home birth you will have to hand all the items you will need.

• You will be concerned about whether you can tell that you are in labour or not. Even for an experienced midwife or doctor, it can be difficult to know when you are in established labour. Don't be afraid to ring your midwife or hospital delivery ward for advice if you're in any doubt.

Baby's clothes and accessories
You should have on hand prior to the birth a selection of baby clothes, nappies, and bedding.

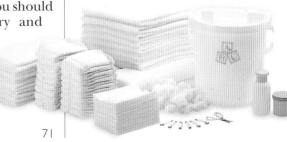

MOTHER

At the end of the first month of pregnancy, six weeks after your last period and four weeks since conception – you probably won't be sure that you are pregnant, although you may have your suspicions. There are some pregnancy kits that will give you a positive result even at this early stage.

Symptoms You will notice few, if any, symptoms at this stage, although you may feel slightly premenstrual and pass urine more frequently than usual. From a very early stage the breasts feel sore and heavy and the nipples tingle. Quite soon after that, veins become visible under the skin on the surface of the breast. You may even feel sick at this stage.

Ovulation cycle Once the embryo has implanted on the lining of your uterus, your normal ovulation cycle ceases. The corpus luteum (see p.28) in the ovary continues to secrete progesterone, which prevents menstruation from occurring and keeps the pregnancy healthy and viable.

Cervix Under the influence of progesterone normal cervical mucus becomes very dense and thick, forming a plug. This mucus plug will remain in place until the end of your pregnancy, when it will be expelled (the show) as your cervix softens and dilates in preparation for labour.

Uterus The wall of your uterus softens so that the embryo can become firmly embedded. Your uterus enlarges almost from the moment of implantation.

First 6 weeks

The fertilized egg becomes a ball of cells (blastocyst), which floats into the uterus and implants itself in the lining. The basis for your baby's future development is now laid down.

YOUR BABY'S PROGRESS

Once it has implanted, the embryo secretes chemicals that have two functions. First, they signal to your body that the embryo has arrived and this triggers off a number of changes in your body: your ovulation cycle stops, the mucus in your cervix thickens, your uterine wall softens, and your breasts begin to grow. Second, your immune system is suppressed so that the embryo is not treated as foreign and rejected, but is allowed to grow. In addition, an outer layer of the blastocyst develops into a protective cocoon around the embryo. This cocoon will create the rudiments of the placenta and the support system in which the embryo will grow – the amniotic sac (the watery balloon in which it will float), the chorion (a safety cushion around the amniotic sac), and the yolk sac (which will manufacture blood cells until the liver takes over). The chorion then grows finger-like projections, the chorionic villi, with which the cocoon burrows firmly into your uterine lining.

The cells specialize Throughout these early weeks, the embryo's cells become more specialized. There are now three layers of them, each destined to create different organs of the body. The innermost layer forms a primitive tube that will later develop into the lungs, liver, thyroid gland, pancreas, urinary tract, and bladder. The middle layer will become the skeleton, muscles (including the heart muscle), testes (or ovaries), kidneys, spleen, blood vessels, blood cells, and the deepest layer of skin, the dermis. The outer layer will provide the skin, sweat glands, nipples (and breasts, if it is a girl), hair, nails, tooth enamel, and the lenses of the eyes. These three cell-layers differentiate to create an entire human body.

THE EMBRYO'S SUPPORT SYSTEM

The villi of the growing placenta intermingle with the maternal blood vessels of the uterine wall in such a way that they eventually become surrounded by "lakes" of blood. Maternal blood flows in and around these spaces and, because it is divided by only a cell or two from fetal blood, exchange of nutrients and waste between fetus and mother can occur in these blood spaces. The placenta is a hormone factory pumping out hormones, such as human chorionic gonadotrophin (hCG), that are designed to support a healthy pregnancy. Until the sixth week, the embryo's blood cells are supplied by the yolk sac; after the end of the third week, his blood circulation is pumped by his own heart.

YOUR BABY AT SIX WEEKS OF PREGNANCY

YOUR BABY

The sixth week
Surrounding layers of chorion and amnion protect the embryo, and blocks of tissue that will become the vertebrae, can be seen to be forming. Between these grow bunches of nerves.

The embryo has gill-like structures that will later become its jaw, neck, and part of the face

The rudimentary heart of the embryo bulges predominantly

The rudimentary spinal cord appears

Before you may know you are pregnant, the embryo reaches a critical stage in development; thus it is vital to plan for pregnancy.

Spinal cord During the second week of life, a dark mark appears on the back of the embryo, marking the position of the spinal cord.

Heart By the end of the third week, there is a heart that is now beginning to beat.

Sensitivity In the third week the embryo enters a sensitive phase of development when all the major organs are forming. Embryos are generally robust but can be harmed by drugs, alcohol, smoking, infections, etc. Many don't survive, largely because of serious chromosomal defects.

BABY'S VITAL STATISTICS

By the end of the sixth week of life, the embryo's length will be approximately 4mm (⅛ in). It will weigh less than a gram (0.03oz).

Changing shape
By the end of this period, the embryo is no longer a hollow cluster of many cells. It is prawn shaped – long and narrow with a slight waist in the middle. It has a top, a bottom, and sides. The bottom is shaped like a pointed tail.

In the middle, the surface layer of cells, which will form the brain and nervous system, creases into two lengthwise folds. The groove that forms between them then closes over to form a tube, which will become the spinal cord. The tube grows at the top and this will become the brain.

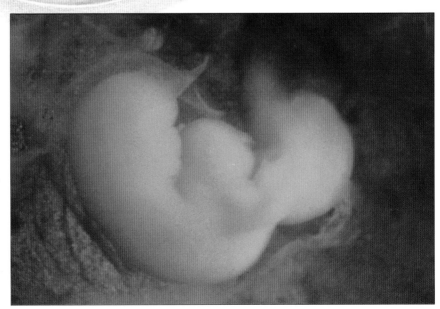

MOTHER

For some, morning sickness is one of the first signs of pregnancy. It can range from mild nausea to severe vomiting and can occur at any time (see also p.210). Other changes happen now that may not be as discernible.

Metabolic requirements Very early in pregnancy the basal metabolic rate begins to increase and therefore a woman who is pregnant requires a greater intake of protein and calories.

Circulatory changes The total blood volume begins to rise; about 25% of this is being used by the placental system.

Genitals The blood supply to the vagina and vulva increases quite rapidly and they develop a purple coloration. The vaginal walls become softened and relaxed, and a watery substance is produced in increasing amounts. This, plus the shedding of vaginal cells, increases the total discharge from your vagina while you are pregnant.

Breasts Your breasts may start to swell or feel tender and heavier than usual. The skin around the areola begins to develop a softer, lighter area known as the secondary areola.

Fatigue You are likely to get tired more easily than usual, and may even feel faint at times.

Skin problems If your face usually breaks out in spots before your period, it is liable to do so again now. Alternatively, your skin may become dry and itchy.

Up to 10 weeks

This is a time of extremely rapid and crucial development as your baby quadruples in size. Lying in the centre of a large placental cocoon, the embryo is still very tiny. Its cells are constantly differentiating to form new structures.

YOUR BABY'S PROGRESS

Within the tube that will ultimately become the brain and spinal cord, the embryo's cells multiply at a phenomenal rate then move away to the areas where they will become active. Nerve cells that will form the brain travel along pathways that are being laid down by glial (glue) cells. These cells enable the nerve cells to move towards each other, connect, and become active.

The head is growing rapidly in order to accommodate the enlarging brain, and the body becomes less curved. A neck begins to develop and the primeval tail disappears.

The skin now starts to differentiate into its two layers, and the sweat glands and sebaceous (oil-producing) glands begin to develop. Hair then starts to grow from the hair follicles so that the skin becomes downy. All the major organs develop. The heart achieves its final form and beats strongly. Stomach, liver, spleen, appendix, and intestine develop. The intestine becomes so long it forms a loop, the circulatory system is established, and most muscles begin to attain their final form.

Facial features Under the skin on its face, a system of primitive facial bones has now emerged and are fusing together. One of these goes down between the eyes and ends on either side of the nostrils, thus forming the nose and the middle of the upper lip. Two others appear under the eyes, forming the cheeks and sides of the upper lip. Two more grow under the mouth, fusing to form the lower lip and chin. All this provides the framework to which the facial muscles become attached, which then enables the face to move.

Some pigment can already be detected in the eyes, which are covered and are very far apart. The internal and external parts of the ears begin to form and the taste buds start developing. The tooth buds of all non-permanent teeth are now in place.

Arms and legs Embryonic limbs continue to develop. Wrists and fingers appear on the arm buds, which lengthen and project forward. The arms become bent at the elbow. Touch-pads form on the fingertips. Leg buds sprout, then develop three distinct sections – thigh, calf, and foot. Toes start to appear. At this stage, your baby's arms and hands develop faster than her legs and feet. This trend will continue after birth – your baby will be able to grasp objects long before she can walk.

YOUR BABY AT TEN WEEKS OF PREGNANCY

YOUR BABY

Colour-enhanced scan
The developing umbilical cord and placenta are clearly visible in the top right-hand corner of the ultrasound scan.

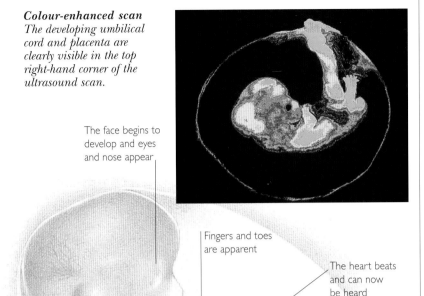

The face begins to develop and eyes and nose appear

Fingers and toes are apparent

The heart beats and can now be heard

The body begins to straighten up

The tail is reabsorbed

Nutrients pass from you into the placenta and the umbilical cord to feed your baby, who needs increasing nourishment to support the rapid growth.

Heart rate The heart beats at 140–150 per minute, which is about twice the rate of yours.

Body shape The embryo's head is still very large in comparison to the body and is bent forward on the chest. The body begins to straighten and elongate.

Internal organs All organs will now be present and most major structures will have been formed.

Reflexes The embryo can respond to touch, although you won't be able to feel it move.

BABY'S VITAL STATISTICS

By the end of this month its crown to rump length will be 2.5cm (1in), and it will weigh approximately 3g (0.1oz).

External features
The embryo's eyes become pigmented and the first visible signs of the nostrils, lips, and ears also appear. The rudimentary ears now divide into inner and outer sections, the eyelids form, and the tip of the nose can be seen. The embryo's muscles start to build and by the seventh week of life the first embryonic movement can be detected using ultrasound. The picture shows the embryo at six weeks of development since conception.

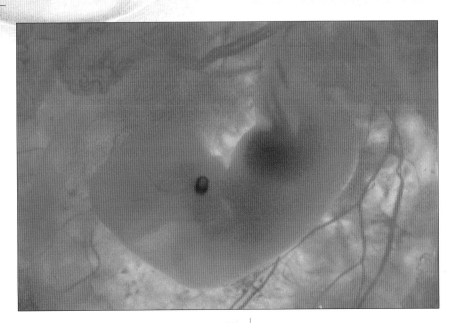

MOTHER

You will probably start to feel better during this month, particularly if you have been suffering badly with nausea and vomiting.

Weight You will probably begin to gain weight as baby and baby's support system grow rapidly.

Hormones Your hormones begin to settle down and you will probably feel much less emotionally unbalanced and vulnerable.

Fundal height Your developing baby is causing the fundus (see External examination, p.178) of your uterus to rise through the pelvic brim where it can be felt. You will probably have an ultrasound scan at this time to confirm the stage of pregnancy.

Outlook If you had been anxious about the pregnancy, you will now feel more relaxed as the risk of miscarriage diminishes to practically nothing.

Circulatory system Your cardiac output has reached almost the maximum level that will be maintained throughout the remainder of your pregnancy. To lower your blood pressure, the arteries and veins in your extremities relax, so your hands and feet are nearly always warm.

Up to 14 weeks

Fourteen weeks after your LMP, all of your baby's major organs have formed and his intestines are sealed in the abdominal cavity. He now starts to grow and mature.

YOUR BABY'S PROGRESS

By the eleventh week of pregnancy, your baby is recognizable as a human being, and he is now called a fetus (offspring) rather than an embryo. His head is very large compared to the rest of his body; by 14 weeks it will be about one-third of his whole length. His eyes are completely formed, although the eyelids are still developing and remain closed. His face, too, is completely formed. His trunk has straightened out and the first bone tissue and ribs appear. The fingers and toes have nails and some hair may have grown. His external genital organs are now growing and the sex of your baby may be discernible by ultrasound. Internally, his heart is beating between 110 and 160 times per minute and the circulatory system continues to develop. The fetus swallows amniotic fluid and excretes it as urine.

His sucking reflex is establishing itself – his lips purse, his head turns, and his forehead wrinkles. The muscles he will use after birth for breathing and swallowing are also being exercised.

In fact, by the end of this month your baby will have discovered movement. He now begins to move vigorously, but you probably won't be able to feel his movements until the fourth month.

Blood-cell production While your baby will continue to rely on the placenta for nourishment, oxygen, and the clearance of waste until he is born, a system of blood-cell formation that will eventually support independent life is essential. Towards the end of this month, the yolk sac becomes superfluous as its task of producing blood cells is taken over by your baby's developing bone marrow, liver, and spleen.

HIS SUPPORT SYSTEM

The placenta is developing very quickly, ensuring that there is a rich network of blood vessels to provide your baby with vital nourishment. Now the layers thicken and grow until the chorion and membranes cover the entire inner surface area of the uterus. The umbilical cord is now completely mature and consists of three intertwined blood vessels encased in a fatty sheath. The large vein carries nutrients and oxygen-rich blood to the fetus, while the two, smaller, arteries carry waste products and oxygen-poor blood from the fetus to the placenta. The umbilical cord is coiled like a spring because the sheath is longer than the blood vessels, and allows him plenty of room for manoeuvre without the risk of damaging his lifeline.

YOUR BABY AT 14 WEEKS

Feet and hands
Your baby's fingers and toes are developing rapidly and becoming fully formed.

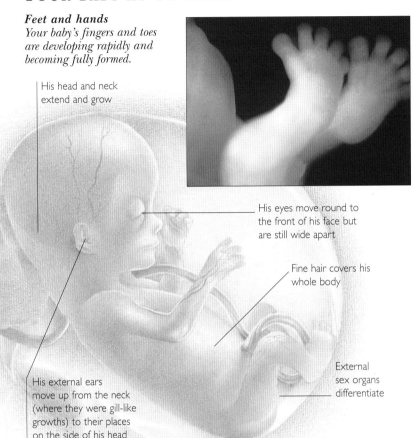

His head and neck extend and grow

His eyes move round to the front of his face but are still wide apart

Fine hair covers his whole body

External sex organs differentiate

His external ears move up from the neck (where they were gill-like growths) to their places on the side of his head

YOUR BABY

Your baby is fully formed; now he needs to mature. He is very active at this stage, although you won't feel him yet.

Bones In the form of flexible cartilage, the bones in his body are rapidly developing.

Movements He jerks his body, bends his arms and legs, and has an occasional hiccup.

Jaws These already show 32 permanent tooth buds.

Amniotic sac The fetus floats comfortably in a warm bath of amniotic fluid (at 37.5°C, the temperature of the amniotic fluid is higher than your own body temperature). He has plenty of space for movement.

BABY'S VITAL STATISTICS
By the end of this month his crown to rump length will be 9cm (3½ in), and he will weigh 48g (1.7oz).

12 week-old fetus
The profile has become more human and the features are much more clearly defined. This fetus now has a definite chin, a large forehead, and a button nose. His eyelids have begun to develop across his fully formed eyes, and he is beginning to respond to external stimuli – if his mother's abdomen is poked, he will try to wriggle away. An ultrasound scan would reveal fetal movements at this stage but these cannot be felt by the mother until next month at the earliest.

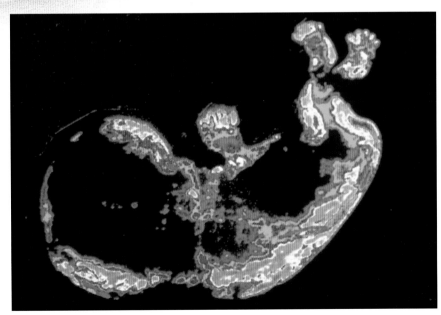

MOTHER

You are showing many signs that pregnancy is advancing well, although you may not have gained much weight. You will probably have extra vitality and energy.

Nipples They are darkening in colour as your skin becomes more deeply pigmented. They may tingle, feel sore, and the surface veins are becoming more prominent.

Heart This is working twice as hard as before, putting out sufficient blood (six litres per minute) to maintain the increasing needs of your vital organs. The uterus and skin need twice as much blood as usual and the kidneys 25 percent more.

Abdomen A dark line, called the linea nigra, may develop down the centre of your abdomen. Your uterus has been forced out of the pelvic cavity into your abdomen by your growing baby and can be felt on examination.

Quickening Towards the end of this month you will probably feel your baby moving – a bubbling, fluttering sensation like butterflies, little fishes, or wind! First-time mothers feel movements later than women in subsequent pregnancies (see also p.194).

Up to 18 weeks

The second trimester starts from the 14th week of pregnancy. Your baby is steadily growing and if you have a scan at this time it is possible to discern the baby's sex. If it is felt necessary, you will be offered various tests to rule out any abnormalities around this time. The length of the femur will be measured, as well as the diameter of the head; this latter measurement will be used to confirm the EDD.

YOUR BABY'S PROGRESS

She is looking more human, with legs longer than arms and the parts of her legs in proportion. The skeleton continues to produce more bone and those parts with sufficient calcium can be seen on X-ray. The fetus now contains the same number of nerve cells as an adult. The nerves from the brain begin to be coated in a layer of protective fat (myelin). This is an important step in their maturation because it facilitates the passage of messages to and from the brain. Connections between nerves and muscles are established so that your baby's well-formed limbs can move around their joints when muscles are stimulated to contract and relax. Now that her arms are long enough, her hands can grasp each other if they touch accidentally, and she can form fists. However, movements are not yet under the control of the brain. Nor do they register with you at first because the fetus is not big enough to activate nerve endings on the uterine wall. Second-time mothers tend to feel fetal activity sooner (see p.194).

The fetus' external genital organs acquire a more distinctive appearance. A girl's vaginal plate, the precursor to her vagina, is clearly developing, and a boy's testes are at the deep inguinal ring, and well on their way to descending into the scrotum.

HER SUPPORT SYSTEM

The placenta is producing the increasing amounts of chorionic gonadotrophin, oestrogen, and progesterone that are needed throughout pregnancy. It also produces an assortment of other hormones that maintain the health of the uterus, and play an essential part in the growth and development of the mother's breasts in preparation for lactation. The placenta forms a barrier against general infection, although not against viruses, such as rubella (German measles) and AIDS, and poisons such as alcohol and nicotine. By the end of the 16th week, the placenta has grown in thickness to about one centimetre (half an inch) and seven to eight centimetres (three and a half inches) across.

Growth will continue until at term it reaches a weight of 500 grams (1lb), a thickness of three centimetres (an inch and a half) and a diameter of 20–25 centimetres (8–10 inches). It is firmly attached to the uterine wall (usually the upper part).

YOUR BABY AT 18 WEEKS OF PREGNANCY

YOUR BABY

Ultrasound scan
At this time, your baby's nose, fingers, and toes can be seen clearly. Her head is still large in comparison to her body.

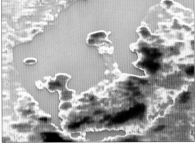

Tiny fingernails
are visible

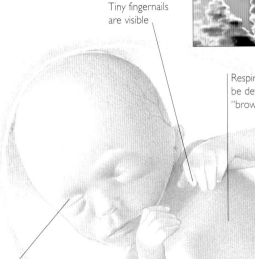

Respiratory movements can now
be detected as can the protective
"brown fat"

Her eyelids have
formed and are fused
shut. They will open in
the sixth month

**Your baby's skin is transparent
and her blood vessels can be
seen clearly, as can her bones,
which are beginning to harden
throughout her body.**

Tastebuds They have begun to
develop on her tongue.

Ears As the tiny bones inside her
ears harden, she begins to hear
sounds – your voice, your heart,
and your digestion rumbling.

Lungs They are developing and
she "breathes" the amniotic fluid.
She will continue to receive
oxygen via the placenta until
she is born.

BABY'S VITAL STATISTICS

*By the end of this month her
crown to rump length will be
13.5cm (5½in), and she
will weigh 180g (6oz).*

Head and face
*Her face is developing and
becoming more human in appearance
and she begins to make her first facial
expressions. She can frown, squint, and
grimace. Eyebrows and eyelashes start
to grow, and the hair on her head
becomes slightly coarser, and is coloured
by special pigment cells. Her ears stand
away from the head, and her eyes now
look straight ahead although they are
still widely spaced. The retinas of her
eyes have become sensitive to light,
although they remain covered by her
eyelids, and she is aware of bright
light from outside of her mother's
abdominal wall.*

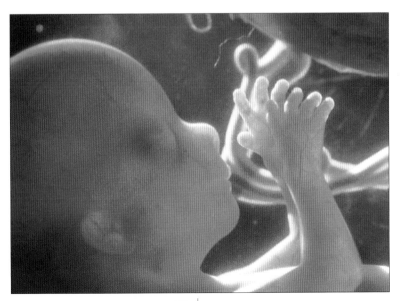

MOTHER

At this time, well into your second trimester, you'll probably notice a mood change. Your energy, and sense of fun should have returned and nausea should have disappeared.

Movements If you did not feel your baby move earlier, you will certainly feel him now. The experience of the baby "quickening" is wonderful.

Abdomen Your waistline has disappeared and you may find stretchmarks.

Skin Dilated blood vessels may cause tiny red marks (spider naevi) to appear on your face, arms, and shoulders. These should fade after the birth.

Minor complaints The gums may become spongy, probably owing to hormonal influences. You may experience constipation and heartburn. The risk of bladder infections increases because of the relaxation of the smooth muscle in the urinary tract.

Metabolic changes Your thyroid gland becomes more active and one result can be a tendency to perspire more heavily than usual. Your breathing will become deeper and there may be some shortness of breath when you exercise.

Up to 22 weeks

Your baby has sufficiently increased in size at this time to have developed a nervous system and muscles capable of allowing him to move. Because he is still so small, he can swim up and down and be in any position at any time.

YOUR BABY'S PROGRESS

Starting now, from 19 weeks after your LMP, your baby's rapid growth rate, except for weight gain, starts to slow down and he matures in other ways. He begins to build up his defence systems.

A sheath begins to form around the nerves in his spinal cord to protect them from possible damage. He also has his own primitive immune system, with which he can partially defend himself against some infections. To produce body heat and maintain his temperature, your baby needs specialized fatty tissue. This is provided by a substance known as "brown fat", which started to form during the fourth month. Now, deposits of brown fat begin to build up in areas of his body such as his neck, chest, and crotch. This will continue until term. One of the reasons that premature babies are so vulnerable is that they have insufficient amounts of brown fat, and so are unable to keep themselves warm.

His skin will continue to grow, although it will be red and wrinkled because there is so little fat underneath it. His body begins to get plumper from this month. The sebaceous glands become active and produce a waxy, greasy substance (known as the *vernix caseosa*), which provides his skin with a protective coating during its long immersion in the amniotic fluid.

Your baby's body is also covered with fine hair called lanugo. Nobody is as yet quite sure of its purpose, but it may help to regulate his body temperature, or it may be there to hold the protective *vernix caseosa* in place.

His movements As his nerve fibres become connected and his muscle development and strength increases, his movements are more purposeful and coordinated. He embarks on his own athletics programme – stretching, grasping, turning – to build up his muscles, improve his motor ability, and strengthen his bones. These movements can make your abdomen sore.

Sex organs A boy's scrotum is solid at this stage. A girl's vagina starts to become hollow and her ovaries contain about seven million ova, which will be reduced to approximately two million at birth. By the time she reaches puberty, between 200,000 and 500,000 ova will be left and she will release only 400–500 of these during her adult life – approximately one per month. Nipples and underlying mammary glands develop in both sexes.

YOUR BABY AT 22 WEEKS OF PREGNANCY

YOUR BABY

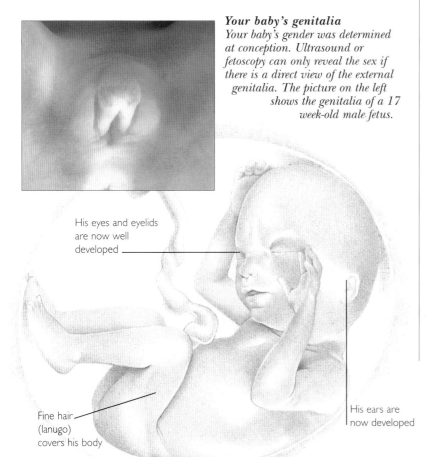

Your baby's genitalia
Your baby's gender was determined at conception. Ultrasound or fetoscopy can only reveal the sex if there is a direct view of the external genitalia. The picture on the left shows the genitalia of a 17 week-old male fetus.

His eyes and eyelids are now well developed

Fine hair (lanugo) covers his body

His ears are now developed

Although he is well developed, your baby cannot yet survive outside your uterus. His lungs and digestive system are not fully formed, nor is he fully able to maintain his own body heat.

Vernix caseosa The waxy coating produced by your baby's oil glands keeps his skin supple.

Taste He can now distinguish sweet from bitter.

Touch His skin is now sensitive to touch and he will move in response to any pressure that is put on the abdomen.

Teeth Hidden in his gums, many of his "baby" teeth have already been formed.

Heartbeat This can now be heard by less sensitive stethoscopes.

BABY'S VITAL STATISTICS

By the end of this month his crown to rump length will be 18.5cm (7in) and he will weigh 0.5kg (1lb).

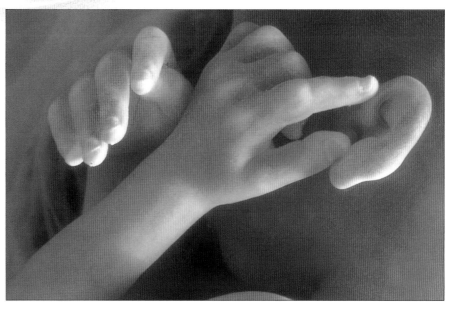

His hearing
He can hear the sounds of your blood flowing through your blood vessels, your heart beating, and your stomach rumbling. He can hear sounds from outside the uterus and will respond to sound, rhythm, and melody from now onwards. You could try singing and talking to your unborn child. After birth, he will probably be soothed by the same songs, finding them reassuring, and he will feel safe and secure when he hears his parents' voices.

MOTHER

Now that fetal movements are well established, you should be feeling some every day. When she hiccups, for example, you will feel a sudden jerk.

Weight You will be putting on weight at the rate of about 0.5kg (1lb) per week. Don't worry if you are told you look externally "small for dates". Your size will depend on many factors such as your build, stature, carriage, and the amount of amniotic fluid inside. It's the size of your growing baby that counts and that will be checked by ultrasound scanning.

Aches and pains As your baby grows, and your uterus along with her, they push upwards against your ribcage so that it will rise by about 5cm (2in) and your lower ribs will spread outwards. This can give you rib pain and, because your baby is now beginning to press up on your stomach, you may also start to have bouts of indigestion and heartburn (see p.208). As your uterine muscle stretches, you may get stitch-like pains down the sides of your abdomen.

Up to 26 weeks

Your baby is growing taller and stronger, while her movements are becoming more complex. She is also showing signs of sensitivity, awareness, and intelligence. A baby is legally viable if born after 24 weeks of pregnancy, and could survive with specialized neonatal intensive care.

YOUR BABY'S PROGRESS

She is still red and skinny but she will soon start to put on weight. Any extensive wrinkling of the skin is due to a lack of subcutaneous fat and a relative increase in the amount of skin.

Her body is growing faster than her head and by the end of this month her proportions are approximate to those of a newborn. Her arms and legs have their normal amount of muscle, her legs and body are in proportion and her bone centres are beginning to harden. The lines start to appear on the palms of her hands. The brain cells she will use for conscious thought now start to mature, and she begins to be able to remember and learn. (In one experiment, babies in the uterus were trained to kick in response to a specific vibration).

The genitals are now completely differentiated; if the baby is a boy, testosterone-producing cells in the testes increase in number.

Her hearing Your baby can hear sound frequencies that are beyond your range; she will move more in response to high frequencies than to low ones and move her body in rhythm with your speech. From this month she will begin to respond to drum beats by jumping up and down. Some mothers report having to leave concerts because their unborn babies would not keep still.

If she hears a piece of music frequently, she may discover that when she is grown up it is familiar to her – even if she can't remember ever hearing it. Some musicians have said that they "knew" unseen pieces of music, and later discovered that these were played to them, by their mothers, while in the uterus.

She can also learn to recognize her father's voice from this month onward. A baby whose father talks to her while she is in the uterus can distinguish her father's voice in a roomful of people immediately after she is born, and will respond to it emotionally – for example, if she is upset, she will stop crying and calm down.

Her breathing Inside her lungs, air sacs are forming in ever-increasing numbers. They will continue to increase until eight years after she is born. Around them, the blood vessels that will help her to absorb oxygen and expel carbon dioxide are multiplying. In addition, her nostrils have now opened, and she is beginning to make breathing motions with her muscles, so that her system has plenty of breathing practice before she is born.

YOUR BABY AT 26 WEEKS OF PREGNANCY

YOUR BABY

Her skin has lost its former translucent quality and has become opaque and reddish-looking. It is still wrinkled because she hasn't yet built up enough fat deposits

Her body is still thin, but is now more in proportion to her head

She continues to grow slowly and steadily. If she is born prematurely, she would have a slim chance of survival.

Lungs The bronchi of her lungs are growing, although they are not yet mature.

Brain The patterns of her brainwaves now resemble those of a full-term newborn child. The source of these brainwaves is thought to be the cortex, the highly evolved part of the brain. She has now developed patterns of sleeping and waking.

BABY'S VITAL STATISTICS

By the end of this month her crown to rump length will be 25cm (10in) and she will weigh just under 1kg (2lb).

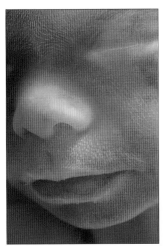

Facial features
The features of this six- month-old fetus are very similar to those of an infant at birth. Lanugo, the downy hair, forms patterns because of the oblique way in which the hair roots are positioned in the skin.

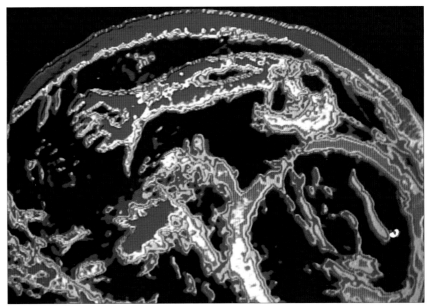

Ultrasound
The baby is growing bigger, gaining weight, and taking up more of the uterus. In the top of the above view, which has

been taken by ultrasound and then colour enhanced, a fully formed arm, hand, and shoulder lie adjacent to the head.

MOTHER

This ends your second trimester. You may start to feel tired and, knowing that your baby just needs to mature, you may now begin to anticipate the birth.

Colostrum This sweet, watery fluid, less rich than breast milk and easier to digest, will probably have formed in your breasts. It will provide your baby with his first few meals before your milk comes through (see also p.326).

Urination Your growing baby will now be pressing against your bladder, causing you to pass urine more frequently.

Sleeping problems Very few positions will be comfortable if you are very big. Lying on your side with one knee to your chest and the other stretched out will probably be most comfortable.

Low back pain Owing to an alteration of your centre of gravity caused by the enlarged uterus plus the slight loosening of the pelvic joints, you may experience backache. Wearing low-heeled shoes and sitting with a straight back on a hard chair or the floor will help. Avoid lifting if you can.

Up to 30 weeks

Your baby is now so big that when your doctor or midwife gives you an abdominal examination, they can assess his position. This is the last month he can turn a somersault.

YOUR BABY'S PROGRESS

Great changes take place in the nervous system this month. The brain grows larger (to fit inside the skull, it has to fold over and wrinkle up until it looks like a walnut), and the brain cells and nerve circuits are all fully linked and active. In addition, a protective fatty sheath begins to form around the nerve fibres, just as a similar sheath formed earlier around the spinal cord, and this fatty sheath will continue to develop until early adulthood. As a result, nerve impulses can travel faster and your baby becomes capable of increasingly complex learning and movement.

Your baby starts preparing himself for birth. (If he were to be born prematurely at this stage, he would have an excellent chance of survival. Even though such a baby may have some breathing problems and difficulty in keeping himself warm, modern special care facilities should help him thrive.) Some fat is beginning to appear underneath his skin, which smoothes out, loses its wrinkles, and becomes more rounded. His coat of hairy lanugo may diminish to a patch on his back and shoulders. The membranes that sealed and protected his eyes during their growth will, by the beginning of this month, have fulfilled their function as his eyes are now fully formed and his eyelids have separated and allowed his eyes to open. He continues to develop his swallowing and sucking skills.

His breathing He has now fully developed his mature breathing rhythm, and the air sacs in his lungs start to prepare for the first breath he will take in the world outside the uterus. They line themselves with a coating of special cells and a fluid (surfactant) that will prevent them from collapsing.

His movements Over the course of this month, he will find he has less room to move about in, and will gradually give up moving around so much. He will wriggle uncomfortably if you have your body in a position that doesn't suit him (see p.194).

Orientation During his weeks of "gymnastics practice", he has done more than increase his muscle tone – he has developed the ability to orientate himself in space. He will probably continue to lie in your uterus with his head upward during this month, although if he is maturing very fast he may turn upside down and settle into place for delivery (engage) rather earlier than usual. This is more common in first-born babies.

YOUR BABY AT **30** WEEKS OF PREGNANCY

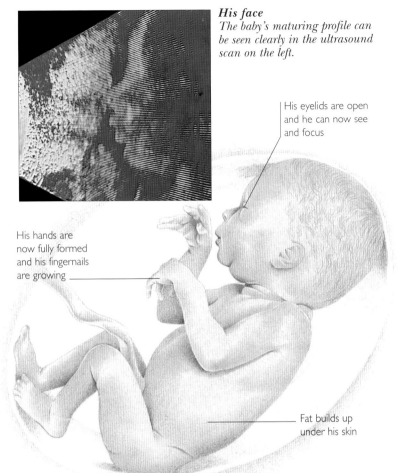

His face
The baby's maturing profile can be seen clearly in the ultrasound scan on the left.

His eyelids are open and he can now see and focus

His hands are now fully formed and his fingernails are growing

Fat builds up under his skin

YOUR BABY

Your baby continues to gain weight and to mature. He communicates with you by wriggling and kicking.

Temperature He now begins to control his own body temperature.

Fat White fat begins to build up under his skin.

Red blood cells His bone marrow has now completely taken over responsibility for the production of red blood cells.

Urine He passes urine into the amniotic fluid at the rate of about ½ litre (1 pint) every day.

Genitals The testes of boy babies descend first into the groin and then into the scrotum (premature boy babies will usually have undescended testicles).

BABY'S VITAL STATISTICS

By the end of this month his crown to rump length will be 28cm (11in), and he will weigh about 1.5kg (3lb).

Your baby grows
His body is now growing plumper as the subcutaneous fat builds up under his skin, filling out the wrinkles. His eyebrows and eyelashes are fully developed, and the hair on his scalp is becoming longer. His eyelids have now opened, and he begins to practise seeing and focusing – the limitations of his field of vision (20–25cm/8–9in) at birth is thought to be related to how far he is able to see while he is in the uterus. As the ultrasound on the right shows, his head and body look more balanced in size. He now has the proportions of a newborn baby.

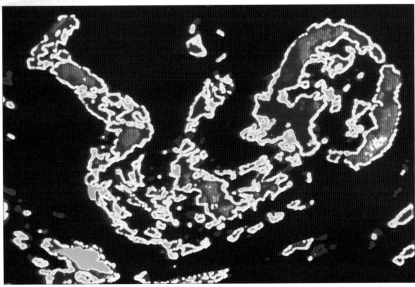

MOTHER

You will probably be having more frequent antenatal checks now. Your doctor will be monitoring your blood pressure and urine and checking the baby's position.

Contractions Your uterus hardens and contracts as a practice for labour. Known as Braxton Hicks' contractions, these only last about 30 seconds and you may not be aware of them.

Pelvis Your pelvis has now expanded. It may ache, especially at the back.

Blood You will probably have a low haemoglobin level at this stage in your pregnancy.

Abdomen Your baby's size is increasing so that the uterus is pushed hard against your lower ribs, and your ribcage may become quite sore. Your abdomen is so stretched that your navel inverts and the increased pigmentation of the linea nigra can make it look very prominent.

Up to 34 weeks

Thirty-four weeks after your LMP, your baby is perfectly formed. All her proportions are exactly as you would expect them to be at birth. Still, she has some maturing to do and some weight to gain before she is ready to be born.

YOUR BABY'S PROGRESS

Her organs are now almost fully mature, except for her lungs, which are still not completely developed, although they are secreting increasing quantities of surfactant, which will keep them from collapsing once she begins to breathe air. She can make strong movements that can be felt on the surface of your abdomen. Almost all of the babies born at this time survive.

Her skin, nails, and hair Her skin is now pink rather than red, due to the deposits of white fat underneath it. Fat deposits build up under her skin in order to provide energy and regulate her body temperature after she is born. The protective *vernix caseosa* that covers her skin is now very thick. Her fingernails now reach the ends of her fingers but her toenails are not yet fully grown. She may have quite a lot of hair on her head.

Her eyes Her irises can now dilate and contract. They will contract in response to bright light, and also to enable her to focus – although she will not need to develop this skill until after she is born. She can close her eyelids, and she has begun to blink.

Her position Some babies assume the head-downwards position about now, but there is still plenty of time – most engage after 36 weeks. However, she may remain in the breech (bottom-down) position until birth, although most babies do turn on their own.

HER SUPPORT SYSTEM

From this month the placenta layers may start to thin. To make oestrogen, the placenta converts a testosterone-like hormone that is produced by your baby's adrenal glands. By this month these glands have reached a size equivalent to those of an adolescent, and every day they produce ten times as much hormone as an adult's adrenal glands. They will shrink rapidly after birth.

The amniotic sac, or bag of waters, contains a large amount of fluid, most of which is the baby's urine; she can void as much as one pint of urine daily. Excess *vernix caseosa*, nutrients, and products necessary for lung maturation, are also present. The umbilical cord is large, strong, and tough. A firm, gelatinous substance surrounds the blood vessels and this prevents kinks or knots in the cord that could affect the baby's blood supply.

YOUR BABY AT 34 WEEKS OF PREGNANCY

YOUR BABY

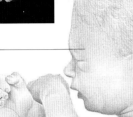

Her head and face
The ultrasound on the left shows very clearly how both the shape of her head and her profile have developed, so she now looks like a "proper baby".

Her face is now smooth with most of the wrinkles gone

Fingernails reach tips of her fingers

There may be a lot of hair on her head

Your baby is putting on weight; about eight percent of her total weight is fat

Your baby's main activity now is to settle into a head-down position and adjust to her lack of space in the uterus.

Eyes She can now focus and blink.

Weight gain She will have gained at least 1kg (2lb) since last month. This is made up primarily of increased muscle tissue and fat.

Lungs Her lungs are still developing so that she can adjust to respiration outside the uterus. If she were to be born at this stage, she would almost certainly have breathing difficulties, although she would stand an excellent chance of survival.

BABY'S VITAL STATISTICS
By the end of this month her crown to rump length will be about 32cm (12in), and she will weigh about 2.5kg (5lb).

Your baby's size
It is now becoming rather a tight fit in the uterus, especially if your baby is large. As a consequence, her movements now tend to decrease in frequency, although you should still be able to feel her moving (see pp.194 & 195). In addition, her body, like that of the baby in the ultrasound scan on the right, will now start to become tightly curled as her elbow and knee space is restricted. Quite a few babies are bottom-down (breech) at the start of this month (see column, p.259), but most will have tipped head-down by term.

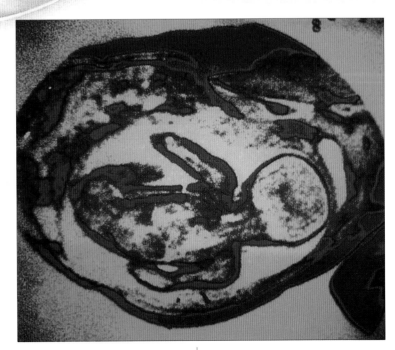

MOTHER

You will be seeing your doctor every week now. He or she will be checking that everything is going well.

Engagement In most first-time mothers, the baby's head drops down into the pelvis at about 36 weeks. You will feel more comfortable and breathing will become easier. It is normal for the baby's head not to engage until later; sometimes not until labour has started.

Posture You may tend to make up for extra weight at the front by leaning backwards. This throws your head back so that your line of vision is different from usual. Your centre of gravity has altered, so you may bump into things or drop them.

Sleeping and resting It may be more and more difficult for you to get a good night's sleep as your large abdomen makes finding a comfortable position difficult. However, rest as much as possible, with your feet up if you can.

Nesting instinct Usually occurring during pre-labour (see p.270), this often seems to manifest itself in an urge to clean the cooker! Try to resist it – you'll need all of your energy for giving birth.

Up to 40 weeks

It can be difficult to calculate the exact date of conception, although most women have their fertile period about 14 days after the first day of their last menstrual period. Because of this doctors set an artificial but convenient timescale of 40 weeks, calculated from your LMP, although a fetus actually reaches "full term", meaning it is fully developed, after about 38 weeks.

YOUR BABY'S PROGRESS

During this month your baby will usually shed almost all of the fine hair (lanugo) from his body. There may be some small patches left in odd places and perhaps some in his body creases.

His skin is smooth and soft, and there is still some *vernix caseosa* left on it (mostly on his back), which will help his passage down the birth canal. He will be almost chubby prior to birth. His fingernails are long and may have scratched his face; they will need shortening after birth. His eyes are blue, although they may change in the weeks after birth; when he is awake they are open.

In these last weeks, your baby produces increasing amounts of a hormone called cortisone from his adrenal glands. This helps his lungs to mature in readiness for his first breath.

Meconium His intestine is filled with a dark green, almost black, substance (meconium). It is a mixture of the secretions from his alimentary glands together with lanugo, pigment, and cells from the wall of his bowel. It will be the first motion he will pass after birth, but he may pass it during delivery.

Immune system His own system is still immature, so to make up for this he receives antibodies from you via the placenta, which will protect him against anything that you have antibodies for, such as flu, mumps, and German measles. After he is born, he will continue to receive antibodies from you via your breast milk.

HIS SUPPORT SYSTEM

The placenta now measures 20–25 centimetres (8–10 inches) in diameter and is three centimetres (just over one inch) thick, thus creating a wide area for the exchange of nourishment and waste products between yourself and your baby. There is now more than one litre (two pints) of water in the amniotic sac.

The hormones produced by the placenta are stimulating your breasts to swell and fill with milk. This also causes swelling in your baby's breasts, whether it is a boy or a girl. This will recede after birth. If your baby is a girl, the cessation of these same hormones following delivery may cause her to have a light bleeding from her vagina (like a period) a few days after her birth.

YOUR BABY AT TERM

YOUR BABY

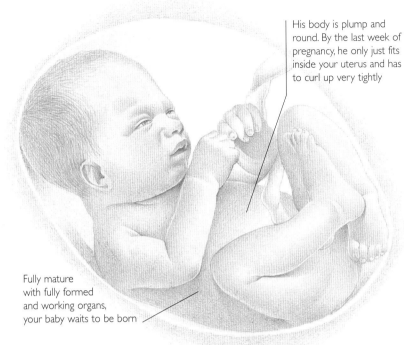

His body is plump and round. By the last week of pregnancy, he only just fits inside your uterus and has to curl up very tightly

Fully mature with fully formed and working organs, your baby waits to be born

Your baby prepares to be born; his lungs mature and the last of his brown fat is laid down.

Reproductive organs The testes of most boy babies will have descended by now. In a girl baby, the ovaries are still above the pelvic brim and do not reach their final position until after birth.

Movements Although his movements will be a fraction of what they were earlier, you should still be able to feel him kick.

BABY'S VITAL STATISTICS

By the end of this month her crown to rump length will be about 35–37cm (14–15in), and she will weigh about 3–4kg (6–8lb).

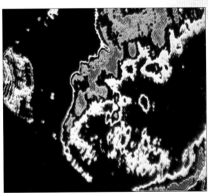

Engaged head
The above ultrasound scan shows the baby lying head down, with his head against his mother's cervix (bottom right-hand corner).

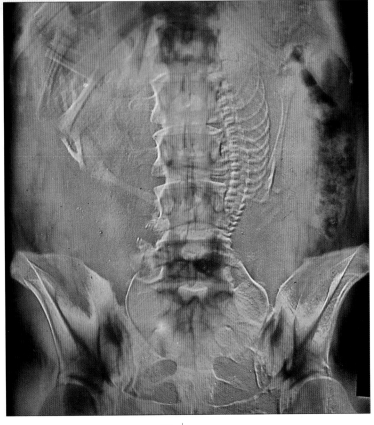

Prepared for birth
As your baby gets heavier and matures, he will tip head-down in your uterus. In the colour-enhanced X-ray on the right, the baby's head can be seen settled deeply into the mother's pelvis.

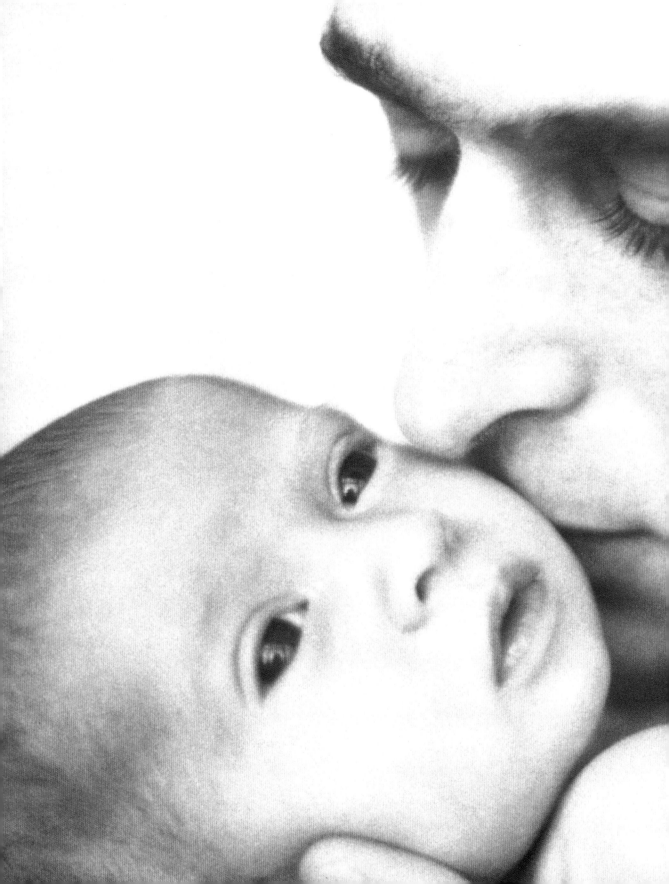

CHAPTER 3

Preparing for
FATHERHOOD

Most men have strong nurturing instincts and most men, given half a chance, make excellent fathers. No one feels confident about becoming a parent and the prospect of fatherhood is understandably daunting. A little thought and preparation goes a long way to boosting morale and to giving a man a sense of fulfilment.

THE MODERN FATHER

Tasks that used to be seen exclusively as a mother's responsibility – like bathing the baby, doing the weekly shop with the children, and taking and fetching from school – are now increasingly shared by fathers.

• A significant minority of fathers are becoming primary carers of their children.

• Many fathers are fitting into their working day activities like the school run, helping in the classroom, or taking their child to the doctor.

• Most fathers love the bedtime bath and story routine, especially if they've been away from their children all day.

Bonding
Fathers and children can form lifelong bonds through their contact during the baby's first weeks of life.

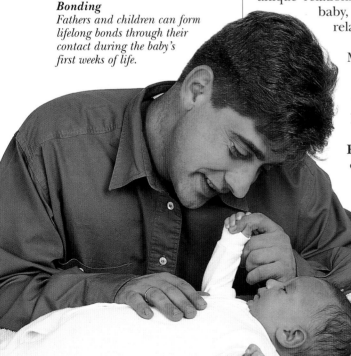

What is a father?

This chapter is addressed specifically to fathers so that they can understand pregnancy, birth, and baby care from their own perspective. Getting pregnant and having a baby, however, should be looked on as a joint venture by parents, even though fathers usually take a back seat in books like this. I want to correct that bias. Men are as good at fathering as women are at mothering and babies love being nurtured by fathers as well as mothers: that fact alone makes a powerful argument for parenting being equal and shared.

MAKING ROOM FOR FATHERS

On the face of it, participating equally in parenting may seem fraught with obstacles, but it needn't be. Parents can share all the elements of baby care with a little planning and a generous heart. After all, baby care means loving your baby, encouraging your baby, teaching your baby, watching your baby grow and develop, and establishing bonds with your baby that in all probability will be the strongest you ever make with anyone. Who in their right mind would miss out on it?

Men should try not to allow themselves to be deprived of this unique relationship. And when they're fully involved with their baby, a little miracle occurs along the way: their relationship with their baby's mother flourishes, too.

No-one has trouble defining a mother's role. Mothers care for children: they feed, comfort, dress, and bathe; they encourage, teach, carry, undress, put to bed, and maybe sing to sleep. We know this because it's what we experienced as children. Defining a father's role is more problematic.

Finding a role model Much as we may love our own fathers, the way we experienced them as children is not necessarily how we hope our own children will experience their fathers. Men are constantly being exhorted to become fully involved in nurturing their children, but few have any role model to demonstrate what this actually means. To put it bluntly, what we want is for fathers to be more like mothers.

Babies don't differentiate Babies and young children don't see any difference in male and female nurturing. They will experience comfort, warmth, and security from two adults and, though they soon learn to tell their mother apart from their father, they don't make value judgments based on a pre-determined notion of what mothers' and fathers' roles ought to be. Apart from breastfeeding, there is nothing a woman can do for a baby that can't be done by a man.

The need for parenting Babies don't need mothering and fathering, they need parenting. They need the most important adults in their lives to be models of what parents do for their children; when this is achieved, the next generation of fathers will not be at a loss concerning what a father's role should be. Care for a child is indivisible; she will only compartmentalize her needs if this is what she learns that she should do from her experiences.

YOUR ATTITUDE TO HAVING A CHILD

However right it may seem at the time, the decision to have a child needs the same reasoned, clear-eyed evaluation you would give to buying a house or a new car. It can be useful to put into words some of the half-formulated thoughts and questions that rest in the corners of the mind. Even if you think you both really want a baby because you love each other and it's the natural thing to do, it's still sensible to think about all the issues. For example, are you both clear about how a baby will affect your way of life? Does it seem instinctively right for your relationship, or are you just reacting to pressure from others, such as the potential grandparents? Do you both have the same desire for a baby?

A NEW KIND OF PARENTING

The composition of the traditional family has changed in recent times, as has the way it functions. Whereas fathers used to be protectors, having little direct involvement in day-to-day child care, their importance as equal partners at home is now being recognized – side by side with women's increasing role as equal or even primary financial provider. In recent years an alternative family arrangement has developed where the father cares for home and family by choice, while his partner earns the daily bread. One reason why such families are often strong and successful units is because they take account of both partners' talents and generally come about after careful discussion and planning. But whatever the practical arrangements within your individual family unit, providing a stable, loving, and open environment in which to bring up children is probably the only important constant.

The caring father
Fathers can help themselves unlock an often hidden side of their nature through nurturing and caring for their children.

93

PRENATAL BONDING

You can never start bonding with your baby too early. Babies can hear sounds outside the womb by five or six months; if you talk to your baby, he will bond to your voice while he is still in the womb and, in fact, he can hear your low-pitched voice more clearly than his mother's. To help you to bond with your baby:

• gently massage your partner's tummy and feel your baby move

• talk and coo softly to your baby, and kiss and nuzzle him through your partner's skin

• listen to the heartbeat – a cardboard tube, such as the inner tube of a toilet roll, can make a good amplifier

• go to scans with your partner and watch your baby develop (see p.180)

• read as much about pregnancy and birth as you can – at least as much as your partner – so that you can talk things over together

• discuss names for your baby together – this gives your unborn baby a personality and you can start relating to him or to her

• plan well ahead to attend antenatal classes for fathers and any lectures your partner goes to on childbirth.

The expectant father

Finding out that you are going to be a father is one of the most exciting moments of your life. The emotional impact of the news will be just as strong on you as it is on your partner. However, the effect on men is often underestimated and you are likely to find that once the initial excitement has worn off, people will stop asking you how you are feeling. It's therefore important to talk about your emotions, especially to your partner, and to get involved in the pregnancy and birth plans. Allow the unborn baby to be as big a part of your life as you can – this, after all, is something that is happening to both of you, not just to your partner.

UNDERSTANDING YOUR EMOTIONS

The pregnancy may not seem real for the first couple of months – not least because your partner will look much the same. Don't worry if you feel differently about the pregnancy from her; it is an internal experience for her and an external one for you, and a couple doesn't suddenly become one person with one set of feelings just because they are having a baby together. However, once you see that your partner's body has begun to change and, later, when you have felt the baby move, the idea of having a baby will become more real.

It is at this time that your feelings of joy and excitement may be replaced by fears and worries; whatever your family set-up, it is normal for a man to begin to worry about being able to provide for his family. Having a child can be an extra financial burden, especially if your partner is going to give up her job, but don't rush into making life-changing decisions, such as getting a new job or seeking promotion. It's difficult to know whether you'll want extra responsibility a year down the line, once you're a parent. Remember, as a father you have more than just material possessions to offer your child.

HOW YOU CAN PARTICIPATE

Being an expectant father is the one time in your life when you are quite likely to feel out of control. This feeling of being an outsider will not be helped by the way other people treat you: well-meaning female friends and relatives may unconsciously push you out of what they see as their territory. You may also find that the professionals, such as obstetricians and midwives, direct their conversations at your partner more than at you.

Take the initiative Don't just step back and allow your female relatives and friends to become more involved than you. Talk to your own friends and colleagues: you may be subject to a certain amount of teasing but, equally, you may find other fathers keen to share their experiences with you. Try to find out as much as you can about the pregnancy so that you can understand the changes taking place in your partner's body. If possible, go with her to the scans so that you can see your baby developing, talk about the fact you are going to be a father, and ask as many questions as you want.

PLAN FOR THE BIRTH TOGETHER

Discuss with your partner the type of birth that she wants (see p.106) and together decide what your involvement will be. Plan to talk to your employer about taking time off to go to the antenatal appointments as well as the birth, so that you can spend some time at home with your partner after the baby is born.

The birth plan Talk over the issues raised by the birth plan (see p.122) with your partner but don't impose your views. If she feels strongly about certain issues, such as trying for a drug-free labour (see p.282), respect her feelings but make sure you discuss the pros and cons. Don't assume you will be squeamish at the birth. Witnessing the birth of your child is probably one of the most moving things you will ever experience, and holding your baby in the first few seconds of life not only helps bond the two of you but is a tremendous emotional experience.

BEING INVOLVED

It's your baby too. There is no need to suppress any of your feelings or thoughts. You can feel perfectly free to:

- be open about your feelings

- express your concerns

- talk candidly to your partner about sex so that it does not become an issue

- be party to all arrangements and plans for the birth

- go to antenatal classes

- go to antenatal appointments to hear your baby's heartbeat and see him move on the ultrasound

- visit the hospital and delivery room with your partner and meet any professionals involved

- be present at the birth.

WHAT TO DO	HOW IT CAN HELP YOU
Talk to your partner	*The best way to understand how your partner is feeling and what is going on in her body is to talk to her. Ask her what it is like to feel the baby move; discuss your plans for the birth together; find out if she's got particular discomforts. She will be pleased to share her experiences with you.*
Go to antenatal classes	*If you go to antenatal classes (especially father-only sessions) you will have an opportunity to learn about the birth and talk through your own concerns. This will help you to work out the best way to support your partner and enable you to be more involved in birth choices.*
Talk to other fathers	*Get to know the other expectant fathers at antenatal classes – they will probably be feeling the same as you and be glad to have someone to talk to. Talk to friends and colleagues who have babies; find out what their experience was like and ask their advice.*
Read about pregnancy and parenting	*Read pregnancy and parenting books and any leaflets you are given. The more you understand about what's going on during the pregnancy the more familiar it will become and it can help you to understand how your partner is feeling. It will also enable you to ask the right questions.*
Ask questions	*Go to antenatal appointments with your partner so that you can meet the professionals and be present at the examinations. As a first-time parent there will be things you don't understand and need to know about. If you ask questions of professionals they are more likely to involve you.*

COPING WITH THE UNEXPECTED

A labour that doesn't go to plan can be scary for both of you. Be prepared in advance for the fact that unexpected interventions may be necessary.

• Well before your baby is due, talk to your partner about what she feels about any special situation that may arise. Make sure you know her views and preferences for any eventuality. Bear in mind, however, that she may change her mind when it comes to the point.

• Unless it's an absolute emergency, make sure that any interventions suggested are talked through properly with you and your partner, and either or both of you ask questions if it isn't clear. But remember that the final decision is hers.

• If something is suggested that you know your partner wants to avoid, try to buy time. For instance, if labour has slowed, suggest a change of position before procedures to accelerate labour are introduced.

• If the medical team decide the labour needs monitoring with high tech equipment, try not to be distracted by it. Concentrate on your partner, not the technology.

• Remember that if something unexpected occurs, and the medical team has to intervene, it's never your partner's fault. These things happen.

• Whatever happens, talk about it afterwards, especially with your partner, but also with friends and, if necessary, health professionals. You'll have a lot of feelings to work through.

Fathers at the birth

In the days prior to due date make sure you can always be contacted easily. If you've got a mobile phone, keep it switched on. You may feel there's not much for you to do at the birth but just being there is a huge comfort to your partner and you have a practical role too. Trust your intuition and judgment as to what's needed and ask for feedback.

DURING LABOUR

Your presence can be a great support to your partner during the labour. You may feel that there is not a lot you can do in comparison with the medical staff, but it is important for you to be there and to be loving and intimate with your partner. Whatever your own emotions, try to be slow and gentle, quiet and reassuring. Don't, on the other hand, try to do too much and get in the way of the medical staff or become an irritation to your partner; give her space when she wants it. Be positive and never criticize in what you say to her; she needs lots of praise, encouragement, and sympathy.

Practical help There are various things you can do to help your partner cope with the discomfort and the pain of giving birth. Offer her practical help such as a warm hot-water bottle if she's got backache, sprays of water or a cool flannel if she's too hot, and sips of water if her mouth is dry. If she wants to go without pain relief encourage her while it seems reasonable but if she asks for it, don't put her off. She's the one who is in pain. You will probably have discussed this beforehand as part of your planning, and she may then have been quite adamant in not wanting pain relief. But if she changes her mind in labour don't argue with her; nobody can know how they are going to feel when giving birth until it happens.

Seeking explanations Talk to the midwife or doctor if you don't understand what's happening, or if you're worried. They are there to help both of you, but remember that they are professionals who have your partner's and your baby's best interests at heart. At the same time, don't let the hospital staff and their machines become the focus of your attention.

Your partner's moods Keep your sense of humour; if your partner shouts – or swears – at you, or seems to get angry or overwrought, take it in your stride. It's her way of coping with a very stressful situation. It is quite a normal occurrence, particularly so at the transition phase of the first stage of labour (see p.273). You can treat it as a positive step towards the birth – it's a sign that the second stage of labour isn't far off.

SECOND STAGE AND BIRTH

Helping your partner and watching your baby being born is an overwhelming experience for all fathers. The second stage is hard work for mothers; it's a real effort, but there are ways you can help your partner during this stage, so that you can feel as involved in your baby's birth as possible.

Practical help If you have been attending antenatal classes you will already have worked out together the positions that your partner thinks will best suit her for giving birth. Now you should help her to get into the position that she feels is most appropriate, and support her there. However, this may not be the one she thought of using, nor even be among the ones you have practised. That does not matter; just support her in whatever position she feels is right at the time. Talk to her and encourage her all the time throughout the second stage, and keep in physical contact so she knows you're with her all the way.

The moment of birth If you can see your baby's head as it crowns, describe it to your partner or hold a mirror for her to see the head – this will be a huge encouragement to her. However, don't get in the midwife's way, as she will need to be able to monitor the baby's progress second by second, and to check the birth of the head. Once the baby is fully out, let your partner know what sex it is, even if you had been told this during the pregnancy. Say that you have a son or a daughter, not just "it's a boy", or "it's a girl"; the words "son" and "daughter" express family feelings. If the midwife agrees, clamp and cut your baby's cord yourself. It's a fantastic moment – the moment your baby really becomes an individual being.

Sharing feelings When the baby is born, share with your partner in the first minutes of your child's life. If you feel like weeping, don't hold back. This is one of the most emotional moments of your life. By all means photograph or video your partner and baby, but don't do this to the exclusion of helping them. They are more important than anything else.

MEETING YOUR BABY

This is the moment for which you've waited nine months, when you can take your baby in your arms together for the first time, the moment that will make everything you've just gone through worthwhile. Your midwife will probably lay the baby on your partner's tummy or give him to one of you to hold while the cord is clamped and cut; let your baby feel and smell your skin by taking your shirt off. Hold him close to your face and let him look up into yours. Share this moment and savour it; this is a meeting that will change both your lives forever. It is also the moment when you claim your new status as parents. You will never forget this experience. It's so emotional that you may well both find yourselves weeping with joy and relief.

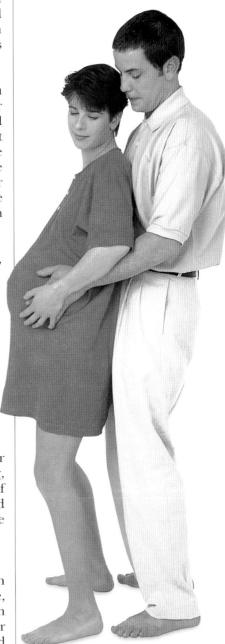

Positions for labour
Support your partner in whatever position she finds best for giving birth. Standing and squatting are favoured by many women, while their partner's contact provides warmth and loving reassurance.

AFTER THE BIRTH

After the birth, you may feel you are as emotionally exhausted as your partner, but it's important not to underestimate the physical effort of labour and birth on a woman. Because of tiredness she may not appear to experience quite the same emotions as you.

Your partner's reactions You will probably experience a wave of euphoria now that your baby is born, but if labour has been long and arduous your partner may be too exhausted to experience this same "buzz" immediately. It doesn't mean she isn't as excited and delighted as you are, but after a lengthy labour, it's not surprising if she finds it difficult to express immediate enthusiasm. Just hold her close and let her know how proud you are of her and of your new son or daughter. Stay with them both for as long as possible after the birth, including settling them in to the postnatal ward.

Valuing your role Congratulate your partner on her achievement, and let her know how much you appreciate her. But in responding to her needs at this time, don't belittle your own contribution and the support you've been able to give. You may think you haven't really been much help – this is a common reaction for fathers who have seen their partners struggling through labour, particularly if it was a long one. However, most mothers will say how beneficial it was to have the emotional support and encouragement from their partner throughout labour and at the birth.

Saying hello Take the opportunity to hold your baby while your partner is being stitched, or checked; go into a quiet corner of the room and get to know the new member of your family. Let her look into your eyes; if you hold her close so she's just 20–25cm (8–10in) from your face, she can see you and smell you, and she'll learn to recognize you from the very beginning (see p.316). Remember too that sight is not her only way of experiencing this new world, and that the sense of touch is very important to babies. Take your shirt off and hold her against your skin or gently stroke her – both strong ways of bonding.

CAESAREAN DELIVERIES

Even if your partner has chosen in advance to have a Caesarean delivery (see p.308) she'll be anxious, because it is quite a major operation. But if the Caesarean is deemed necessary after labour has started because of an emergency she is quite likely to feel distressed, bewildered, and helpless. However, there's much you can do to smooth the way for her. If she is finding it difficult to talk to the doctors make sure you find out exactly why they want to perform the operation. Although she has to give her permission for it your partner may still not be quite clear afterwards what the reasons were, and it is important that you will be able to help her understand them.

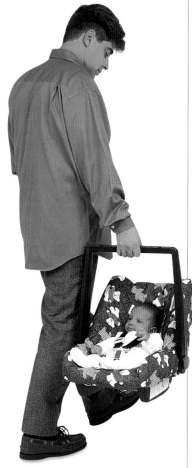

Helping after a Caesarean
If your partner has had a Caesarean delivery, she'll need plenty of rest in order to heal and will need your help with lifting and carrying in the first weeks after the birth.

A Caesarean under local anaesthesia Unless your partner wants a general anaesthetic or the operation is too urgent, see if it can be done under epidural anaesthesia. This means you can share the experience and meet your new baby together. During the operation, sit by your partner's head and reassure her that all is well. You don't have to watch what is going on; you'll both be shielded by the surgical drapes. But if you find the operation distressing or you feel faint – and many people do, even nurses – leave the room quickly. Don't hang on, or you may cause further difficulties for the medical staff.

A Caesarean under general anaesthetic If the Caesarean is being done under general anaesthetic, your partner may not regain consciousness for an hour or more, and you'll probably be given your baby to hold for much of this time. You should cherish this time with your baby: father-child bonding can often be at its best following a Caesarean section birth, because the early time you have together is so precious.

Sudden birth – the father's role

Occasionally labour comes on with such speed that the mother is overwhelmed by the desire to push before her partner has access to professional help, let alone getting to hospital! Although second stage can take a couple of hours, it may not, and babies have been known to be born after a couple of pushes. If it looks as if this is about to happen, neither of you need panic – babies who come quickly are almost always strong and vigorous and most emergency births are perfectly straightforward with no complications.

What to do first On no account leave your partner alone for more than a minute or two; she needs to know that you are right by her. You should help her position herself where she feels most comfortable. Telephone the doctor or midwife and explain the situation. If it's difficult to get hold of them call the emergency services and ask for an ambulance as soon as possible. Wash your hands well and have a heap of clean towels ready. Fold one and put it to one side for the baby. If you've got time find some old sheets or plastic sheeting to cover the floor or furniture.

During the birth Watch for the top of the baby's head appearing at the vaginal opening. When it's visible, ask your partner to stop pushing and just pant. This will give the vagina a chance to stretch fully without tearing. Feel around the baby's neck to see if the cord is looped round it. If it is, hook your finger under the cord and draw it over her head. Hold the baby firmly as she emerges – she'll be slippery – and give her straight to her mother to hold. Wrap her immediately in the spare towel so she doesn't get cold. Don't touch the cord. If the placenta is delivered before medical help arrives, put it in a dish or plastic bowl so it can be checked by the midwife or doctor.

HOME ALONE

When you go home after the birth you may feel a bit lonely and possibly a bit "flat", but don't worry there is still plenty that you can get on with.

• Share the good news with everyone. Use the time to telephone people; you'll find your relations will want all the details.

• Make sure you catch up on sleep. You've had an exhausting time too during the labour, and you can't support your partner fully when she comes home if you're worn out as well.

• Fit the straps for the baby seat in the car, if you haven't already got round to this.

• Use your time at home to do the washing and cleaning. Stock up on groceries and other household items, so that everything is ready and welcoming for when your new baby comes home.

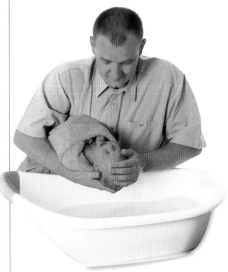

Bathing your baby
You and your partner will be shown in hospital how to bathe your new baby. Giving your baby a bath helps you to bond with her and is something that most fathers enjoy.

WHAT A NEW FATHER NEEDS

New fathers may think that the relationship with their partner is one-way traffic at this time, with him giving all the support. However, you're right to have expectations of your partner too. Your partner should try to:

- **recognize your difficulties** – she should be ready to accept that this is also a confusing and emotional time for you

- **give you some of her time** – the baby may be time-consuming but it is good for your relationship as a couple and as new parents for her to reserve some of her time and attention for you

- **allow you to make mistakes** – if she gave birth in a hospital, she will necessarily have had more time to get used to your baby, but she needs to allow you to handle and care for him too, and not criticize if you fumble

- **be open about when to resume sex** – you will probably want to before her but be understanding as it's probably better to experiment with non-penetrative sex until after the six week postnatal visit and she's discussed contraception with her doctor.

Learning about your new baby

The first few weeks with your baby are important in getting comfortable with your new role as a father. The contribution you make while your baby is still small and vulnerable is vital for the whole family.

IN THE FIRST FEW DAYS

As a new father you may feel rather cut off at first from your partner, particularly during her time in hospital. At the same time, you may feel an intense elation that you want to share with her, but she may seem a bit distant as her body recovers from the birth and she tries to establish breastfeeding. However, there is a lot you can do that will involve you with both mother and baby.

Take the initiative Don't wait to be asked to share your baby's care. Take the opportunity to learn how to do all the practical things your baby needs while your partner is still in hospital.

Get to know your baby Use these early days to establish a close relationship if you are going back to work in a week or two. Even if your partner is in hospital, change the baby, learn to handle him, talk to him, hold him close so that he can focus on your face, or simply hold him if he's asleep. Bring him to your partner when he needs to be fed, and try to be there for the first bath.

Be ready for your partner's mood swings At some point during the first week your partner may get the "baby blues". They come about as a reaction to the sudden withdrawal of the pregnancy hormones and to all her new responsibilities. Your partner will be very tired if the labour was prolonged. These "baby blues" are temporary and subside after a week to ten days. Your partner may try to hide her feelings so as not to worry you or because she fears you won't take her seriously. Never belittle or make light of her feelings: she has a lot to cope with. If her baby blues last more than two weeks make sure she sees her doctor to exclude PND (see p.361).

THE NEW RELATIONSHIP

Concentrate on building a relationship with your baby from the start. Your own feelings as a parent will be enormously enriched if you spend as much time as possible with him. Don't isolate yourself or just see yourself as the breadwinner. Being an equal partner in your baby's care will be rewarding and beneficial to you and to your family as a whole.

Give your baby love Babies need as much love as they can get, and there's no difference between the love of a father and that of a mother. If your baby is being breastfed, then obviously he'll need his mother when he's hungry, but at all other times he'll benefit just as much from your closeness and attention. This closeness from you will mean that he learns to be secure with both of you, which will help him to settle and will also help to take the pressure off your partner.

Support your partner Your partner will be very tired to start with as a result of going through labour and birth, and from the physical and emotional responsibility of breastfeeding. Provide her with the time and space to meet your baby's nutritional needs, and reassure her constantly that she's doing a difficult job well. Your support can make all the difference. If you're back at work, your time will be limited during working hours, but relish the opportunity to do as much as you can for your partner and your baby when you're at home.

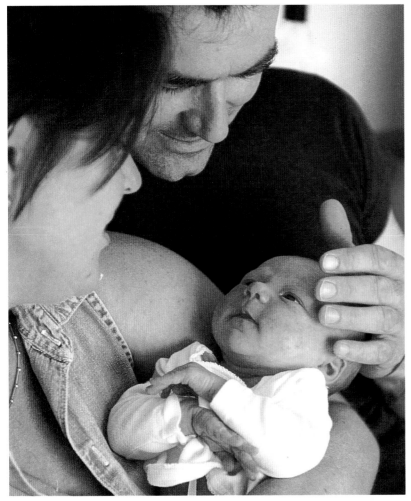

WHAT A NEW MOTHER NEEDS

As a new father you may be tempted to concentrate only on the practicalities of looking after the baby. But remember that your partner has strong emotional needs too. Try to:

• **recognize her vulnerability** – a new mother feels very exposed, both physically and emotionally, in the days after the birth

• **appreciate the depth of her feelings** – you should accept the strength of a mother's overwhelming involvement in the baby. If this seems to exclude everyone else, do not construe it as a rejection of yourself

• **protect her privacy** – one of your most important roles is to make sure that she is not overwhelmed by visitors. Ensure that she has the time and space to establish breastfeeding and to recover from the labour and birth.

Spending time together
For a working father, time spent with your new baby and your partner is irreplaceable. You should spend as much time together as you can, especially in the early days.

SLEEP ROUTINES

Understanding the way your baby's sleep patterns work will help you to tune into his needs, particularly during the night. It will also help you adapt to what could be an unsettling routine.

Being realistic You need to be realistic about how much time your new baby will sleep – I'm afraid it's probably less than you think. He spends 50–80 percent of the time in light sleep, when he wakes very easily. His sleep cycle – light, deep, light – is shorter than an adult's, and he's vulnerable to waking each time he passes from one sleep state to another. Your baby isn't waking to spite you; he's programmed to wake up for all kinds of reasons – when he's wet, hot, cold, unwell – because his survival depends on it.

Having a sleep routine Your baby has to be deeply asleep before he'll settle so try a tranquillizing sleep routine – gentle rocking, quiet songs, and talking softly. When he first falls asleep lay him down and gently pat his shoulder at about 60 beats a minute for a few minutes. He's deeply asleep when his eyelids don't twitch and his limbs feel limp.

Getting home late If you find when you get home from work your baby is usually asleep, ask your partner if he can nap in the afternoon so that he's awake when you arrive. Be patient if this isn't possible; it's not your partner's fault. If this is the case, try getting up earlier to spend time with your baby before work.

NIGHT DUTY

WHAT TO DO	HOW IT CAN HELP YOU
Prepare yourselves for broken nights	*Many babies continue to wake once or twice during the night well beyond 12 months of age. If you're both prepared for this, you'll find it much easier to adjust.*
Share the burden	*Taking turns to get up is important. You may have followed the traditional pattern of father going to work, while mother stays at home, but remember that looking after a baby is also a full-time job.*
Change your sleep pattern	*Broken nights are not necessarily sleepless nights. By developing a new sleep pattern, you'll find that you're able to wake, attend to your baby and then go back to sleep immediately.*
Keep your baby close	*If your baby's cot is by the side of your bed, you don't have to disturb yourselves too much when he wakes for a feed. Put him back in his cot when you're ready to go back to sleep.*
Stay together	*Sleeping separately from your partner could undermine your relationship with her and with your baby. Only sleep in separate rooms as a last resort, for example because of illness or extreme fatigue.*
Avoid sleep deprivation	*Long-term sleep deprivation can have serious consequences, so it's better that you both lose some sleep than that one of you alone takes all the burden and becomes completely exhausted.*

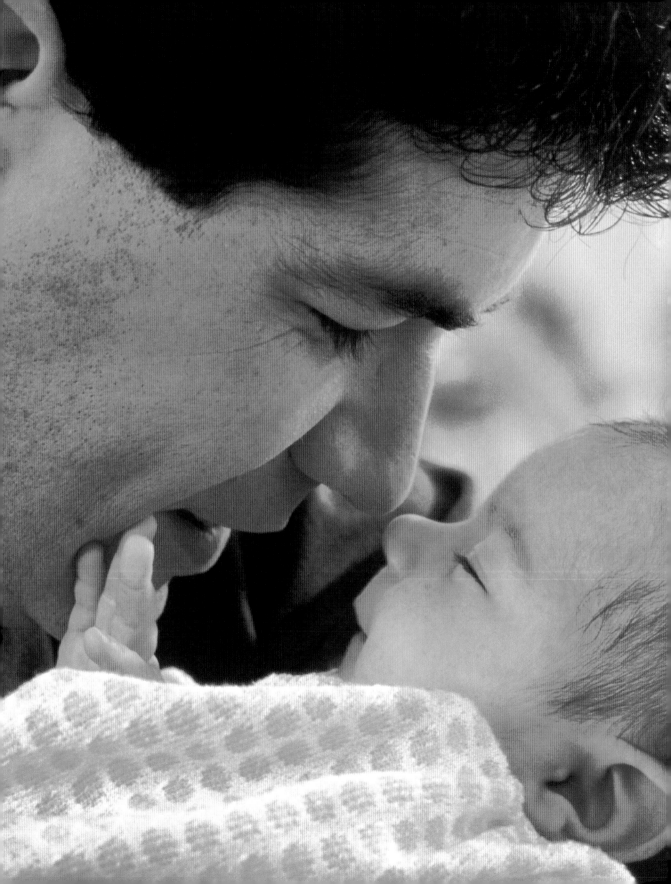

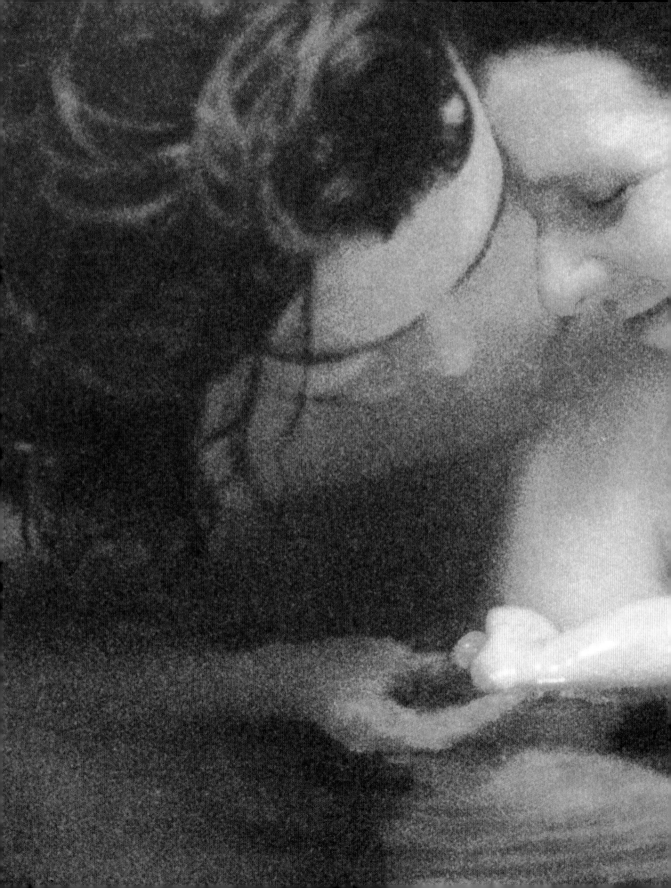

CHAPTER 4

The birth of your CHOICE

There are many choices surrounding labour and birth and you should be aware of all your options. In theory it's possible to have exactly the kind of birth you want, but it's up to women and their partners to take an assertive, informed part in the way their labour and delivery will be handled.

ACTIVE BIRTH

Whether you're in hospital or at home, you'll be encouraged to have an active birth in which your partner or another birth assistant is also actively involved.

An active birth is basically one in which you are not in bed and you don't lie down for delivery – you keep moving. Supported by their partners, mothers are encouraged to move about and become more actively involved in the process of childbirth, adopting whatever positions feel comfortable for labour and birth.

Methods of preparation for an active birth are widely incorporated in childbirth classes, as it has been proven that movements and positions that enable contractions to be aimed downwards, thus pushing the baby towards the floor, make labour more efficient. Squatting, kneeling, sitting, or standing can all help to reduce pain and ensure greater comfort and an easier and shorter progress through labour. A mother who is free to move around may reduce her risk of needing to have an episiotomy, forceps being applied, or a Caesarean section performed.

Your birth assistant
Every woman going into labour should have with her someone other than medical and nursing professionals to offer support and encouragement. The best assistant is your partner, especially if he has attended your antenatal classes with you. However, it doesn't have to be your partner. Your mother, sister, or best friend could also be an excellent choice, particularly if she's had children of her own. Studies have shown that the full emotional and physical support of a trusted individual can help reduce a labouring woman's need of pain-relieving drugs.

The choices in childbirth

Over the past few decades, women have been taking greater control of their health and the medical profession has generally responded enthusiastically to the changing desires and needs of women; the "choices" in childbirth have never been greater, nor our wishes more paramount. Today most of us ask to have our children more naturally, and this option is available, both at home and in hospital.

THE MODERN NATURAL BIRTH

It is reasonable for most women to want natural births: where there is no fear because the process of birth and delivery is familiar; there is no unnecessary medical intervention; there is a calm, homely atmosphere; where mothers are allowed to do what they desire – to take up the most comfortable positions; and there is no undue pressure to take pain-relieving drugs. Female bodies are well designed for giving birth; the soft tissues of the birth passage open so that a baby is gently squeezed out. Breathing and relaxation techniques can make birth even easier to manage, and many natural childbirth philosophies advocate these techniques.

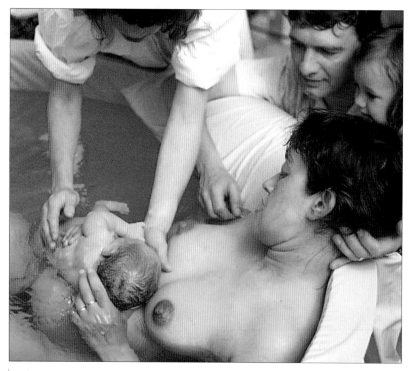

Most of the philosophies of childbirth adopt some form of a psychological re-learning so that your pain expectation is reduced, and your pain threshold raised. In many cases, breathing techniques are central to the philosophy. There are slight differences in the type that each teaches, but all emphasize intense concentration on breathing patterns and the learned ability to relax your body at will. The best way to experience a totally natural birth is in a dedicated centre or at home (see below). However, increasingly, general hospitals also offer the use of water pools and the opportunity to give birth out of bed and in whatever position the mother finds most comfortable.

THE MODERN MANAGED BIRTH

Normal pregnancies and uncomplicated births are almost entirely managed by teams of midwives and, although they may be hospital-based, the trend is towards less intervention. In a managed birth, labour is actively controlled for the safety of both mother and baby. A highly-controlled birth in hospital is essential for some women who may have complications during pregnancy, labour, and birth – an anticipated breech birth, for example.

However, in a hospital setting you are more likely to experience some of the modern obstetric procedures. Epidural anaesthesia is literally on tap and continuous electronic fetal monitoring may be necessary. Consequently, medical intervention is more common: there are more inductions and Caesareans, and more use of forceps. Although these practices do indeed confer a benefit on a percentage of births where intervention is needed, it is now recognized that the routine use of them is not justified (see Childbirth's Contentious Issues, p.108). However most women find a hospital setting makes childbirth the event they expect it to be, and they feel more secure in this environment.

HOME BIRTH

In many European countries healthy women may opt for a home delivery if their pregnancy has been straightforward. In the United Kingdom and the United States it is more difficult. In order to consider a home birth, most doctors would like to see an obstetric history of one normal child, by a normal delivery, before agreeing to a home birth for a second baby. Arranging a home birth can be difficult, and you must be very sure that it is the best option for you. Always keep an open mind about transferring to hospital if things are not progressing well.

Your doctor may suggest to you that a home birth is not as safe as a hospital birth, that it presents too many risks. But there is always some risk attached to giving birth, and statistics have proved that in some circumstances a hospital birth can actually be less safe than a planned home birth (see p.114). However, unplanned out-of-hospital births can be extremely dangerous, whether it is a teenager trying to conceal an unwanted pregnancy, or a couple who do not make it to hospital and whose baby is born en route.

BIRTHING POOLS

The use of water to aid an active birth has gained steadily in popularity.

Birthing pools are used primarily as a means of pain relief during labour, not for the birth itself. There can be some danger if the baby is delivered under water and the head is not lifted out right away.

Many hospitals now offer birthing pool facilities, or you may be able to hire a portable pool (see **Addresses**, p.370). Water births must always be supervised by a qualified attendant.

THE CASE FOR HOME BIRTH

A planned home birth can be one of the safest ways you can give birth.

A recent British all-party report concluded that although 94 percent of all births take place in hospitals, they are no safer, and may be less safe, than home births.

In Australia, a study of 3,400 home births found that there was a lower perinatal mortality rate, and less need for Caesareans, forceps, and suturing for an episiotomy or a tear, than in women delivering in hospitals. The mothers were not all "low risk": the figures included 15 multiple births, breech deliveries, women who had previous Caesareans, and women with previous stillbirths. The group as a whole was older than the national average. Less than 10 percent had to transfer to hospital.

CHILDBIRTH'S CONTENTIOUS ISSUES

Certain procedures historically associated with childbirth are being re-evaluated. Some have been found to be unnecessary, others unjustified. On the other hand, most of today's obstetricians believe that they can guarantee that childbirth is a safer and happier experience for the mother and the baby with the help of all the modern technology available. For example, in the first stage of labour this may include effective analgesia including epidural anaesthesia; monitoring of the fetal heart with a rate meter and the uterine contractions with a tocograph; recording cervical dilatation on a partogram to make sure that progress is being made, and the occasional use of an oxytocin drip to ensure that uterine contractions are sufficiently strong, frequent, and regular.

   While a fuller discussion of certain of the following subjects is given in other parts of the book, this is a good place to preview certain issues. By drawing your attention to arguments against some of these medical practices, this will help you question them if necessary with your medical and nursing attendants. More often than not, your wishes will be complied with, but occasionally you will be told that to continue with a particular option will put your baby and you at serious risk – for instance, if your baby is showing signs of distress and you fight to continue with totally natural childbirth. In this situation you should be prepared to change to your alternative birth plan (see column, p.123). This happens rarely, however, so don't accede to medical intervention unless you secure adequate answers to your questions. Intervention sometimes occurs because of the desire of midwives and doctors to get the baby out quickly. An episiotomy, for instance, is often made necessary when you're encouraged to deliver your baby's head before the skin and muscles in the perineum have been given a chance to stretch. Given time very few women need an episiotomy – as Michel Odent has proved.

Nothing by mouth In cultures other than our own, a woman in labour is encouraged to eat and drink to keep up her strength. There is no medical nor scientific rationale for starving a woman during labour. In fact, quite the opposite. Sometimes a labouring woman has a sudden demand for energy and needs sugar. Other women don't wish to eat but they certainly need fluids; the hard work of labour uses up much energy, which causes sweating, and a woman must replace the fluids that she has lost through her skin. The only time you may be asked not to consume anything is if there is a high risk of an emergency Caesarean.

Moving to a delivery room In most hospitals you labour and deliver in the same room, but depending on the unit you may be moved to an operating theatre if you need an emergency Caesarean. Ideally, labour should proceed smoothly in peaceful surroundings, in a room equipped with good lighting, oxygen, and a suction apparatus to clear out the baby's air passages.

Induction Artificially starting labour is not a new idea, but it only became an easy procedure in the latter half of the twentieth century. Labour is only induced for medical reasons such as pre-eclampsia, high blood pressure, or post-maturity, when induction can save the lives of mothers and babies.

Amniotomy This is when the membranes (the bag of waters) surrounding the baby are artificially ruptured. It is now fairly routine practice in a high-tech birth, but is not done early in labour unless the fetal heart-rate is abnormal. Amniotomy is performed for three reasons. The first is so that electronic fetal monitoring equipment can be set in place; the second is to check if the amniotic fluid contains meconium (this is the baby's first bowel movement and its presence may indicate fetal distress); the third reason is that once the bag of waters has been removed, the baby's head can then press hard on the mother's cervix, facilitating dilatation of the cervix and completion of the first stage of labour.

Fetal monitoring Electronic fetal monitoring, where equipment is strapped to the mother's abdomen (see p.275) is becoming routine for a short time – about 20 minutes – on admission, so there is a permanent record of the baby's heart rate in case of problems later. Obviously having a "window" into the uterus during labour is of great value, but it is hard to change positions while the equipment is attached (although a portable type is becoming more widely used), and this may slow labour. Also, machines can go wrong, and need trained staff to use them correctly. If machines are incorrect, or interpreted incorrectly, then unnecessary intervention can occur. In addition, using a machine to monitor the baby may switch attention from the mother to the machine, which can be very upsetting for the labouring woman.

Forceps These are tong-shaped instruments (like large sugar tongs) used to ease the baby's head out of the birth canal. Forceps have saved the lives of many babies and their mothers, and can reduce the need for a Caesarean section for a baby that is stuck up in the pelvis. The use of forceps means that an episiotomy must be performed. Ventouse extraction (see pp.306 & 307), in which a cup is attached to the baby's head by suction, is increasingly being used instead of forceps to avoid the necessity for episiotomy (see below).

Episiotomy This is a surgical cut to enlarge the vaginal outlet at delivery, and is the most commonly performed operation in the West. Episiotomies are employed in order to avoid tears, which have ragged edges and are difficult to stitch together. Additionally, healing is less efficient. Tears, however, can be avoided if a woman stops pushing while the head is being born, and allows the uterus to ease out the head very gradually rather

THE UNKINDEST CUT?

An episiotomy is an incision that helps deliver a baby's head; it isn't always needed (see p.110).

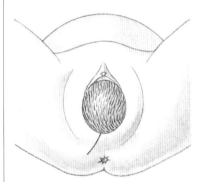

The medio-lateral cut
This cut is angled down and away from the vagina and the perineum into the muscle.

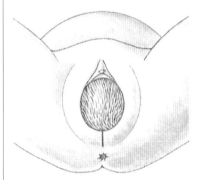

The mid-line cut
This is performed by cutting straight down into the perineum, between the vagina and anus.

If you have already had an epidural, you will probably not need any further anaesthetic. Otherwise, a local anaesthetic in your perineum, known as a pudendal block, will be necessary.

WHEN YOU NEED AN EPISIOTOMY

There are certain circumstances when the safe delivery of your baby's head and body will require an episiotomy.

• Birth is imminent and your perineum hasn't had time to stretch slowly.

• Your baby's head may be too large for your vaginal opening.

• You aren't able to control your pushing so that you can't stop when necessary and then push gradually and smoothly.

• Your baby is in distress.

• You are going to need a forceps delivery (see p.306).

• Your baby is a breech presentation and there is a complication during delivery.

than suddenly. If the head is delivered suddenly, a tear is usually inevitable, so an episiotomy will be done if the perineum is under stress.

If an episiotomy is done too early, before the perineum has thinned out, muscle, skin, and blood vessels are damaged and the bleeding may be profuse. Also, tissues are crushed by the scissors as they are cut and this leads to bruising, swelling, slow healing, and accounts for a perineum that is stitched too tightly. This tightness causes great discomfort in the postnatal period, and may even lead to a painful scar, which may prevent you engaging in intercourse for months afterwards. If you wish to avoid an episiotomy, it's as well to have it clearly stated on your notes that you wish an episiotomy not to be done unless entirely necessary. You must have a local anaesthetic in the perineum before an episiotomy is performed. It is your right and you must insist that you get it.

Breech birth Many women and midwives believe that a gentle and unhurried approach to birth, coupled with skilled midwife care, enables a breech baby to be born vaginally with the minimum of risk. However, research has shown that vaginal delivery is riskier than Caesarean delivery for a breech birth, and most breech babies are delivered by Caesarean section, but usually with epidural anaesthesia.

Time What is considered to be the normal length of labour varies from hospital to hospital – for example, the "right" length for the second stage can be two hours or 30 minutes, or somewhere in between, depending on the obstetrician or midwife. The normal length of labour varies between women, and from birth to birth, and it is the marrying of what is normal for you with what is considered right by the hospital that may cause problems.

In most cases where the first stage is considered to have gone on too long, the membranes are ruptured (if they haven't done so already), or an oxytocin drip is set up to increase the rate and strength of contractions. Where the second stage is considered to take too long, episiotomies and forceps deliveries are often performed. However, many midwives say that it is usually obvious when labour is proceeding well but is just taking some time, as opposed to when it is slow because something is wrong.

Being together It is uncommon for babies to be separated from their mothers after birth unless they need special care or the mother requests it. However, your partner won't be able to stay with you in the hospital as there aren't usually facilities for partners, which can leave him feeling very depressed after the excitement and emotion of the birth. In addition, most women say that they were too excited to sleep afterwards, and wished that they had someone to talk to. Before you go into hospital, ask how long your partner can stay with you after the birth.

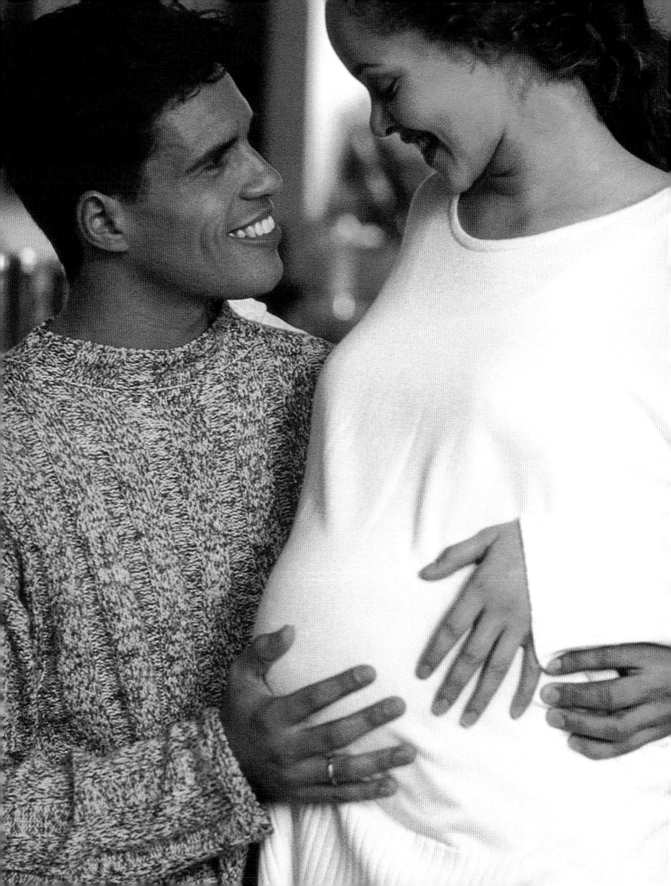

THE BRADLEY METHOD

This refinement of birth preparation was initiated by Dr. Robert Bradley and is also known as husband-coached childbirth.

The Bradley method teaches women to accept the pain, and to go with the flow under the guidance of the husband or partner, friend, or counsellor. The coach attends the antenatal classes with the mother, helps her with her exercise and breathing routine, and comforts, coaxes, and coaches her through labour and delivery.

The danger of this is that most women need to be distracted from the pain, to focus outside of themselves, in order to cope, and that going into the pain can be totally overwhelming.

In addition, each labour is completely individual and may be very dissimilar to what you have practised, and a woman often reacts to giving birth in a different way than she imagined. Some birth partners can become so enthusiastic about the coaching that they lose sight of the woman and her needs.

Childbirth philosophers

A number of people have influenced the way women and their carers approach birth in the late twentieth century. Their teaching and ideas have altered antenatal and postnatal care, thus making childbirth an ever-evolving experience, and they are beginning to have an effect on the atmosphere and procedures surrounding childbirth in the Western world. Most seek to enable the woman to follow the lead of her body, in a loving and intimate environment.

DR. GRANTLEY DICK-READ

The first obstetrician to realize that fear of giving birth was a main cause of pain in labour, Dr. Dick-Read, brought the principles of natural childbirth to the attention of not only the medical world, but to mothers as well. He was the doctor who introduced proper education of mothers through antenatal classes and careful teaching, and also emotional support, in the hope of eliminating fear and tension. His teaching was so basic that it is now taken for granted by all centres, and there is no method of childbirth which does not rely on his teaching, including breathing exercises, breathing control, and complete relaxation. Dick-Read's watch-word was preparation – not only with information, but also by seeking help, reassurance, and sympathy.

FREDERICK LEBOYER

The Leboyer method of delivery works best if it's seen as an attempt to help people understand what the newborn baby sees, hears, and feels. Leboyer was influenced by the psychiatrists Reich, Rank, and Janov, who shared the belief that later problems in life stem from birth's trauma. Leboyer's concern, therefore, is not primarily with the mother, but with the baby's experience of labour and delivery, and how this affects the baby in adulthood.

In order to minimize this trauma he suggests, in his book *Birth Without Violence*, that the birthing room have soft lighting, and that noise and movement be kept to a minimum. Leboyer also believes that immediate skin-to-skin contact is essential to calm the baby, and that she should be laid on her mother's stomach as soon as she is born. He further suggests that the newborn should then be bathed in warm water as this is the closest she can get to the nurturing environment of the uterus.

Not all of this fits in with the physiology of what actually occurs at birth. A baby needs to feel air on her face to stimulate her lungs to breathe for the first time: placing her in a warm liquid may not be sufficiently stimulating for her to continue breathing. Many professionals say that there is no proof that his theories work. However, it is only right that every baby be welcomed into the world with reverence, so even if you don't agree with all of Leboyer's theories, you can still be interested in a gentler birth.

DR. MICHEL ODENT

As a general surgeon, Dr. Odent was extremely shocked when he first witnessed women pushing their babies up hill against the forces of gravity because their feet were held in stirrups. Consequently, stronger contractions were needed, which were more painful, labour was much slower and exhausting, and there were more complications because mothers were in a position where the baby was held back from being delivered.

This initial shock led him to devise his own methods of childbirth, broadly based on traditional midwifery, at Pithiviers in France. Odent believes that, given the opportunity, women in labour return to a primitive biological state, where they function at a new level of animal awareness, losing inhibitions, and entering a state of consciousness where they will follow their basic instincts. He believes that the body's natural narcotics, endorphins, are responsible for this.

Pithiviers has the lowest rate in France for episiotomy, forceps delivery, and Caesarean section, and all interference is kept to a minimum. By no means all of the mothers have been low risk. Many have been women for whom a complicated delivery was foreseen (a breech baby, for example), who then go on to have a successful natural birth at Pithiviers.

SHEILA KITZINGER

A very highly respected birth practitioner, who has an enormous amount of influence in the West, Kitzinger believes that birth is a very personal experience, and that the labouring mother should be an active "birth-giver", rather than a passive patient.

She has likened the modern, managed birth in a modern, managed hospital to giving birth in captivity; in essence, to being in a zoo. She says that the zoo may be humanely and scientifically managed; the keepers may be kind and considerate, and pride themselves on a low mortality rate and the good condition of their charges; the visiting times may be frequent and the premises friendly and welcoming; there may be space to move around in the cage; those in charge may have tried to re-create the natural habitat, but the zoo still dictates the behaviour of the captives.

She believes that the challenges facing the maternity services today are firstly to enable parents to have a real choice, whether for a totally managed birth, a totally natural birth, or somewhere in between, and to respect their wishes concerning where, and how, their child is born. Secondly, she believes that birth is not an illness, and that a labouring mother and her partner should not be treated as patients, but as intelligent adults whose right it is to have the final say in decisions surrounding the birth of their baby.

THE LAMAZE METHOD

This method of psychological counselling was pioneered in Russia, and was then adopted in France by Dr. Lamaze.

Over 90 percent of women in Russia and 70 percent of French women are now taught variations of the Lamaze method of childbirth. It has become equally popular in the United States, and still forms the basic teaching of the National Childbirth Trust in Britain.

Lamaze felt that no matter how relaxed a woman was, she almost certainly would experience some pain, and that she would have to cope with it.

Following the reporting of Ivan Pavlov's research into stimulus-response conditioning in dogs, Lamaze saw the value of conditioned learning in helping women to cope with the pain of childbirth.

It has three mainstays. The first is that fear of labour is reduced or eliminated by information and understanding. Secondly, you learn how to relax and become aware of your body, and therefore how to cope with pain. Thirdly, you consciously use rhythmic breathing patterns through each contraction in order to distract your mind from the pain.

Home birth

At home, pre-labour (see p.270) will shift imperceptibly into full labour, without any changes of attendants.

• You will remain in familiar surroundings with no need to travel while in labour.

• Once notified, your midwife will come to your house and stay with you throughout.

• You will be encouraged to take your own time during labour.

• Your membranes normally will be left to rupture spontaneously.

• You will be encouraged to seek relief of pain without the aid of drugs (see p.282). However, pain relief will be available from your midwife in the form of gas and air or pethidine if it is prescribed by your doctor in advance.

• Your midwife will try hard to help you retain an intact perineum thus avoiding an episiotomy.

• Your partner and family can be an integral part of the birth.

• After the birth you will be free to celebrate as you choose.

The main difference between home and hospital birth is that at home the birth is your responsibility, and you lead the way. You are the team captain, and everyone else supports you. The major drawback is that if anything does go seriously wrong, medical backup is not immediately to hand although the chances of this happening are very small because of the relaxed environment. The "birthing" room should be properly prepared with your midwife's guidance and necessary supplies should be available in advance.

WHAT TO EXPECT

During the early stages of labour, you will probably find it is more comfortable if you move around. Many women feel a burst of energy and some get an overwhelming urge to clean the kitchen or sort out a cupboard. This is an expression of nesting and is a subconscious urge to prepare for the imminent birth. Use this time to arrange your birthing room, gathering sheets and newspapers and getting ready all the things you, your midwife, and the baby will need. Once labour has become really established, you or your partner should phone the midwife if she isn't already on her way, as well as anyone else you want present.

Throughout labour your midwife will be with you continuously and she will monitor the baby every five minutes with a hand-held ear trumpet or sonicaid (see p.178). She and your partner will encourage you and help you into the most comfortable positions; some pain relief will be available if you need it.

As the baby is being born you will probably find it helpful to squat. Your partner may "catch" the baby before putting him to your breast and your baby may breastfeed immediately. His cord will be clamped and cut once it has stopped pulsating, he will be quickly checked over (see Apgar score, p.292), and the midwife will help you deliver the placenta. The baby will then be given a thorough examination and weighed in a spring scale. You will be cleaned up and, if necessary, sutured. Then you will be ready to become intimately acquainted with your new family member.

THE ADVANTAGES

There are certain clear advantages to having your baby at home, such as the security of knowing you are in familiar surroundings with all the privacy you require. Your partner can play an integral part in the birth and your other children may also be present. You will have the major say in your labour, avoiding routine medical intervention. At home you don't have to perform according to preconceived medical ideas of what is normal. You create your own normal labour in your own home. You will have the same midwife throughout and you will not be separated from your baby or your partner afterwards. You will avoid the possibility of cross-infection from medical staff and other mothers and babies: bonding and breastfeeding usually happen spontaneously. One of the biggest bonuses of this type of delivery is that your partner can be an integral part of the birth – holding, cuddling, and looking after the baby while your needs are being attended to.

THE DISADVANTAGES

Rest assured that the vast majority of home births go without a hitch. However, if something does go seriously wrong, you will have to go into hospital – the midwife will always accompany you. The three main problems that can occur are your baby getting "stuck" during the delivery; your baby having difficulty breathing at birth (although breathing difficulties in the newborn are often due to pain-killing drugs – one risk which does not usually occur at home); you having retained some or all of the placenta.

Not all of these problems require immediate emergency hospitalization. Most breathing difficulties, for example, can usually be eased by clearing the airways, giving oxygen, and massage; midwives carry oxygen just in case. A retained placenta will mean that you and your baby will have to travel into hospital.

A very few babies will be too weak or disabled to fend for themselves. They will need the attention of a special care baby unit. If your baby is needy, you and he will have to travel to the nearest obstetrical unit – although special care seldom affects the final outcome for newborns with severe birth defects. Some mothers feel that if their babies are too handicapped to survive, they would rather they died peacefully at home.

You should also bear in mind that childbirth is very messy and noisy, and some preparation is needed in advance (see p.264).

YOUR BABY'S EXPERIENCE

Your baby will benefit from the relaxed atmosphere at home and will have exactly the same care from your midwife as if he'd been born in hospital.

• Your baby's heart rate will be monitored by a fetal stethoscope or a hand-held sonicaid.

• He will emerge into the skilled hands of the midwife, or be caught by your birth partner.

• Once breathing he will be given to you immediately after his birth and may suckle spontaneously.

• His umbilical cord will be clamped and cut once it has stopped pulsating.

• The skin-to-skin contact your baby experiences as you give him a welcoming cuddle may help him to start breathing.

• The midwife will weigh and examine the baby; there will be no hurry to clean him up.

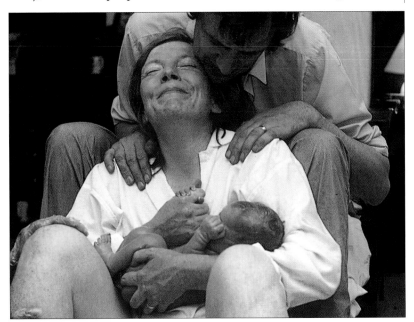

Birth at home
The birth of your baby will be a private celebration as he is born into the intimate environment of his family. The absence of bright hospital lights and noise will allow you to greet your baby calmly and gently. If you have other children they can get to know this new member of the family immediately and you can have them present at the moment of birth if you wish.

Hospital birth

Most babies are born in hospital. Although more and more women are choosing to have babies at home, the majority of women, encouraged by their medical advisers or their own preference, will give birth in hospital.

WHAT TO EXPECT

The unfamiliarity of hospital surroundings can add to the drama of the occasion but here are some tips on making the experience more pleasurable. You probably will have been advised to leave all valuables at home, but on entering hospital you may be asked to remove your remaining personal effects, including jewellery. This can be depersonalizing so ask if you can keep your personal belongings with you in a bag. If you wear contact lenses ask about the hospital's policy as they may prefer you to bring spectacles.

After admission   On arrival, your midwife will ask you about the progress of labour – the frequency of contractions and whether your waters have broken, for example. Then she'll examine your abdomen to confirm the situation, the baby's position will be felt and the baby's heart checked. (You're unikely to be examined by a doctor unless the midwives feel there is a problem about which they want a second opinion.) Your blood pressure and temperature will be taken and you'll be given an internal examination to see how far your cervix has dilated. You will probably be asked to be attached to a fetal monitor for about 20 minutes, after which you'll be free to move about as you want.

Giving birth   If you have decided that you want to manage without drugs for as long as possible during labour, the midwives will usually be more than happy to help you cope using other methods of pain relief (see p.282). Drug relief, however, is available and you can ask to start with smaller doses if you don't feel you need the full measure.

Once the baby is descending you will be assisted into a semi-reclining position. If you are in any danger of tearing, an episiotomy (see p.109) is usually performed as the baby's head is crowning. The use of forceps always necessitates an episiotomy (see p.306). Your baby will be delivered on to your abdomen and while you take your first look at each other you will be given an injection of Syntometrine into your thigh; this ensures that your uterus will contract firmly, thereby reducing the chance of severe bleeding after the delivery of the placenta.

Your baby will then be given an Apgar score (see p.292) while you are cleaned up. You are usually sutured by the midwife at this point, although in some hospitals you may have to wait for this procedure until a doctor arrives.

YOUR EXPERIENCE

Your experience of giving birth in hospital will vary depending on your choice of hospital and professional attendants (see p.120), but will probably include the following procedures. If you wish your experience to be different, you must talk to your doctor or midwife.

• You will probably travel to hospital while you are in labour.

• You will go through brief hospital admission procedures.

• Your membranes may be ruptured and fetal monitoring equipment set in place (see p.275).

• If labour slows down, or stops, you will probably be given oxytocin to stimulate uterine contractions.

• Pain-relieving drugs of different types will be available.

• Your birth partner will usually be allowed to stay with you during labour and the birth.

• You will probably be attended by shifts of different midwives and doctors, especially if you are in labour during the night.

• An episiotomy may be performed to ease the delivery of the baby's head and prevent possible injuries to your perineal or vaginal tissues.

• You will probably be given Syntometrine (see p.291) to reduce the risk of bleeding after the placenta is delivered.

• You will be given your baby to hold after birth and be encouraged to start breastfeeding.

THE ADVANTAGES

In certain situations a hospital birth offers the best chance of a successful and happy outcome. Having your baby in hospital is the safest option if you suffer from a medical condition such as heart disease or diabetes, if you are expecting twins, if your baby is known to be breech, or if as a first-time mother, your obstetrical history just presents too many unknown factors.

Should anything go wrong during the labour and birth, emergency medical assistance will be at hand and a wide range of pain-relief medication during labour is readily available. You may feel more confident knowing that your baby can be given treatment in a special care baby unit if the need arises.

By staying in hospital after the birth you may be able to have a more complete rest which could be difficult to arrange at home, especially if you have other children.

THE DISADVANTAGES

Once you enter hospital it's easy to feel overpowered by the atmosphere, although some are getting more relaxed. Bear in mind that everybody in hospital is following rules and routines and that you're going to have to fit in with them. That doesn't mean, however, that you have to do anything you aren't happy about. Your partner may feel a bit in the way and separate from the birth of his child, so try to include him in whatever way you can. It is a good idea to find out as much as possible about the hospital procedures and set-up while you are pregnant, so that you are more prepared once you go into labour.

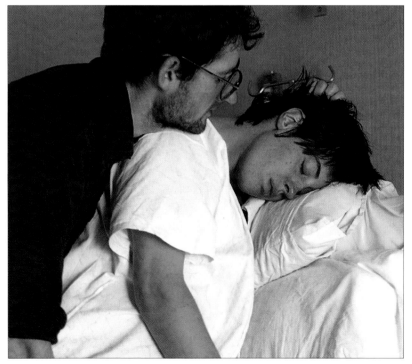

YOUR BABY'S EXPERIENCE

Your baby will be born surrounded by medical staff with the expertise to handle any problems that arise.

• An electrode to measure her heart rate may be attached to her scalp during labour.

• With the exception of epidural anaesthesia she will experience any drugs that you are given, and this may mean that she feels drowsy or is slower to feed once she is born.

• She will be handed to you to cuddle and get acquainted with for a few minutes.

• Her umbilical cord will be clamped and cut as soon as she has been born.

• She may have her mouth and nose suctioned routinely to clear them of any mucus.

• She will be weighed and examined (Apgar score) by the doctor or midwife (see p.292).

• She will be returned to you, possibly cleaned and wrapped in blankets, to begin bonding and breastfeeding.

• At a later time she will be thoroughly examined by a doctor for any abnormalities.

Birth in hospital
As far as possible, you should be allowed to assume positions that are comfortable and to have your birth partner close at hand.

There are many things that you will need to think about or investigate when you are choosing a hospital in which to give birth. Here are some questions to ask yourself or others, before you decide.

• What sort of birth do I want?

• What birth facilities are on offer in my area?

• Am I prepared, or able, to travel for antenatal care? Can it be provided by my doctor?

• What sort of reputations do the hospitals in my area have? Have I got as many different opinions, from as many different sources, as I possibly can?

• What are the staff at the different hospitals actually like? What are their views on labour and birth? Do I agree with them? There may be a difference between a hospital's policies and the way the staff actually approach childbirth.

• Do I want a special care baby unit to be immediately on hand?

• How long do I want to be in hospital for, and what sort of rooming-in facilities are on offer?

• Do I want to feed my baby when and how I feel like it?

• Do I want my baby with me at night? All night?

• What are the visiting hours?

• Can my partner (and children) be with me whenever I want?

• Can my partner stay with me the first night after the birth?

The care on offer

Information about the hospitals in your area is available from your doctor, antenatal clinic, social worker, friends, and acquaintances. However, the only way to find out what a hospital can offer you and whether you feel that it is right for you, is to go and visit it and to ask questions. There may not be more than one maternity hospital in your area, but if you do have a choice, make sure you get satisfactory answers so that you can come to a confident and wholehearted decision about which one to choose.

TYPES OF HOSPITAL

There are various kinds of hospitals most of which cater for maternity care. Without question the most modern facilities are found in teaching hospitals. Here, doctors are always on duty so if you run into any complications one would attend you. As a rule doctors at teaching hospitals are usually more experienced in dealing with complicated births. The smaller community hospitals tend to be more friendly and flexible. There is much less red tape because there are fewer staff and patients; it's easier to meet the people who can help you, and there's no doubt that you will be able to arrange for a more personalized childbirth.

VISITING HOSPITALS

To help you make your final choice, the first thing to do is to tour one or more hospitals with your partner. Most maternity units offer a formal tour, sometimes as part of general antenatal preparation classes, otherwise as part of the general welcome made to mothers booking in. Ask about when these tours take place and see if you can join one before your book in.

GETTING TO KNOW YOUR HOSPITAL

Hospitals can be intimidating, although much less so when you get to know them. It is a good idea to visit the hospital of your choice at least once, more if possible, so that you can meet the staff who will be looking after you, get the feel of the routine, and look at the delivery room and other facilities. The more chance you have to walk around, the more accustomed you'll become to the surroundings and the more relaxed you'll be. Familiarizing yourself does pay dividends. You and your partner should do this together so that you both get to know the place and the people and therefore will feel confident when you are actually there for the birth itself. However, don't visit without prior arrangement. Security considerations now mean that postnatal wards and maternity units are carefully monitored and unannouned visitors are likely to be challenged.

Make sure that you and your partner scout around the outside of the hospital and find the night entrance. Many women go into labour at night and it won't help if you have to search for the entrance in the dark.

CHANGING YOUR HOSPITAL

If you find that your hospital is not living up to your expectations, you don't have to abandon the system altogether. A hospital is there to serve you; health care is a consumer issue and you do have the right to refuse certain procedures. If you are very unhappy with any aspect of the care at your hospital, you can arrange for a transfer to another one.

You could also contact the head of the clinic or your obstetrician and explain your feelings, describing the clinic's shortcomings. You may get on so well with a sympathetic obstetrician that you don't want to leave anyway, although you should bear in mind that he or she is highly unlikely to be there for your delivery. But if you insist on changing hospitals, your obstetrician will almost certainly recommend another doctor at a centre of your choice.

BIRTHING ROOMS

The majority of hospitals have birthing rooms which are unclinical and more like your own home with comfortable chairs, low lighting, soft music, piles of cushions on which you can arrange yourself, with drinks and snacks on hand.

The whole aim of a birthing room is to help the mother relax, overcome fears, and relieve tension. A normal routine prior to birth makes for a normal delivery, and once you're in a birthing room you will not be moved unless an emergency occurs that requires immediate attention. This ensures there are no uncomfortable breaks with a jarring change of movement, mood, and surroundings. It's not necessary to lie down to have your baby, or to be surrounded by rather intimidating technological paraphernalia. In a birthing room you can take up whatever position you want in order to have your baby.

For many women, a birthing room provides the ideal compromise between home and hospital births because it provides similar surroundings and facilities to home, but with emergency expertise on tap if the need arises.

MATERNITY CARE UNITS

Family-centred maternity care is offered by some of the more progressive hospitals and larger medical centres. It is a philosophy aimed at nurturing the family unit during labour, delivery, and after birth. A hospital that has adopted this kind of maternity care respects the social, personal, and family importance of childbirth, and should offer the optional elimination of certain routine procedures and addition of others.

Some aspects of hospital maternity care may appeal to you greatly such as a Leboyer-type delivery, non-separation of parents and baby, rooming in, early discharge, etc. However, this varies from hospital to hospital and you'll have to visit the unit to discuss your options with the staff. A hospital may say that it has family-centred care but you may find that it doesn't fulfil your prerequisites, so find out just what they are offering.

QUESTIONS TO ASK

Once you have chosen a hospital, find out as much as you can by asking questions.

• Will I be able to wear my own clothes and personal effects (rings, contact lenses, spectacles)?

• Can my partner or friend stay with me all the time? Will they ever be asked to leave?

• Will I be able to move around freely during labour, and give birth in any position I choose?

• Will I be able to have the same carers throughout labour?

• Can I bring in my own midwife to attend to me throughout labour?

• Are beanbags, birthing chairs, and stools provided?

• Does the hospital offer birthing pools? If not, will I be able to use a hired one?

• What is the hospital policy on pain relief, electronic monitoring, and induction?

• What kind of pain relief is available and is it available at all times?

• Will I be able to eat and drink if I want to?

• What is the hospital policy on episiotomies, Caesareans, and the expulsion of the placenta?

• If I tear or have an episiotomy, are the midwives allowed to suture me, or will I have to wait for a doctor to attend to me?

There are many different approaches to birth, so ask your GP, obstetrician, or midwife the following questions to find out exactly what to expect.

• What are your views on inducing labour and birth?

• Under what circumstances would you consider it necessary to rupture the membranes?

• Do you believe electronic fetal monitoring is a valuable aid in every birth?

• Would you be concerned if labour was slower than normal?

• What are your views on freedom of movement, the use of water or a birth pool, and breathing techniques to help relieve pain? What drugs do you normally give to control pain?

• Would you be concerned if the lights were dimmed during labour?

• How often do you perform episiotomies?

• Under what conditions would you consider a Caesarean section to be necessary?

• Will we be able to have some time alone with our baby immediately after his birth?

Professional attendants

There are a number of options open to you regarding who attends your labour – it does not have to be a straight choice between hospital expertise or a home midwife. Wherever you decide to have your baby, the system can usually be tailored to suit your individual needs and requirements. Of course, the professional attendant is not the only one you should think about. Most women are supported by their partners or a friend during childbirth, and hospitals now welcome this.

YOUR DOCTOR

Your general practitioner will probably be the first professional person that you see. You may already have an idea about his or her views on birth – especially if you are interested in having a home birth. A few doctors are happy to attend a home delivery of a normal pregnancy, many are not so willing, some fall somewhere in between – preferring to see at least one straightforward delivery in hospital first. Many doctors provide antenatal care if you are having the baby in the hospital to which they have referred you. Occasionally you may be able to attend your doctor's clinic even if you are booked into another hospital – try to explore all of the options.

OBSTETRICIANS

An obstetrician is a consultant who specializes in medical problems in pregnancy and childbirth. When you book into a hospital you will be assigned to an obstetrician. You can ask to be referred to a particular obstetrician although that consultant is not obliged to take you.

Obstetricians tend to be male and although the number of women coming into the profession is rising, male obstetricians still outnumber their female colleagues by a ratio of five to one. If you feel strongly that you want a female obstetrician to attend you, it would be worth checking to see that the hospital of your choice employs any. If it does, you should make your preferences clear on your birth plan. There is, however, no guarantee that the obstetrician of your choice will be on duty when you go into labour and at the birth.

You will be unlikely to see your consultant unless you have any problems during your pregnancy. Most of the routine care is provided by the junior doctors who work alongside the midwives in the obstetrics team.

MIDWIVES

The modern, professional midwife is a specialist in childbirth, qualified to take responsibility for you before, during, and after the birth. She has specific skills to care for you during labour and delivery, and knows when to call for obstetric advice and assistance. Unlike the obstetrician, her focus is the normal not the abnormal – she is interested in the whole of you, not just your uterus and how it may misfunction. Midwives working outside hospitals tend to be more flexible than hospital carers.

Domino midwives   Midwives working under the "domino" (DOMiciliary IN and Out) scheme are community midwives who come to your house when labour starts, and then take you to hospital for the delivery; your GP and hospital staff are rarely involved. If all is well, you may be discharged in a few hours.

Independent midwives   These midwives provide continuous care in a variety of situations. They will deliver you wherever you choose, whether at home or in hospital and undertake to be with you throughout the labour and delivery.

Hospital midwives   In most hospitals midwives now take the lead in the care of labouring women, although they are nominally subordinate members of teams headed by obstetricians. Members of the midwife teams you will have met during your antenatal care will deliver you with the minimum of obstetric intervention. Some members of the team could be male.

INDEPENDENT MIDWIVES

Because she will be your primary caregiver you will need to get to know her. You may like to ask the following:

• What training and experience has she had?

• Does she work alone, or with other midwives? Will you be able to meet them?

• What are her considerations in managing labour?

• What is her back-up system? Does she work closely with any doctors?

• What equipment, drugs, and resuscitation equipment for the baby does she carry?

• What antenatal care does she provide? Are there home visits?

• Under what conditions would she transfer you to hospital?

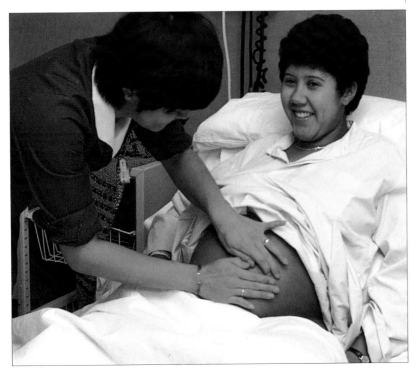

Your birth attendant
The professional attendant who assists you to give birth should be someone you know and trust, and who will give you the kind of support and attendance that you and your partner need. The best attendant is someone who helps to create an intimate atmosphere within which you can work with your body to bring a new life into the world.

COVERING YOUR ALTERNATIVES

Although you will make your plan according to the kind of birth you would like to have, it is a good idea to have another one on stand-by.

This alternative plan can set out the procedures that you would prefer to be followed should complications arise. On rare occasions, labour may become unexpectedly prolonged or difficult, or the baby may need special attention. By considering all the possibilities, you enable your birth attendants to take care of any situation as you wish.

Planning your labour
Make a note of all of the issues that are important to you, and then discuss them with your GP.

Birth plan

Making a plan of your baby's birth will help to ensure you have active involvement in the way he is born and what happens to you as a family after the birth. By carefully considering all your ideas and preferences, and by discussing them with your birth attendants and partner, you will be able to establish a bond of trust and create a happier and more comfortable labour.

A CONSENSUS PLAN

Think about the issues that are important to you and then find out as much as you can to see if what you want is feasible (see pp.118 & 120, and column, right). There is no point in making a plan that cannot be used once you are in labour.

Discuss your birth plan with your GP early in your pregnancy so that he or she can refer you to a hospital that would be most likely to accord with your wishes, if that choice is available to you. You should also discuss your wishes with your midwife, antenatal teacher, and other members of your antenatal team because they will be able to advise and inform you about the kinds of experiences mothers have had locally.

Hospital response Your hospital team will be pleased to see how well you have prepared yourself for the labour and your full participation will be encouraged. Occasionally mothers used to experience negativity from some hospital staff on the grounds that a birth plan might interfere with their standard practices. That is unlikely to happen now – in fact your hospital notes will have a space within the folder for your preferences to be recorded in consultation with your midwife.

Working together Cooperation is an important feature of the birth plan. By working it out in detail with all your attendants, including your partner, you should be able to alleviate any anxieties and feel more in control of your baby's birth. Make sure staff are aware of any alternative scenarios and maintain a friendly relationship with your carers who will want to follow your wishes as far as they can provided you and your baby are not at risk. Once you have discussed the issues that are important to you, give a copy of the plan that is kept with your notes to each of your birth partners or carers. This will be important if, during labour, you are attended by someone who doesn't know your wishes.

Special considerations Make a note on your birth plan of any special needs, such as diet for example, which may be applicable during your time in hospital.

PRESENTING YOUR BIRTH PLAN

*These two examples of a birth plan outline different choices of birth – there are many variations. The plan may be laid out as a list, a letter, or a document such as that from the Chelsea and Westminster Hospital, London (see **Addresses**, p.370).*

Thank you for all the information that you have provided in the antenatal classes and at the childbirth classes. I have thought carefully about how I would like my labour and delivery to be.

My partner, John, will be my companion during labour. He has attended childbirth classes with me.

I understand that electronic fetal monitoring is routinely used and I am happy for this to be done.

If I need pain relief I would prefer an epidural, with as low an epidural dose as possible so that I still have feeling in my legs and am aware of contractions. I would prefer for it to wear off for the second stage, as I would like to push out the baby myself.

If everything goes well and I do not need pain relief, I would prefer to be able to walk around and give birth using a birthing stool, which I will provide myself.

If I have to have a Caesarean section I would like my partner, John, to be with me throughout the operation.

I intend to breastfeed on demand and want the baby to sleep next to me if at all possible. I would also like my partner, John, to be able to stay with us for the first night.

Jenny Lewis

I am looking forward to coming into Central Hospital. I would like to record a few points about the birth as the midwives have suggested. They are:

Support person	I will be accompanied by my sister, Sarah.
Shaving and enemas	I would prefer not to be shaved or to have an enema.
Monitoring	I would prefer to be monitored by a sonicaid or Pinnard stethoscope.
Positions	I will probably want to deliver the baby in a semi-upright position, as this is how I had my other two babies.
Pain relief	It is likely that I will need gas and air, as I did last time.
Episiotomy	I would prefer not to be cut if it can be avoided. I would welcome help in order to help prevent it.

Paula Bell

When? *Make sure you've discussed your plan with your carers by your eighth month.*

IT'S YOUR CHOICE

Look at all the possibilities that will help you to approach your labour with confidence. Don't feel that it has to be totally managed, or natural; it can be a blend of many things. Here are some alternatives:

• hospital/home birth

• medical induction of labour if necessary/spontaneous start

• amniotomy if necessary/ spontaneous rupture of membranes

• fetus monitored electronically for a short time only/continuous fetal monitoring

• nothing by mouth only if high risk of Caesarean/eat and drink as and when desired

• types of pain relief: Pethidine, epidural, gas and air, breathing exercises, TENS, diversion

• catheterization only with epidural/empty own bladder as necessary

• commanded pushing/ spontaneous pushing

• deliberate breath-holding/no deliberate breath-holding

• elective episiotomy/episiotomy only if absolutely necessary

• mother not touching vaginal area/touching baby's head as it crowns, lifting baby out

• use of Syntometrine to speed delivery of placenta/natural expulsion of placenta.

CHILDBIRTH TEACHERS

You'll probably choose a childbirth teacher fairly early in your pregnancy; make plans to start classes in your seventh month or earlier.

Both the quality and approach of classes can vary – some are tightly structured with little question-and-answer time, others allow plenty of time to practise techniques. Some depend mainly on lectures, others on class participation. The teacher is very often the determining factor, so do check with other couples you know who have attended classes before you make your final choice.

Try to select a teacher whose philosophy of birth fits in with the type of birth you'd like to have. Conflicts and confusion can arise if what you learn in class does not accord with your later experience in hospital or at home.

Find out how many couples are taught in each class. Half a dozen couples is ideal as you will receive plenty of attention from the teacher while being intimate with your fellow participants.

Childbirth teachers are, by their very nature, aware and sensitive to the needs and problems of pregnancy. Yours will probably be more than happy to talk to you – even if you are not yet attending childbirth classes.

Childbirth classes

As an enthusiastic proponent of prepared childbirth, I believe that everyone can benefit from childbirth classes. These classes are tremendously enjoyable. The camaraderie is wonderful and you may find the other members of the group act as a substitute for your extended family as you exchange folklore; certainly they will make you feel less alone and isolated. It's a great help to be able to share feelings and experiences with people who are in the same position and it helps to relieve tension and anxiety. Strong personal bonds are often formed with others in the class that can be the basis of lasting friendships.

PARENTCRAFT CLASSES

These are particularly useful for first-time parents because they're designed to give you information that will make you both feel more confident. They work in three ways:

First, the classes cover the processes of pregnancy and birth, including female anatomy and physiology, and the changes that occur to you and the baby throughout the pregnancy. This is done so you will have a clearer understanding of what is involved and why things are happening. The teachers will also talk to you about the sort of medical procedures that you can expect, and why these will be done.

Second, they provide instruction in relaxation, breathing, and exercise techniques that will help you to control your own labour, reduce pain, and give you the confidence that only comes with being familiar with what's happening. Bear in mind that bodies, not brains, give birth, so anything that helps you tune into your body is going to be useful. Your partner should learn how to give you a massage to help relieve your pain (see p.283).

Third, the teachers will talk you through the stages of labour and birth, advise on breastfeeding, and will offer practice in bathing and dressing the baby, changing nappies, bottlefeeding, and making up formula. This will help you cope with the practicalities of caring for your newborn.

EXERCISE CLASSES

Strengthening the muscles used in childbirth often results in an easier and more comfortable delivery. With this is mind, many hospitals offer antenatal classes that incorporate exercise and relaxation classes, and there are independent organizations as well – some are even for specific types of birth. If you tell your instructor that you would like to have your baby while you are standing or squatting, you will be given specific exercises to help strengthen your back, hips, pelvis, and thighs.

YOGA

With its emphasis on muscular control of the body, breathing, relaxation, and tranquillity of mind, yoga is an excellent resource to use as a preparation for pregnancy. However, yoga is a philosophy that pervades the whole of life and, though special exercises for pregnancy exist, they are only a small part of the system. Consequently, it is not something that you can do casually – to have any benefit it must be practised regularly, preferably starting long before you conceive.

TECHNIQUES OF CHILDBIRTH CLASSES

Many studies have shown that taking a childbirth class shortens the length of labour. In one study, the average duration of labour for a group of women who had taken classes was 13.56 hours, compared with the average labour of 18.33 hours in the control group, which had no training. This is probably because knowing how to deal with pain produces a more relaxed labour. Strategies taught by childbirth classes to deal with pain include:

Cognitive control You disassociate your mind from the pain by visualizing a pleasant scenario in which to experience the pain. For example, you will feel happier about experiencing contractions if, every time you have a pain, you imagine your baby moving further down the birth canal, closer to emerging. In this way, you will concentrate on the non-painful part of the sensation.

You can also use distraction to cope with pain during labour, although this works best in the early stages. Counting to 20, going through a list of possible names for your new baby, or concentrating on a beautiful picture or piece of music, should enable you to take your mind off the pain, and keep it from completely filling your consciousness and overwhelming you. Focusing your attention on your breathing techniques and becoming consciously aware of your breathing pattern is another way of forcing your mind away from focusing on pain.

Systematic relaxation In order to decrease your fear of pain and thus increase your tolerance for it, you will be taught exercises to relax the various muscles of the body. In this way you will be able to isolate pain from the contracting uterus rather than allowing it to pervade other parts of your body.

Hawthorne rehearsal You receive enhanced attention from a birth assistant. Psychological research has shown that the more attention you are given, the less pain you feel.

Systematic desensitization You gradually become more tolerant of pain. An example used in many classes is your coach pinching your leg very hard to illustrate how painful a contraction will be. This pinching is repeated every time you attend an antenatal class, and by the end of the course you will be able to tolerate harder squeezing for longer periods.

FATHER'S ROLE

In an antenatal class you can show your partner for the first time just how central a role he is going to play.

Classes will make a supportive man a more effective birth assistant by familiarizing him with the processes of labour and delivery.

Some courses have father-only sessions where the men can talk freely about any problems or anxieties they have about the forthcoming event. A worried man should find security and support in the teacher, as well as in the company of other fathers-to-be.

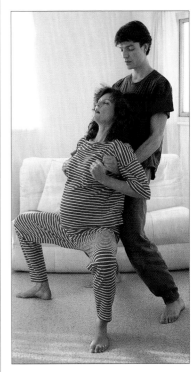

Team effort
Childbirth classes give a couple a unique opportunity to work together as a team towards a common goal – the birth of their baby, and very often this teamwork results in a special closeness.

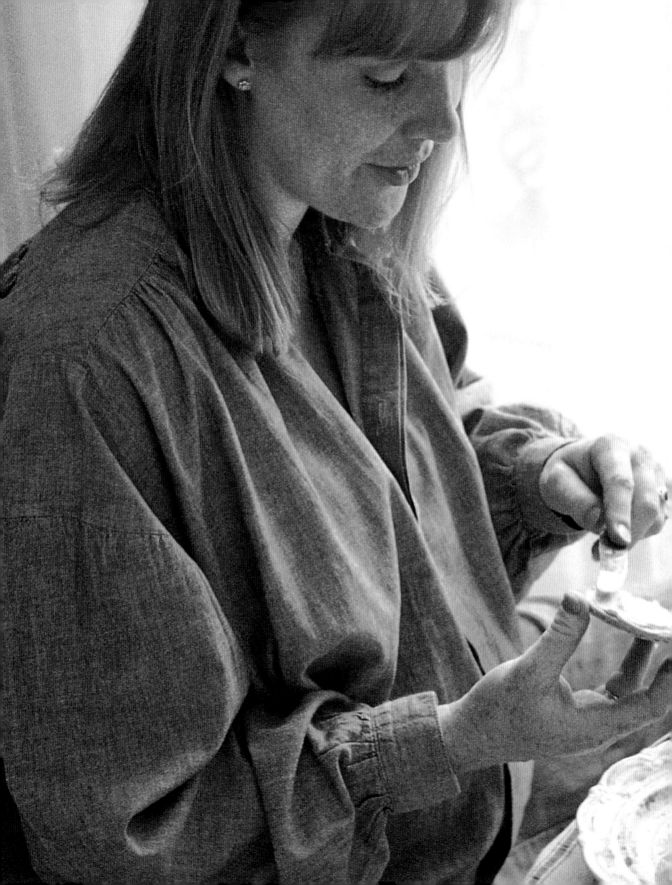

CHAPTER 5

Food and eating in
PREGNANCY

*Eating healthily in pregnancy is mainly a
question of eating a wide variety of the right
kind of foods – those rich in essential nutrients.
Concentrating on fresh fruit and vegetables,
whole grains, organically reared meat, and
low-fat dairy produce will ensure a healthy
environment in which your baby will develop.*

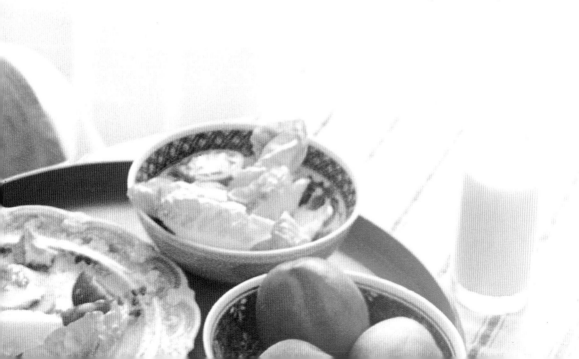

EATING FOR YOURSELF

Your body will never work harder than it does during pregnancy and childbirth. To cope with the increased demands, maintain your strength, and enjoy your pregnancy, you must eat well.

• Increase your intake by 500 calories per day.

• Start to eat 5–6 small meals a day instead of 2–3 big ones.

• Make certain you get sufficient protein and carbohydrates (see p.132); the former supplies essential nutrients for your developing baby, the latter meets your energy needs.

• Eat foods that contain vitamins, such as vitamin C, and minerals, particularly iron (see p.133). These are essential for the healthy functioning of all your organs.

Food in pregnancy

Pregnant women, like most people, rarely have the time to sit around measuring ounces and portions and assessing calorific values. In fact, there's no need to do this as long as you follow some basic guidelines about healthy eating in pregnancy. An important rule is that the nearer food is to its natural state, the more nutritious it is. So fresh is best, frozen is next best, and make tinned foods your last choice. In many ways, good nutrition is common sense.

EATING FOR TWO?

As your pregnancy progresses your appetite will increase; this is nature's way of making certain you eat enough for you and your baby. Your energy requirements will increase only by 15 percent, or 500 calories per day, far less than if you ate twice your normal amount of food. (Certain mothers-to-be, however, such as those who previously ate an inadequate or unbalanced diet, may be nutritionally at risk and have special requirements – see also column, p.138.) The saying "eating for two", therefore,

AVERAGE WEIGHT GAIN DURING PREGNANCY

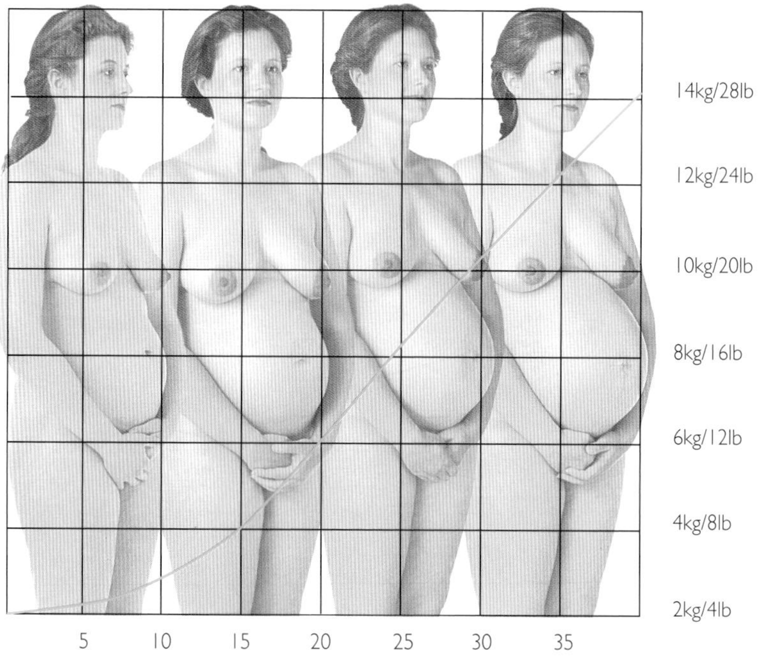

Gaining weight
Doctors recommend that a woman of average weight, experiencing an average pregnancy, ought to gain around 10–15kg (20–30lb) in the total 40 weeks gestation as shown in the chart on the right. This allows about 3–4kg (6–8lb) for the baby and about 7–12kg (14–24lb) for the baby-support system (placenta, amniotic fluid, increased blood, fluid, fat, and breast tissue). It is usual to gain very little, if anything, during the first trimester, around 0.5–1kg (1–2lb) each week between months four and eight, then very little, or none at all, in the last month. A steady gain like this means that your body can adapt more easily to your increasing size, and your baby is provided with a continuous flow of nourishment.

14kg/28lb

12kg/24lb

10kg/20lb

8kg/16lb

6kg/12lb

4kg/8lb

2kg/4lb

5   10   15   20   25   30   35

underlines your responsibility to provide for the nutritional needs of your developing baby. Everything you eat should be good for you and your baby; more problems develop if you eat too little rather than too much. Pregnancy is not the time for dieting. Research has shown that when mothers-to-be eat poor diets, there is a higher incidence of spontaneous abortions, neonatal death, and low birthweight babies than normal.

However, you do need to beware of really excess weight gain; fat that is deposited at the tops of the arms and the thighs is very difficult to get rid of after pregnancy. Junk food, from chocolate bars to hamburgers and fries, tends to be made up mainly of fat and sugar, which are of little value to your growing baby, and your body converts it to maternal fat.

A quite substantial amount of fat will be lost by breastfeeding your baby, as it is accumulated specifically to be converted to milk during lactation. However, some will remain and this will be difficult to lose once you have finished breastfeeding.

You therefore owe it to yourself, as well as your baby, to eat a diet that is best for both of you. While you should adhere to the nutritional recommendations on pages 134 & 135, you can balance your food intake over a 24- to 48-hour period rather than at each meal. Make sure that you don't miss meals – your baby grows all day, every day, and suffers if you starve.

BABY'S REQUIREMENTS

During pregnancy, you are your baby's only source of nourishment. Every calorie, vitamin, or gram of protein that your baby needs must be eaten by you. You are the sole manager of your unborn child's nutrition; you, and only you, can make sure that the best quality food reaches her.

You will fulfil all of your baby's requirements if you eat lots of fresh fruit, vegetables, beans, peas, wholemeal cereals, fish, fowl, and low-fat dairy products. (A Danish study showed that eating oil-rich fish – salmon, herring, sardine – may help lessen the risk of preterm birth.) Make your diet as varied as possible, choosing from a wide range of foodstuffs.

DON'T FORGET MUM

The other important person you must eat for during pregnancy is yourself. A good diet will mean that you have better reserves to cope with, and recover from, the indisputable strain of pregnancy and the hard physical work of labour. Anaemia and pre-eclampsia (see p.224) are much more common in those mothers who have a poor diet, and some problems, such as morning sickness and leg cramps, may be exacerbated by what you do or don't eat – not eating enough salt, for example, is thought to cause leg cramps.

Overall, good nutrition will help minimize excessive mood swings, fatigue, and many common complaints (see pp.206–213). In addition, a sensible eating regime that cuts out or restricts the amount of empty calories you consume will mean that you will be left with less excess fat to lose after your child has been born.

EMPTY CALORIES

The following foods should be avoided in pregnancy; they usually contain nothing more than sugar or sugar substitutes and refined flour.

• Any form of sweetener – and this includes white or brown sugar, golden syrup, treacle, and artificial products such as saccharine and aspartame.

• Sweets and chocolate bars.

• Soft drinks, such as cola and sweetened fruit juices.

• Commercially produced biscuits, cakes, pastries, and pies, as well as jam and marmalade.

• Tinned fruit in syrup.

• Artificial cream.

• Sweetened breakfast cereal.

• Ice cream and sorbets that contain added sugar. Freeze fruit juice or puréed fruit instead.

• Savouries that contain sugar, such as peanut butter, relishes, pickles, salad dressings, spaghetti sauces, mayonnaise, and many others – read the label.

YOUR OFFICE SUPPLIES

The average nine-to-five job can wreak havoc with your nutritional intake. However, forward planning and a few strategically situated supplies can help.

In the office refrigerator:

• mineral water

• unsweetened fruit juice

• plain live-culture yogurt

• Dutch or Swiss cheese

• hard-boiled eggs

• fresh fruit

• "snack" vegetables – carrot and red pepper sticks, tomatoes

• wholemeal bread

• jar of wheatgerm.

In your desk drawer:

• wholemeal crackers, crispbreads, or breadsticks, perhaps with seeds

• dried fruit

• nuts or seeds

• decaffeinated instant coffee and decaffeinated tea bags

• powdered skimmed milk for extra calcium in drinks.

In your handbag:

• wholemeal crackers, crispbreads, or breadsticks, perhaps with seeds

• dried fruit, nuts, and seeds

• fresh fruit or "snack" vegetables

• small thermos of unsweetened juice or milk

• glucose sweets for emergencies.

Make sure everything is securely wrapped and sealed.

THE BEST FOOD TO EAT

Quality food is as close to its original state as possible and offers you and your baby good nutritional value. Eating quality food should be your goal throughout, as well as after, pregnancy.

When shopping, select fresh produce; seasonal fruit and vegetables will be fresher as well as cheaper. Always select sound fruit and vegetables; reject any that look tired or are going bad. Buy your meat and fish from reputable shops – don't run the risk of contracting a food-related illness (see p.139). If you can afford it, opt for free-range or organic foods to avoid pesticides and growth hormones (used particularly in beef and intensively farmed poultry), but do make sure that organic foods have been properly approved (by the Soil Association, for example). You should also check labelling of processed foods for the inclusion of genetically modified (GM) ingredients. Until the scientific research into the safety of these foods has been completed and fully debated, it is sensible to avoid GM foods during pregnancy.

Frozen packets of vegetables are good standbys, particularly when vegetables are out of season. Avoid tins, except for plum tomatoes and fish. Always read labels – the nearer an ingredient is to the top of the list, the more there is of that one ingredient. Bear in mind that sugar has many different names (see p.132) and can appear on a list more than once.

Foods that have been over-refined, such as white flour and white sugar, have had all of the natural goodness stripped out of them and can offer you and your baby nothing but excess calories. Instead, choose wholemeal bread, pastry, and flour, rather than "enriched" refined products, as it is highly unlikely that the enrichment puts back in all that has been taken out. The two "waste" products of refining are bran (the fibre) and wheatgerm (the heart of the wheat) and these contain most of the goodness. Bran is probably an unnecessary addition for the average pregnant woman (although it will help prevent constipation), but everyone can benefit from the multitude of vitamins and minerals in wheatgerm. Wheatgerm is crunchy and nutty and can be added to salads and sandwiches, as well as to cooked and baked dishes; it is available from health food shops.

GOOD EATING HABITS

Willpower alone will probably not be enough to achieve your aims; it has a habit of letting you down in the face of temptation. The first step is to avoid temptations like biscuits and a cup of tea in the afternoon, or take-aways. Have a homemade, sugar-free fruit-and-nut bar, and a decaffeinated tea bag to hand. Cook a batch of meals at the weekend that you can store and have when you're too tired to cook. Banish junk food from your kitchen.

Learn to snack on nutritious foods and eat little and often if your appetite is quickly extinguished. Towards the end of pregnancy, eating substantial amounts will become a bit of a problem, so you really have to make every mouthful count. Eating a burger and chips, for example, washed down with coffee will fill you up to the extent that you won't be able to compensate nutritionally with a tuna fish salad and a glass of milk later on.

Think before you eat – a high protein chicken and lettuce sandwich on fibre and folic acid-rich wholemeal bread is much better for you than fat-rich bacon and avocado on fibreless white! Invest in a healthy-eating cookbook and learn how to make dishes that are lower in fat and sugar but still taste delicious.

VEGETARIANISM

A large number of people do not eat meat; many more limit their intake of meat, particularly red meat. If you fall into one of these categories, you need to take special precautions to ensure you eat enough protein, vitamins, and iron to meet your own and your baby's needs (see also p.136).

There are complementary plant protein sources such as dried beans and grains. These, if eaten in combination, will provide you with most of the necessary amino acids normally found complete in animal forms of protein (see below).

Vegetarians should ensure they take sufficient iron as there is relatively little in vegetable matter and certain substances interfere with its absorption (see p.133). If you eat no animal products at all, you have to work harder to make sure that you are not deficient in any nutrient – particularly calcium and vitamins B6, B_{12}, and D, all of which are provided by dairy products. Although very little B_{12} is needed, lack of it will eventually lead to pernicious anaemia, so if your diet contains no animal products you should take vitamin B_{12} supplements.

COMPLEMENTARY PROTEINS

SHORT CUTS

When time, energy, or money are short, eating nutritiously can often seem to be too much hassle. Here are some tips that will help you do the best nutritionally for you and your baby, without too much effort:

• keep a supply of various frozen vegetables

• buy meat and fish in bulk, and freeze in meal-size portions

• cook ahead and freeze

• buy ready-made fresh salads

• a microwave cooks food quickly and retains nutrients

• keep it simple – eat raw fruit and vegetables; steam, stir fry, or grill for speed, or bake so you can leave food to cook on its own

• enlist help – many grandparents-to-be will undoubtedly be keen to give you a hand.

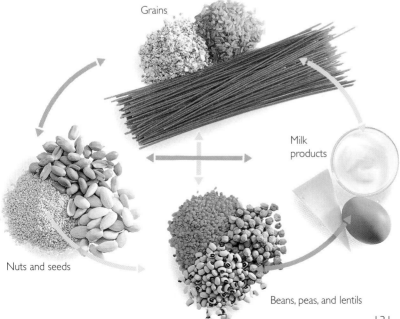

Grains

Milk products

Nuts and seeds

Beans, peas, and lentils

Combining proteins
All animal products contribute first-class proteins, so called because they contain all the essential amino acids that the body needs in the right proportions. Plant products contribute second-class proteins because the amino acids that they provide are not of the right proportions. To receive the full complement of necessary amino acids, you would have to eat certain foods in combination. For example, peas could be served with rice or corn; a handful of nuts could be added to rice and sweetcorn salad.

◁ ▷ Generally complementary

◀ ▶ Sometimes complementary

Due to the intensive development of your growing baby, your protein requirement increases by 30 percent from the onset of pregnancy.

This means your needs jump from 45–60g (1¾–2¼oz) to 75–100g (3–4oz) of protein daily, depending on how active you are.

Proteins are made up of amino acids, which are vital to individual body cells and tissues. A total of 20 different amino acids are required by the body. The body can synthesize 12 of these, the non-essential amino acids, but eight others, the essential acids, must be supplied by food you eat. These latter are first-class proteins and are found only in animal products such as meat, dairy products, fish, poultry, and eggs. Always choose organically reared produce, especially poultry, eggs, beef, and offal, whenever possible.

Your choice of proteins, however, also needs to be guided by what else you are getting from protein-rich food. Offal and meat are the richest sources of first-class proteins and contain vital B vitamins. However, some meat, particularly red meat, can be very high in animal fat, while liver shouldn't be eaten in pregnancy as it is high in vitamin A, which may be toxic to the fetus, so you could choose fish instead.

Fish is a first-class protein that is high in vitamins and nutritious fish oils, and is low in saturated fat.

Equivalent amounts of protein are one egg, one slice of hard cheese, two tablespoons peanut butter, two tablespoons cottage cheese, half a cup of peas or beans.

Essential nutrition

Research has found that what you eat when you are pregnant not only affects your baby at birth, but also appears to have a long-term effect throughout your child's life – even into old age.

PROTEIN

Protein is probably the most essential nutrient for your baby; the amino acids that make up protein are literally the building blocks of the body. Proteins form the main structural elements of the cells and tissues that make up muscles, bones, connective tissues, and many of your organ walls.

The type and quality of protein in food varies (see column, left). Generally, the more expensive foodstuffs like meat, fish, and poultry are the best sources, but less expensive products eaten together can also supply you with adequate protein. Wholewheat bread or noodles with beans, cheese, or peanut butter; or cornmeal or noodles with sesame seeds, nuts, and milk are cheaper ingredients that will keep your protein intake high. You need at least three servings of protein foods (see p.134) daily.

CARBOHYDRATES AND CALORIES

These should provide the largest part of your daily calorie intake. As you need to increase your calorie intake by 500 calories during pregnancy, you should make certain that you eat the best kind of carbohydrates you can and avoid empty calories (see p.129).

Simple carbohydrates are sugars in various forms. The most common types and sources are sucrose (cane sugar), glucose (honey), fructose (fruit), and maltose, lactose, and galactose (milk). Because these carbohydrates are absorbed quickly from the stomach, all are a source of "instant energy", which is useful when you are in dire need. Glucose sweets may also be helpful in the case of nausea.

Complex carbohydrates are the starches contained in grains, potatoes, lentils, beans, and peas. The body has to break them down into simple carbohydrates before it can use them, so they provide a steady supply of energy over a period of time. In addition, complex unrefined carbohydrates (wholemeal oats and brown rice) are good sources of vitamins, minerals, and fibre.

VITAMINS

Good sources of many vitamins (and minerals) are vegetables and fruits. Some are rich in vitamin C; others contain vitamins A, B, E, minerals, and folic acid; you must include all in your daily diet. Vitamins are quickly destroyed by exposure to light, air, and heat. Many cannot be stored by the body, so good levels are necessary daily. Leafy green vegetables, yellow/red vegetables and fruit supply vitamins A, E, B6, iron, zinc, and magnesium. Choose broccoli, spinach, watercress, carrots, tomatoes, bananas, apricots, and cherries.

Some vegetables, such as watercress, are rich in many vitamins so you can do yourself and your baby a lot of good if you eat them. Others may not give you a big dose of any individual vitamin, but they will provide a selection of vitamins and minerals, as well as fibre. In particular, you must maintain iron and calcium at high levels to support your baby's development.

Although some B vitamins are supplied by vegetables and fruit, the bulk of our vitamin B intake is usually supplied by meat, fish, dairy products, grains, and nuts. Some are entirely animal-sourced and so vegetarians must take extra care to provide enough B vitamins in their diet. If you don't eat dairy products you should definitely take vitamin B_{12} supplements. Get these from your doctor; never self-prescribe in pregnancy as vitamins can be toxic in large quantities.

Folic acid This vitamin is essential for the production of red blood cells and plays an important part in fetal growth especially during the first 12 weeks of pregnancy. Folic acid is particularly important to the development of the nervous system and research has shown that folic acid supplements taken up to three months before conception and for the first 12 weeks of pregnancy significantly reduce the incidence of neural tube defects such as spina bifida. If you have not started taking folic acid before conception, start as soon as you know you are pregnant. Folic acid is available in tablet form, and is also present in green leafy vegetables, cereals, and bread.

MINERALS

A good diet should supply you with sufficient amounts of minerals and trace elements, those essential chemicals that contribute to the proper functioning of the body but cannot be synthesized by it. Two in particular, iron and calcium, must be maintained at high levels to support your baby's development.

Iron Essential for the production of haemoglobin (the oxygen-carrying part of the red blood cells), its intake must not only be adequate (see column, right) but continuous throughout pregnancy. It's vital to support the large increase in your blood volume and you should bear in mind that iron is cleared from your baby's blood in seconds. However, iron can block the absorption of zinc, which is essential for brain and nervous system development so you need to eat zinc-rich food such as fish and wheatgerm separately from iron-rich food.

Calcium A baby's bones begin to form between four and six weeks, so it is important to maintain a high calcium intake both before conception and during pregnancy. Dairy products, leafy green vegetables, soya, broccoli, and any fish containing bones are rich in calcium. If you don't eat dairy products you may need supplements. Vitamin D is needed for calcium absorption so try to eat eggs or cheese daily.

FLUID CONSUMPTION

During pregnancy your blood volume expands by nearly 50 percent, so you need to keep up your fluid intake.

Water is best, though fruit juice is also good. A good fluid intake also helps to avoid the risk of urinary tract infections. Do not restrict fluid intake if you experience swelling of the hands or feet, as this won't make any difference to this type of fluid retention.

MAINTAINING IRON INTAKE

Normal necessary iron intake varies from woman to woman but your iron levels will be monitored.

If you're iron-deficient when you become pregnant, or develop iron deficiency later, iron tablets or injections may be prescribed by your doctor to prevent you developing anaemia.

VITAMIN D

Vitamin D is manufactured by the body when it is triggered by the action of light on the skin.

• Most light-skinned people need about 40 minutes of light (it is not necessary for it to be sunlight) a day to produce adequate amounts of vitamin D.

• Dark-skinned people who live far from the equator need progressively more depending on their skin tones.

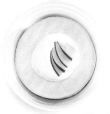

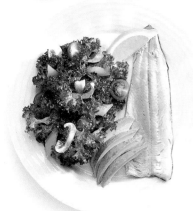

A balanced meal
The above meal of trout and salad, melon with yogurt, and nectarines, and a glass of milk is tasty and nutritious.

Nutritional values

Although there is no need for you to devote the whole of your pregnancy to measuring out portions and calculating your intake, it is good to have a guide so that you can be sure you are eating as well as possible. You can balance your nutritional intake over the course of one or two days, rather than balancing each meal.

DAILY REQUIREMENTS

To give you and your baby the best possible diet, try to eat the following portions each day – each of the suggested sources represents a single portion. You should vary the food you choose.

- First-class proteins – three servings
- Vitamin C foods – two servings
- Calcium foods – four servings in pregnancy, five during lactation
- Green leafy and yellow vegetables and fruits – three servings
- Other fruit and vegetables – one or two servings
- Whole grains and complex carbohydrates – four or five servings
- Iron-rich food – two servings
- Fluids – eight glasses a day, not coffee or alcohol. Water is best.

REQUIREMENTS	SUGGESTED SOURCES	
Calcium foods	50g/2oz hard cheese 100g/4oz soft cheese 325g/13oz cottage cheese 250ml/9fl oz yogurt	200ml/⅓ pint milk or milk made up from powdered milk 75g/3oz tinned sardines, with bones
First-class protein foods	75g/3oz hard cheese 100g/4oz soft cheese 500ml/1 pint milk 340ml/12fl oz yogurt 3 eggs size 1	100g/4oz fresh or tinned fish 100g/4oz prawns 75g/3oz beef, lamb, pork, poultry, offal (not liver), without the fat
Green leafy and yellow/red vegetables and fruit	25g/1oz spinach, broccoli florets 13g/½oz carrots 250g/10oz peas, beans 25g/1oz sweet pepper 150g/6oz tomatoes	50g/2oz melon 6 plums 1 mango, orange, grapefruit 2 apricots 4 peaches, apples, pears
Whole grains and complex carbohydrates	75g/3oz cooked barley, brown rice, millet, bulgar 25g/1oz wholemeal or soya flour 1 slice wholemeal or soya bread 6 wholemeal bread sticks	75g/3oz kidney beans, soya beans, chick peas 100g/4oz lentils, peas 1 wholemeal pitta or tortilla 6 wholemeal biscuits
Vitamin C foods	25g/1oz sweet peppers 225g/9oz tomatoes 200g/8oz blackberries or raspberries 100ml/4fl oz citrus juice	25g/1oz blackcurrants 75g/3oz strawberries 1 large lemon or orange ½ medium grapefruit

VITAMIN AND MINERAL SOURCES

We are dependent on food sources for all our vitamin and mineral needs, except for vitamin D. The chart below is a guide to the best sources of essential vitamins and minerals. These tend to be fragile, so try to eat foods that are as fresh as possible. As you can see some foods contain a variety of vitamins and minerals.

NAME	FOOD SOURCE
Vitamin A (retinol & carotene)	Whole milk, butter, cheese, egg yolk, oily fish, offal, green and yellow fruit and vegetables
Vitamin B1 (thiamine)	Whole grains, nuts, pulses, offal, pork, brewer's yeast, wheatgerm
Vitamin B2 (riboflavin)	Brewer's yeast, wheatgerm, whole grains, green vegetables, milk, cheese, eggs
Vitamin B3 (niacin)	Brewer's yeast, whole grains, wheatgerm, offal, green vegetables, oily fish, eggs, milk, peanuts
Vitamin B5 (pantothenic acid)	Offal, eggs, peanuts, whole grains, cheese
Vitamin B6 (pyridoxine)	Brewer's yeast, whole grains, soya flour, offal, wheatgerm, mushrooms, potatoes, avocados
Vitamin B12 (cyanocobalamin)	Meat, offal, fish, milk, eggs
Folic acid (part of B complex)	Raw leafy vegetables, peas, soya flour, oranges, bananas, walnuts
Vitamin C (ascorbic acid)	Rosehip syrup, sweet peppers, citrus fruits, blackcurrants, tomatoes
Vitamin D (calciferol)	Fortified milk, oily fish, eggs (particularly the yolks), butter
Vitamin E	Wheatgerm, egg yolk, peanuts, seeds, vegetable oils, broccoli
Calcium	Milk, cheese, small fish with bones, peanuts, walnuts, sunflower seeds, soya, yogurt, broccoli
Iron	Kidneys, fish, egg yolks, red meat, cereals, molasses, apricots, haricot beans
Zinc	Wheatbran, eggs, nuts, onions, shellfish, sunflower seeds, wheatgerm, whole wheat

PREPARING FOOD

Try to develop some good cooking habits that will promote healthy eating habits.

• Trim off any fat from meat before cooking.

• Skim fat off the surface of casseroles and soups.

• Bake, steam, microwave, or grill rather than fry.

• Stir-fry in a teaspoon of olive oil, plus a little water, or with a stock cube dissolved in a cup of water.

• Use non-stick pans and the minimum of fat when cooking omelettes or scrambled eggs.

• Use flavoured vinegars, such as raspberry, basil, thyme, or garlic (home-made ones are better than shop-bought), or yogurt for salad dressings, rather than mayonnaise, salad cream, or sour cream.

• Add dried skimmed milk to milky drinks, or when baking, for extra servings of calcium.

• Always choose low-fat, rather than full-fat, dairy products.

• Eat fruit and vegetables raw whenever possible.

The vegetarian mother

Anne had a number of anxieties about her vegetarian diet being unable to maintain her baby's healthy growth and development. We looked at her various concerns and, having identified possible protein and calcium deficiencies, I offered advice on how she would go about obtaining sufficient supplies.

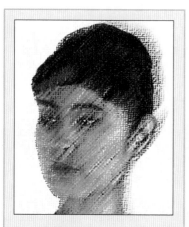

Name **Anne Watkins**

Age **31 years**

Past medical history
Nothing abnormal

Obstetric history **Two full-term pregnancies, normal deliveries, boy aged five, girl aged three**

Anne became a vegetarian two years ago, a year after the birth of her second child, Katie. Although she feels very healthy eating a vegetarian diet that includes dairy produce and eggs, she is concerned about the additional nutritional needs of pregnancy. She is worried that her obstetrician might encourage her to eat meat, and she turned to me for advice and reassurance.

SPECIAL NEEDS FOR VEGETARIANS?

Having had two previous babies, Anne was aware that certain dietary changes might have been necessary even with her previous eating habits, but now that she was a vegetarian, she wanted to clarify certain things. For example, she had heard that a vegetarian diet might be short of vitamin B_{12}; if so, would that harm her baby? She had also read something about folic acid and spina bifida. Was her diet short in this nutrient, and should she take supplements? She knew that some pregnant women are given iron supplements; would she be a candidate?

Anne knew that the main change she had to make to her diet would be to increase the protein content, but what kind of protein and which foods provide it? Pregnancy demands increased calcium intake, should she take calcium tablets or could she get enough from calcium-rich and calcium-fortified foods?

EASY WAYS TO MEET HER INCREASED NEEDS

Opinions on vegetarianism in pregnancy are widely divergent and encompass those of vegans who believe that women taking in no animal protein can carry a healthy baby to term without even vitamin B_{12} supplements, to inflexible doctors who preach that meat and fish are essential ingredients to a pregnant woman's diet. Both of these views are wrong.

In the case of veganism, where no animal products, including dairy products, are eaten, vitamin B_{12} supplements are absolutely mandatory. B_{12} is vital to the healthy growth and development of the fetus, as well as that of a breastfed baby. Therefore, vegan mothers have to add milk and eggs to their diet, or take synthetic B_{12}, during pregnancy and while they are breastfeeding.

A vegetarian diet in which dairy products are also eaten can properly support a pregnancy, and later breastfeeding, as long as calcium and protein intake is increased. All pregnant women should increase their milk intake to a pint a day (choose skimmed rather than whole milk). Anne can also boost her protein and vitamin intake by drinking vitamin-fortified soya milk and eating lots of other soya and dairy products. However, the simplest expedient in increasing the protein and vitamin content of Anne's diet would be if she ate at least four eggs a week. Eggs will provide iron too, although not as much as red meat. While some vegetarians claim that they can get the same amount of iron that red meat provides by eating more green leafy vegetables, they would, in fact, have to eat almost five pounds of these vegetables per day to do so!

I advised Anne to accept her obstetrician's advice if he prescribed vitamin, iron, and calcium supplements, but told her that if he presses her on eating meat, she should contact the Vegetarian Society (see **Addresses**, p.370) for support and further information.

SUGGESTED DAILY VEGETARIAN MENU

Breakfast
Two slices of wholemeal toast with yeast extract and peanut butter. Cup of decaffeinated tea with skimmed milk. One banana

Mid-morning snack
Selection of raw vegetables with hummus (chick-pea dip) and wholemeal pitta bread

Lunch
Baked potato, topped with cottage cheese, red bell pepper, tomatoes, and watercress. Glass of tomato juice. Chopped nuts and dried fruit

Afternoon snack
Broccoli and cheese soup (preferably fresh) with chopped walnuts and low-fat fromage frais. Two slices of rye bread

Dinner
Mushroom and tofu lasagne, spinach, steamed mangetout, and wholemeal garlic bread. Fresh fruit with low-fat yogurt. Grapefruit juice

Bedtime snack
Boiled egg and wholemeal toast "soldiers" with yeast extract. Glass of skimmed milk

Your baby's lifeline
The umbilical cord links your baby with the placenta. Everything, including all the necessary nutrients for growth and development, passes to your baby through the cord.

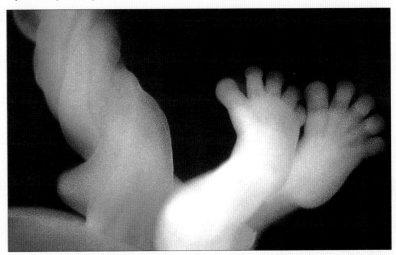

TAKE CARE

B_{12} is frequently deficient in vegetarian diets, as it only exists naturally in animal products. Supplements may be necessary to ensure the healthy growth and development of the fetus.

ANNE'S BABY

As with all babies, nature provides preferentially for the nutritional needs of Anne's baby by ensuring he receives what he needs from her body's stores. The baby, therefore, could be better nourished than Anne.

• **Iron** A baby's iron needs are high in order to support blood formation and organ growth. This can be supplied by eating iron-rich foods

• **Calcium** This mineral is the foundation stone of healthy bones and teeth, a diet that is rich in calcium is necessary to support the needs of Anne's baby as well as her own

• **Protein** To nourish fast-growing muscles, bones, skin, and vital organs, Anne should eat a variety of protein-rich foods

• **Vitamin B_{12}** The development of the baby's brain and nervous system depends on sufficient supplies. Therefore Anne, like every other mother, cannot afford to be deficient

• **Folic acid** The development of the brain, spinal cord, and spine also depend on sufficient intake

• **Calories** The blood sugar of the fetus is always lower than that of its mother because it is used so quickly. A constant supply is needed for healthy growth

ARE YOU
NUTRITIONALLY
AT RISK?

If you fall into any of the following groups, then you could be nutritionally vulnerable and your baby may be at risk. You will need special advice and help from your doctor or antenatal clinic before and during pregnancy.

• If you've had a recent stillbirth or miscarriage, or your children are coming very quickly after one another (a minimum of 18 months between babies is recommended to maximize your health).

• If you either smoke, or drink alcohol heavily.

• If you're allergic to certain key foods, such as cow's milk or wheat.

• If you suffer from a chronic medical condition that means you are regularly taking long-term medication.

• If you are under the age of 18, your own body is growing quickly and you have more than average nutritional requirements.

• If you are carrying more than a single baby.

• If you have been subjected to a lot of stress or any physical injury.

• If your job entails hard labour or is in a potentially dangerous environment (see p.168).

• If before conception you were generally run-down, underweight, or eating an inadequate or unbalanced diet.

Nutritional and food-related problems

A pregnant woman can put herself and her developing baby at risk if she eats insufficient good food to fulfil her nutritional needs; she is nutritionally at risk. Quite apart from this, the food itself may constitute a hazard to her and her baby if it is contaminated with bacteria that cause disease; an example would be chicken or eggs contaminated with salmonella.

MALNUTRITION

Inadequate food intake by a mother can have serious consequences for her baby. There is a higher risk of miscarriage, and having a premature or low birthweight baby that will be more vulnerable at birth and throughout its life. (Having a low birthweight baby does not mean labour will be easier.) Maternal malnutrition also retards the growth of the placenta, and low placental weight is related to a higher infant mortality rate. The most rapid brain development takes place in the last trimester of pregnancy (and in the first month of life after birth) so a severely undernourished mother may prevent optimal brain function.

Inadequate nutrition during pregnancy can have a continuing effect throughout your child's life, and may be a contributory factor to such middle-aged diseases as high blood pressure, coronary artery disease, and obesity. If nutrition is restricted, the fetus diverts what is available to those cells that are immediately important, and away from those cells that will not be important until later in life – in effect, the fetus trades long life for survival.

On the other hand, where a mother is adequately nourished and produces a good-sized baby, such larger babies prove easier to care for and are more vigorous, active, mentally alert, and suffer less from colic, diarrhoea, anaemia, and infection.

The foods necessary for a healthy pregnancy and baby are rarely expensive, but there is help available if you have financial difficulties; your health department can help with unborn-child allowances and supplements. Generally, fresher foods are better, so we can all lower risks of poor nutrition by avoiding foods that contain high levels of chemicals, such as processed foods, and those that contain additives, flavourings, and colourings.

Processed foods A great many of these foods contain chemicals to improve flavour, nutritional value, and shelf life. As a general rule, these should be avoided – in particular, processed cheese and meats, cheese spreads, and sausages. Additives in foods can be easily identified when ingredients are listed on labels. Food colourings and preservatives are represented by E numbers. Always read the labels on packaging to ensure the food is well within the use-by date, and avoid foods that don't list their ingredients. It is a good rule to avoid highly salted foods, particularly those containing monosodium glutamate (MSG), which can cause dehydration and headaches.

Preserved food Smoked fish, meat and cheese, pickled food, and sausages often contain the active agent nitrate. These should be avoided because nitrates can react with the haemoglobin in your blood and reduce its oxygen-carrying power.

Drinks Caffeine (in tea, coffee, and chocolate) is a stimulant and drinks containing it should be avoided in pregnancy. The tannin in tea interferes with iron absorption, so organic herbal teas should be drunk instead. Soft drinks always contain sugar or sweeteners so limit your intake of them. Mineral water is fine.

FOOD HAZARDS

We now know that certain foods are contaminated with large enough numbers of bacteria to cause illness, particularly in vulnerable people – such as pregnant women and babies.

Listeriosis Foods found to contain large numbers of listeria bacteria include soft cheese, unpasteurized milk, ready-prepared coleslaw, cooked chilled foods, pâtés, and improperly cooked meat. The listeria bacteria is normally destroyed at pasteurizing temperatures, but if food is infected and refrigerated, the bacteria may continue to multiply. For this reason, chilled food should not be eaten after the "best-by" date. Listeriosis can spread through direct contact with infected live animals, such as sheep. Symptoms are flu-like: a high temperature and aches and pains, and also sore throat and eyes, diarrhoea, and stomach pain. An unborn child affected through its mother's blood may be stillborn, and listeriosis may be a cause of recurrent miscarriage.

Salmonella Infection with salmonella can often be traced to eggs and chicken meat so it is advisable to avoid foods that contain raw eggs, cook eggs and chicken well, and choose free-range eggs and fowl. Symptoms, including headache, nausea, abdominal pain, diarrhoea, shivering, and fever, develop suddenly from 12–48 hours after infection and last about 2–3 days. If the infection has spread into the bloodstream, antibiotics will be required.

Toxoplasmosis This is a common infection that can be picked up by eating raw or undercooked pork or steak, or by coming into contact with the faeces of infected cats and dogs (see p.169).

Dysentery Carried in the faeces of an affected person, this causes severe diarrhoea and abdominal pain. It is dangerous for pregnant women, causing dehydration. Amoebic dysentery is rare outside tropical areas, but bacterial dysentery is more common. It is usually passed on when an infected person fails to wash his hands properly after going to the toilet and then handles food.

FOOD SAFETY

Never take unnecessary risks when handling and storing food; bacteria can multiply rapidly.

• Always use clean utensils between jobs, or tastings.

• Always wash hands after going to the lavatory and before touching food, and take good care to seal off any infections or cuts.

• Defrost and cook food thoroughly, especially poultry.

• Never let raw meat or eggs come into contact with other foods.

• Avoid dented and rusty tins and any food that looks or smells "off".

• Make sure dairy products have been well pasteurized.

• Do not refreeze food that has already been defrosted.

• Reheat food thoroughly only once, then throw away.

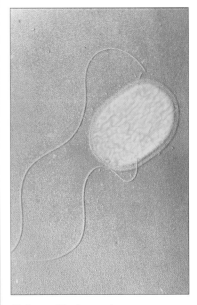

Salmonella bacteria
The above picture shows one of the many hundreds of different strains of the potentially hazardous salmonella bacteria.

139

The diabetic mother

Having or developing diabetes during pregnancy should not be seen as making pregnancy difficult, or as a deterrent to producing a normal, healthy baby. As long as diabetes is carefully managed, with the obstetrician and diabetic physician in close cooperation, the outcome should be very satisfactory.

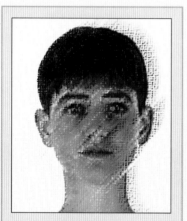

Name **Jill Dalton**

Age **27 years**

Past medical history **Developed insulin-dependent diabetes at age 25 after having had two children**

Obstetric history **A son at age 23, normal delivery, weight 4.82kg (10lb 10oz). Second son at 25, normal pregnancy, normal delivery, weight 5.1kg (11lb 4oz)**

Jill first developed diabetes relatively late, at 25 while she was pregnant with her second child, and has had the disease for only a couple of years. Both these factors give a good prognosis for her pregnancy. Nonetheless, she is highly motivated to attend her antenatal clinic frequently. She realizes that uncontrolled diabetes would lead to complications for her and to far more serious ones for the baby.

PREGNANCY AND DIABETES

As well as being 50 percent more likely than men to become diabetics, women have a tendency to develop the disease during pregnancy. Certain women are recognized as potential diabetics. They usually have had at least one heavy baby or have a family history of diabetes in parents or siblings. Other women, known as gestational diabetics, develop diabetes during pregnancy. Some may remain diabetic after pregnancy but others revert to normal. All these diabetics are treated in the same way.

Pregnancy can complicate established diabetes. While most sufferers will have been treated with insulin, some women with diabetes may have been treated with diet alone or with diet and blood sugar lowering (hypoglycaemic) tablets. The extra demands of pregnancy may lead to insulin having to be prescribed or the prescribed dosage being increased.

JILL'S PREPARATIONS FOR PREGNANCY

Having been an insulin-dependent diabetic for two years, Jill was meticulous about her pre-pregnancy preparations. She planned this present baby and made sure she had a full assessment of her diabetes well before she fell pregnant. In particular, she was concerned about controlling blood sugar levels, the functioning of her kidneys, and the health of her eyes. In the months before conceiving she maintained careful control of her diabetes.

KEEPING CONTROL DURING PREGNANCY

Jill knows that good control of her diabetes during the first trimester should greatly reduce the risk of her baby having any kind of abnormality (see **Possible prenatal complications**, see p.18). Therefore, she came to seek my advice very early in the pregnancy.

I told Jill that now she is pregnant, she may need less insulin for the first three months. Then her body will start to produce hormones with an anti-insulin effect, so she will need more insulin than before. Ketosis is more apt to occur during pregnancy, so Jill has to test for ketones in her urine every day.

KETONES

When carbohydrates are not available for energy, fatty acids are burned instead. This produces ketones. Ketones are chemically related to acetone, which is found in solvents such as nail varnish. The presence of ketones (ketosis) can be detected by urine testing. Ketosis is a rare but dangerous condition, which can occur in uncontrolled diabetes. Ketosis can lead to vomiting, stomach pains, and ultimately to loss of consciousness and death.

However, urine testing will no longer be a reliable way to monitor her blood sugar, because the level at which the kidneys allow sugar into the urine tends to be lower in pregnant women, so that a urine test can give a false result. I advised Jill to buy a blood-glucose meter, which she can use in her own home. She is aware that maintenance of normal glucose concentration in her blood brings the best results for herself and her baby, but that this may occasionally be difficult. I told her that she may require hospitalization, perhaps more than once, in order to stabilize her diabetes, but that she shouldn't let this worry her unduly.

POSSIBLE PRENATAL COMPLICATIONS

As an established diabetic, Jill is prone to a number of disorders while she is pregnant, owing to fluctuations in her blood-sugar levels. She may suffer from urinary tract infections, thrush (see p.212), high blood pressure, pre-eclampsia (see p.224) and polyhydramnios (an excess of amniotic fluid, present in one out of five diabetic pregnancies). She may also go into premature labour.

Her baby, too, may be subject to several problems if the diabetes gets out of control. If maternal blood sugar levels get high, sugar crosses the placenta and is converted into fat, muscle, and enlarged organs. The resulting baby is overweight. The baby produces large quantities of insulin to cope with the high sugar levels. At birth, when he is suddenly cut off from the source of sugar, the baby experiences a sudden, severe drop in blood sugar, while his insulin production remains high. If left untreated, this causes profound hypoglycaemia (shortage of blood sugar), which can ultimately result in coma and death. This situation, however, is never allowed to happen with good antenatal care.

A GOOD OUTLOOK

The good news for Jill is that her careful control of her diabetes will make a big difference. Diabetic women didn't used to be warned of the risks of having babies at all. Now they are helped to exercise control of their condition, with specialist assistance from both their obstetrician and their diabetic physician, to ensure a healthy and normal baby.

Unless there are obstetric complications, such as high blood pressure or pelvic disproportion, and as long as her diabetes remains under control, she can hope for a normal vaginal delivery. She'll probably be advised to allow an induction at 40 weeks if the baby isn't born by then, to avoid the baby growing too big. I advised that she would have a glucose and insulin intravenous drip to control the diabetes during labour, and continuous fetal heart monitoring and fetal blood sampling to detect any fetal distress. After thorough checks in a neonatal special care unit to rule out the need for immediate treatment, her baby should be returned to her so she can breastfeed him.

JILL'S BABY

As long as Jill remains under constant care, the risks to her baby will not be too great. Her doctor will be aware of the following:

• At birth, Jill's baby may be very large so he may have to be delivered with the help of forceps or by Caesarean section

• He may suffer from mild hypoxia (low oxygen supply to the tissues) shortly before birth, and this can lead to neonatal jaundice (see p.342) – a condition that can be treated after birth

• He will be carefully checked after birth for any complications

• Jill should breastfeed him as soon as possible in order to counteract any hypoglycaemia (shortage of blood sugar) in her baby after birth

• In some diabetic mothers there's a tendency to have bigger and bigger babies, and they can be very heavy at birth: 4–5kg (10–11lbs) for instance. While delivery of such a large baby may go without a hitch, some obstetricians prefer to induce labour well before term (at 36 weeks, say) or opt for a Caesarean section before the baby has reached its maximum size or outgrown its food supply.

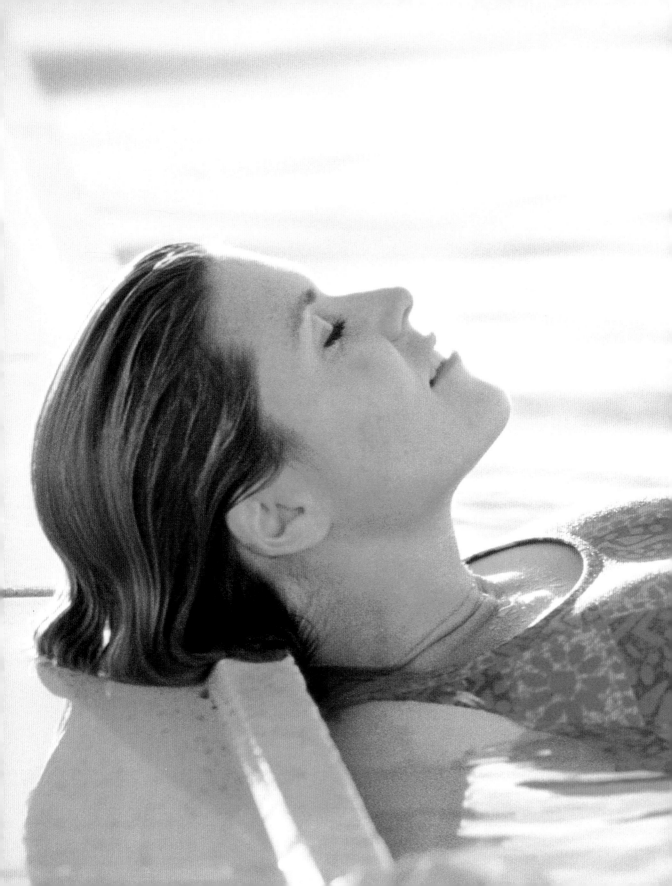

CHAPTER 6

A healthy
PREGNANCY

Keeping fit during pregnancy, both physically and mentally, is of prime importance. Exercising will help you do both. Everyone is exposed to certain levels of stress and anxiety, and even to potentially hazardous situations and substances. Learning how to cope with and avoid problems will ensure a truly fit pregnancy.

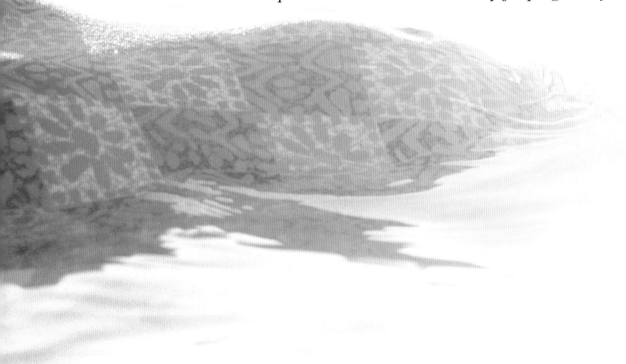

Exercising regularly can be emotionally as well as physically satisfying. It's an enjoyable way of preparing for the months of change ahead.

• You will receive an emotional lift from the release of internal hormones like endorphins.

• You will feel more contented, as the release of tranquillizing hormones that follows exercise aids relaxation.

• You can improve your self-awareness as you learn how to use your body in new ways.

• Backache, leg cramp, constipation, and breathlessness can be alleviated by regular exercise.

• Your energy level will be increased.

• You will be better prepared for the work of labour.

• You will regain your shape more quickly after delivery.

• You can make new friends by meeting other mums at antenatal exercise classes.

• You can share the exercise routine with your partner or other members of your family.

Exercise for a fit pregnancy

The physical benefits of exercise – improving your stamina, suppleness, and strength – will help you face the extra strain placed on your body as it adapts to meet the demands of pregnancy and childbirth. By exercising you can also develop a better understanding of your body's capabilities and learn different ways of relaxing.

Psychologically, exercising counteracts the tendency to feel clumsy, fat, or ungainly, particularly in the last three months. It increases your circulation, and that can help to ease tension. Labour may be easier and more comfortable if you have good muscle tone, and many of the exercises taught in antenatal classes, combined with relaxation and breathing techniques, will help you trust your body during labour. Staying in condition during pregnancy will also mean that you should regain your normal shape within a shorter time of your baby's birth.

YOUR EXERCISE PROGRAMME

Incorporating a daily exercise routine into your busy schedule may not be very appealing. But many of the exercises recommended during pregnancy, as shown on the following pages, can usually be performed while you carry on with other activities: pelvic floor exercises may be performed while cleaning your teeth; foot and ankle exercises while sitting at your desk or on the bus; and tailor sitting while reading or watching television.

Begin your routine at a gentle pace, gradually building up to what feels right for you. Before each exercise, try a few deep breaths. This gets the blood flowing around your body and gives all your muscles a good supply of oxygen. If you suffer any pain, cramping, or shortness of breath, stop exercising; when you resume, make sure it is at a slower pace. If you are out of breath, your baby is also being deprived of oxygen.

A little bit of exercise several times a day is better than a lot of exercise all at once, and then none at all. Normally a woman can restore her energy by lying down for half an hour, but it can take a pregnant woman half a day to recover properly from fatigue. So be kind to yourself and choose an activity that you will find both enjoyable and relaxing.

RECOMMENDED ACTIVITIES

You are free to be involved in most sports during pregnancy (until the last trimester), as long you have been doing that sport regularly beforehand, and you pursue it regularly once you are pregnant so that your body remains in condition. See below for activities that are particularly recommended during pregnancy and for those to avoid.

Swimming This tones most muscles and is excellent for improving stamina. Because your weight is supported by the water, you're unlikely to strain or injure muscles and joints. Some sports centres offer special antenatal classes.

Yoga This has many benefits, such as increasing suppleness and reducing tension. It also teaches you to control your breathing and concentration during labour, which is very useful.

Walking Even if you are not usually an active person, you could at least take up regular walks of a mile or more. Walking is good for the digestion, the circulation, and your figure. Try to walk tall, with your buttocks tucked under your spine, your shoulders back, and your head up, not hanging down. Towards the end of pregnancy, however, you may find that the cartilage in the pelvic joint softens so much that you will get backache if you walk more than a short distance. Always wear well-cushioned flat shoes.

Dancing As long as you are not too energetic, you can dance as often as you wish throughout pregnancy.

PRACTISE WITH CAUTION

Some sports, such as cycling, skiing, and horseback riding, should not be engaged in once you get big because your balance is thrown off by the new weight in front. Other activities, including those listed below, should be avoided because they put your body under unnecessary stress that could harm both you and your baby.

Jogging This is very hard on your breasts and jarring for your back, spine, pelvis, hips, and knees. Don't jog while pregnant.

Backpacking Weight-bearing activities like this one are harmful because they put a severe strain on the ligaments in your back. Bear in mind that during pregnancy, progesterone relaxes your ligaments, and unlike muscles, which can go back to their old shapes, ligaments remain stretched.

Sit-ups Any exercise that pulls on the abdominal muscles is a very bad idea. The longitudinal muscles of the abdomen are designed to separate in the middle to allow room for the enlarging uterus, and sitting straight up from a lying position encourages them to part even further. The strain may slow down the recovery of abdominal tone after delivery. Leg lifts while you are on your back can have the same effect. In order to sit up from a lying position (see also p.161), you should always roll over on to your side and use your arms to push you up sideways. This way your abdomen will not be working and stretching as you get up.

GOOD FOR YOUR BABY

Every time you exercise within your limit, your baby gets a surge of oxygen into her blood that sets her metabolism alight and gives her a real high. All her tissues, especially her brain, function in top form.

• The hormones that are released during your exercise pass across the placenta and reach your baby. At the beginning of exercise, therefore, your baby receives an emotional lift from your adrenaline.

• During exercise, your baby also experiences the positive effect of endorphins, our own natural morphine-like substances, released while exercising, that make us feel extremely good and happy.

• After exercise, endorphins have a profound tranquillizing effect that can last up to eight hours and your baby also experiences this.

• The motion of exercise is extremely soothing and is good for your baby as he feels comforted by the rocking movements.

• As you exercise your abdominal muscles exert a kind of massage on your baby that is comforting and soothing.

• During exercise, blood flow is optimum and so your baby's growth and development proceeds apace with all its benefits.

WHY WARM UP?

A gentle warm-up routine prepares your body for more demanding exercises and can be fitted into your daily life.

Warming up helps to relieve tension. It gently warms up muscles and joints and prevents muscles from overstretching, thus reducing the risk of injury. You may suffer from stiffness and cramp if you don't warm up.

Stretching

Before beginning any exercise routine always warm up gently (see left) with these few stretching exercises. They will stimulate your blood circulation, giving you and your baby a good supply of oxygen. Repeat each exercise five to ten times; make sure you are comfortable and that your posture is good.

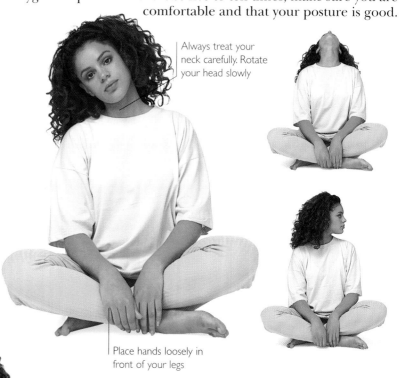

Always treat your neck carefully. Rotate your head slowly

Head and neck
Gently tilt your head over to one side, then lift your chin and rotate your head gently over to the other side and down. Repeat, starting from the other side. Keeping your head straight, turn it slowly to the right, back to the front, and then back to the left. Return to face the front.

Place hands loosely in front of your legs

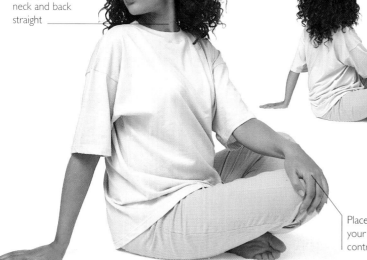

Keep your neck and back straight

Waist
Sitting comfortably with your legs crossed, straighten your back and gently stretch your neck upwards. Breathe out and turn your upper body to the right, placing your right hand behind you. Place your left hand on your right knee and use this hand as a lever to twist your body a little futher, gently stretching the muscles of your waist. Repeat in the other direction.

Place your hand on your knee to help control the stretch

TAKE CARE

- Work on a firm surface

- Always keep your back straight. Use a wall or cushions to support your back, if necessary

- Start your routine slowly and gently

- If you feel pain, discomfort, or fatigue, stop at once

- Always remember to breathe normally – otherwise you reduce the blood flow to your baby

- Never point your toes – always flex your foot to prevent cramps

Arms and shoulders

Sitting with your legs tucked underneath, lift your right arm up and slowly stretch it to the ceiling. Bend it at the elbow and drop your hand down behind your back. Put your left hand on your right elbow, pushing it further down your back. Put your left arm down behind your back and reach up to grasp the right hand. Stretch for 20 seconds, then relax. Repeat with other arm.

Clasp your hands together lightly if you can; if you can't reach, don't worry

Legs and feet

Sit with your back straight and your legs stretched out in front of you. Place your hands on the floor next to your hips to support your weight. Bend your knee slowly and then straighten. Repeat with other leg. This will tone the muscles in your calf and thigh and helps to alleviate cramp.

Keep your back straight and your weight central

Improving circulation

Raise your foot off the floor and flex it outwards. Then draw large circles in the air by moving only your ankles.

Bend your foot towards you to make the muscles work harder; take care not to strain

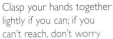
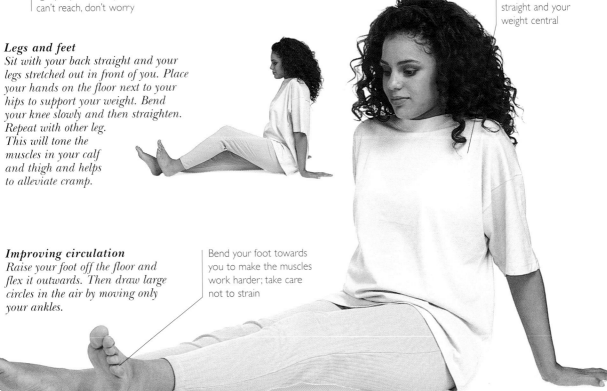

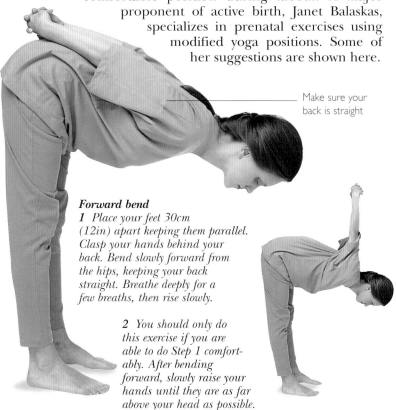

YOUR PELVIC FLOOR

The pelvic floor muscles form a funnel that supports the uterus, bowel, and bladder, and close the entrances to the vagina, rectum, and urethra.

The pelvic floor muscles lie in two main groups, forming a figure of eight around the urethra, vagina, and anus. Muscle fibres orginate front and back from high up on the pubic and sacral bones. The layers of muscle ovelap and are therefore thickest at the perineum.

During pregnancy, an increase in progesterone causes the muscles to soften and relax, and pressure from the enlarging uterus can cause the pelvic floor to become stretched and weak. As many as 50 percent of women who have had babies develop weakness in the pelvic floor. As a result they may experience discomfort or so-called "stress" incontinence – slight leakage of urine when laughing, coughing, or sneezing.

To counter this, physiotherapists have developed exercises you can do to keep the pelvic floor toned.

Pull in and tense the muscles around your vagina and anus, as if you were stopping the flow of urine. Hold as long as you can without straining. Relax. Repeat 25 times or more each day.

Restart this exercise as soon as you can after delivery to minimize the risk of a prolapse. Early exercise will tone up the vagina for sexual intercourse too. Try to make the exercise part of your daily routine.

Body exercises

By performing exercises for your whole body, you will relieve the strain caused by your extra weight and strengthen important muscles. Also, if you learn to move your pelvis easily during pregnancy, you will be better able to find the most comfortable position during labour. A major proponent of active birth, Janet Balaskas, specializes in prenatal exercises using modified yoga positions. Some of her suggestions are shown here.

Make sure your back is straight

Forward bend
1 Place your feet 30cm (12in) apart keeping them parallel. Clasp your hands behind your back. Bend slowly forward from the hips, keeping your back straight. Breathe deeply for a few breaths, then rise slowly.

2 You should only do this exercise if you are able to do Step 1 comfortably. After bending forward, slowly raise your hands until they are as far above your head as possible.

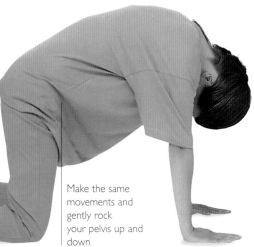

Pelvic tuck-in
Kneel down on all fours with your knees about 30cm (12in) apart. Clench your buttock muscles and tuck in your pelvis so that your back arches upwards into a hump. Hold for a few seconds, and then release, making sure you do not let your back sink downwards. Repeat several times.

Make the same movements and gently rock your pelvis up and down

148

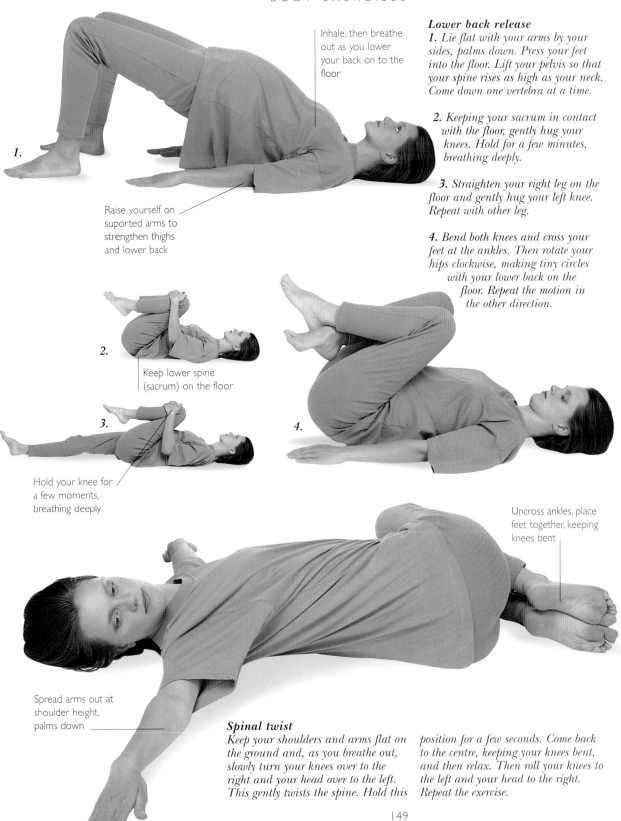

Inhale, then breathe out as you lower your back on to the floor

Raise yourself on suported arms to strengthen thighs and lower back

1.

2.

Keep lower spine (sacrum) on the floor

3.

Hold your knee for a few moments, breathing deeply

4.

Lower back release

1. Lie flat with your arms by your sides, palms down. Press your feet into the floor. Lift your pelvis so that your spine rises as high as your neck. Come down one vertebra at a time.

2. Keeping your sacrum in contact with the floor, gently hug your knees. Hold for a few minutes, breathing deeply.

3. Straighten your right leg on the floor and gently hug your left knee. Repeat with other leg.

4. Bend both knees and cross your feet at the ankles. Then rotate your hips clockwise, making tiny circles with your lower back on the floor. Repeat the motion in the other direction.

Uncross ankles, place feet together, keeping knees bent

Spread arms out at shoulder height, palms down

Spinal twist

Keep your shoulders and arms flat on the ground and, as you breathe out, slowly turn your knees over to the right and your head over to the left. This gently twists the spine. Hold this position for a few seconds. Come back to the centre, keeping your knees bent, and then relax. Then roll your knees to the left and your head to the right. Repeat the exercise.

Shaping up for labour

Your labour may be more comfortable if you have prepared your body and mind in advance. The following exercises are very useful during pregnancy. You may find it easier to give birth while squatting, and tailor sitting will strengthen your thigh muscles and increase circulation to your pelvis, making the joints more supple. By performing this exercise you will also fully stretch your pelvis and help to relax the tissues of your perineum.

After every exercise programme, spend 20–30 minutes relaxing, and, if possible, arrange a routine break during the day. Five or ten minutes with your eyes closed and your feet up can be sufficiently refreshing (it is not necessary actually to sleep), and learning relaxation techniques will be particularly beneficial during labour, when tension can exacerbate the pain. By concentrating on the rhythm of your breathing, you will be able to alleviate anxiety and conserve your energy.

If, as below, you find it difficult to pull your feet close to your groin, start with them about 30cm (12in) away from your body and gradually bring them nearer. Continual practice will loosen the muscles

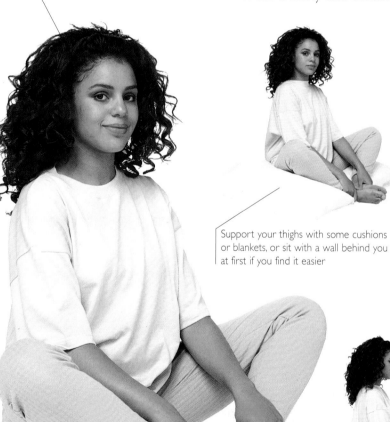

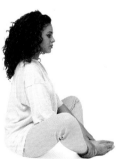

Support your thighs with some cushions or blankets, or sit with a wall behind you at first if you find it easier

Tailor sitting
Sit on the floor, and stretch your legs out in front. Make sure your back is straight. Bend your knees and bring the soles of your feet together then pull them as near as possible towards your groin. Open out your thighs and lower your knees towards the floor. Relax your shoulders and the back of your neck. Breathe deeply. Concentrate on breathing down towards your pelvis resting on the floor, relaxing as you breathe out. As you breathe in, lift up and stretch your spine while keeping your pelvis on the ground.

Correct   Incorrect

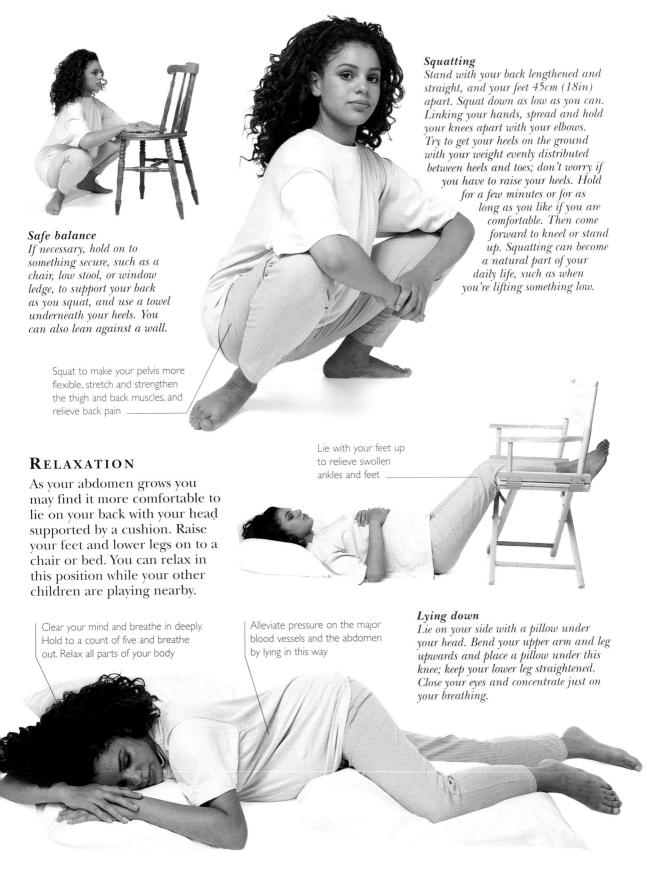

Squatting

Stand with your back lengthened and straight, and your feet 45cm (18in) apart. Squat down as low as you can. Linking your hands, spread and hold your knees apart with your elbows. Try to get your heels on the ground with your weight evenly distributed between heels and toes; don't worry if you have to raise your heels. Hold for a few minutes or for as long as you like if you are comfortable. Then come forward to kneel or stand up. Squatting can become a natural part of your daily life, such as when you're lifting something low.

Safe balance

If necessary, hold on to something secure, such as a chair, low stool, or window ledge, to support your back as you squat, and use a towel underneath your heels. You can also lean against a wall.

Squat to make your pelvis more flexible, stretch and strengthen the thigh and back muscles, and relieve back pain

RELAXATION

As your abdomen grows you may find it more comfortable to lie on your back with your head supported by a cushion. Raise your feet and lower legs on to a chair or bed. You can relax in this position while your other children are playing nearby.

Lie with your feet up to relieve swollen ankles and feet

Clear your mind and breathe in deeply. Hold to a count of five and breathe out. Relax all parts of your body

Alleviate pressure on the major blood vessels and the abdomen by lying in this way

Lying down

Lie on your side with a pillow under your head. Bend your upper arm and leg upwards and place a pillow under this knee; keep your lower leg straightened. Close your eyes and concentrate just on your breathing.

MASSAGE AIDS

A variety of different items can add greatly to the experience. Make sure you have everything ready before beginning the massage in order to avoid breaking the rhythm.

Scented oils are available that will help your hands glide over the skin, and leave it soft and smooth. Their fragrance will add to the atmosphere, making each occasion special.

Feathers, fabric, and other soft-textured materials can be rubbed against the skin to leave it tingling.

Warm, fluffy towels are ideal for covering areas of exposed skin.

Use spinal rolls for firm, smooth counter-pressure (see p.296).

A soft bristle hairbrush applied to the hair with light strokes is very relaxing.

Massage for relaxation

A massage from a partner, or one that you give yourself, is an ideal way to relax and unwind. It stimulates the nerve endings in your skin, improves your circulation, and soothes tired muscles, creating an overall sense of peace and well-being.

SOOTHING TOUCH

Use a good-quality massage oil (one with a vegetable oil base) to reduce friction between hands and skin and make the massage more pleasurable. Try to create a comfortable atmosphere: dim the lighting, put on some soft music, and place pillows or cushions around and underneath yourself. In the later months, you may find it more comfortable to lie on your side supported by pillows, or to sit astride a chair.

Apart from your back, you can massage most parts of your body quite effectively yourself. Work clockwise around each breast, stroking with the palms and fingers of one hand, from the base

SELF MASSAGE

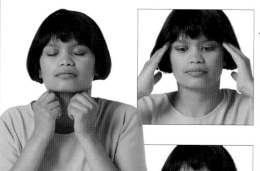

Soothing your forehead
Cover your face with your hands. Place your fingertips on your forehead and rest the heels of your hands on your chin. After a few seconds, draw your hands towards your ears.

Toning your chin
Stimulate the blood circulation under your chin with brisk movements. Using the back of both hands, one after the other, gently slap upwards.

Firming your neck
Make gentle pinching movements around your jawbone. Softly squeeze the skin between your thumb and the knuckles of your index finger. Be careful not to drag the skin.

towards the nipple; gently knead the nipple between your fingers and thumb. Massage your abdomen, hips, and thighs, with the palms of your hands, using a smooth, circular motion.

If you are to be massaged by a partner or a friend, make sure the masseur's hands are warm before starting the massage, and he or she should remove any rings, bracelets, or watches. When you are both in comfortable positions, take a few deep breaths to help you relax. The masseur should begin the massage gently and gradually increase the pressure if it is comfortable for you, but he or she should always keep the movements slow.

Circling Use the palms of both hands simultaneously to make circling strokes in the same direction away from the spine. Lighten pressure when massaging over the abdomen and breasts.

Effleurage Make light, feathery, circular movements with the fingertips as though tickling the skin. This can be done all over the abdomen during pregnancy.

Gliding Place the palms of both hands on either side of the sacrum, with the fingers pointing to the head. Push the hands up to the shoulders, without exerting body weight on to the hands. Slowly glide the hands down the sides of the body back to the starting point.

MASSAGE BY A PARTNER

ESSENTIAL OILS

Aromatic oils can greatly enhance your massage, helping you feel relaxed and refreshed. Their diverse scents also help conjure up wonderful images.

These oils are distilled from flowers, trees, and herbs, and are said to have therapeutic qualities. For example, lavender oil relieves headaches and insomnia. Some essential oils should be avoided in pregnancy, so always take the advice of an experienced aromatherapist before use, and blend the oil with a carrier oil such as almond or olive before applying it to your skin.

Gently press your fingers against the temples to ease tension

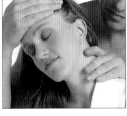

Supporting her head
Kneel behind her to massage her neck muscles. Gently turn her head, keeping it well supported. With the heel of your hand slowly massage downwards from her face.

Relaxing her neck
Slowly stroke up the back of her neck with both thumbs. Make circular movements away from the centre of the neck. Massage all around the base of the skull.

Stroking her brow
Gently massage her forehead and temples with both hands, simultaneously. Using your fingers, make light, circular movements from the centre of her forehead outwards. Run your fingers out over her hair.

Emotional changes

It is not only your body that alters during pregnancy, your emotions will fluctuate rapidly and you will experience feelings you have never had before. It is important to recognize that you will feel upset from time to time, that all pregnant women do, and that there are things that you can do that will help with your mood swings.

Your swinging hormone levels lead to mood changes from elation to depression. Your changing body shape disturbs your self-image. And we are all occasionally beset by fears about our suitability as parents. Emotionally, pregnancy can be very difficult.

HORMONAL CHANGES

Enormous changes occur in your body during pregnancy and, because of this, your mood is likely to swing frequently. It is not unusual to find yourself becoming hypercritical and irritable, your reactions to minor events will be exaggerated, you will feel unsure of yourself and panicky sometimes, and you may even have bouts of depression and crying.

It is normal to feel all of these things, because you are less in control of your feelings than usual. The swinging levels of hormones have taken over and are controlling your moods the way a conductor controls an orchestra. So there is no reason to feel guilty or ashamed if you show irritation, anger, or frustration. If you explain the situation, most people will be understanding. At work, you may have to struggle to preserve a veneer of calm. This effort will definitely pay off, especially if you plan to return to your job after the birth of your baby.

CHANGING BODY SHAPE

Under normal circumstances it takes quite a long time to adjust to a change in body image, such as going from blond to brunette or losing or gaining weight. In pregnancy you are not given time to adjust to the shape of your body, and you may feel strange, even unrelated to the body in which you find yourself. You may also worry that you are putting on too much weight and that you will become fat and unattractive during or after pregnancy.

Thinking of pregnant women as fat, and therefore ugly, is essentially an Anglo-Saxon attitude: many cultures see pregnant women as sensuous and beautiful. Rather than view your increasing curves with despair, think of them as a reaffirmation of life; see the roundness as ripeness, and glory in your body's fertility. Feel confident and proud of your shape and fertility.

Your changing shape
A positive attitude to your appearance is important because it will help keep you buoyant.

CONFLICTING FEELINGS

Even with the most positive attitudes about pregnancy it is normal to have conflicting feelings. One moment you are thrilled at the prospect of a new baby, the next minute you are terrified of your new responsibilities. Becoming a parent is a time of reassessment and change, worries and fears.

The first and most important psychological task you have is to accept the pregnancy. This may sound obvious but there are women who blithely sail through the early months of pregnancy giving it as little thought as possible, which is especially easy until the baby begins to show.

You and the baby's father have to come to terms with the pregnancy and begin to think about the reality. Until now your thoughts about a baby and parenthood would have probably all been in soft focus, a pastel picture of a loving threesome.

Conflicting feelings are sure to surface once you begin to accept the pending realities. Let me reassure you that it's good to have conflicting feelings. It is normal to feel this way and you shouldn't worry about it. It means that you are genuinely coming to terms with the situation. You won't have the horrible shock some people do, who wait to face all this until the baby is at home.

FEARS

You may be worried about labour – whether you will be able to cope with the pain, whether you will scream or defecate, or lose control, or need an episiotomy or emergency Caesarean. Most women worry about these things, but there's really no need. Labour is usually straightforward and how you behave will be of little or no importance. You may be surprised at how calm you are; you may not be calm at all, and that's okay too. Just remember that your birth attendants have seen it all before, so there is nothing for you to feel embarrassed about.

You may worry about how good a parent you'll be, whether you will hurt or harm your baby, or not care for her properly. These are quite common feelings and represent legitimate fears. Like many modern women, you probably do not know much about baby care and are worried about doing a good job. The answer is to get some hands-on experience – handle and care for a newborn baby if you can. Perhaps you could babysit for a friend's baby, or spend some time with her. If you change and feed her, you will probably gain confidence. Try to get these fears into perspective – you probably had similar worries about starting a job.

DREAMS

Dreams may become more frequent, and even frightening, in the last trimester. There are many common themes reported by pregnant women and all express deep feelings and concerns that are entirely natural – everybody worries at one time or another that something will be wrong or go wrong with their baby. You may have dreams about losing the baby; and this is usually an expression of fear about miscarrying or having a stillborn baby.

WILL MY MOOD AFFECT MY BABY?

You may worry that your swinging emotional changes will somehow affect your baby.

Although your baby reacts to your moods, such as kicking when you are angry or upset, your changeable emotions appear to have no detrimental effect on your baby (see **A mother's influence**, p.192).

Dreams and nightmares can be very vivid, and you may find that you wake up abruptly – hot, drenched in sweat, and with your heart racing. Be reassured that this will not harm your baby.

On the other hand, your baby really enjoys your good moods – your excitement, your happiness, and your elation. When you feel good, your baby feels good. When you're relaxed, your baby is also feeling tranquil.

If some activity makes you content and happy – listening to music, dancing gently, painting – do as much of it as you can and share the feeling with your baby.

KEEPING A DIARY

Keeping a diary at any time of your life can give you information and insights about yourself that you might not have the time to recognize.

It is a place where you can let go of those thoughts and feelings that you may not want to share, and it will also help you to focus on yourself. Your child will also enjoy reading it herself – especially when she is about to start her own family.

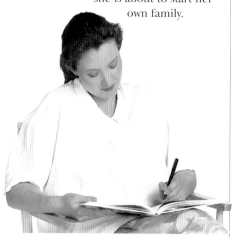

Pregnancy journal
Taking the time to keep a pregnancy journal means that you will have a cherished record of this special time in your life.

Dreams like these may be a psychological preparation for an unwanted outcome and also a way of bringing these feelings to the surface. In a way, they act as a release for your anxieties.

Dreams, nightmares, and thoughts in general may be a way of expressing hostility to your unborn child. She is going to overtake your life, disrupt your privacy and comfortable routine. They may express feelings you may not be able to cope with or may not be consciously aware of. Again, don't make the mistake of taking dreams literally and then feeling guilty or frightened.

SUPERSTITIONS

It is likely that you may be more superstitious than normal. Superstition and old wives' tales were, in the past, ways of explaining an inexplicable world. With the excellent medical care now available, your chances of having a damaged child are very low, and what you might interpret as a bad omen certainly does not mean that anything will go wrong with your baby.

COPING WITH EMOTIONAL CHANGES

Try to see the emotional turmoil you are experiencing as a positive force as you adjust to being pregnant and becoming a mother. Don't imagine that having second thoughts or fears means that you've made a mistake. You're tossing this around in your head the way one wrestles with any big life decision. Yet social conditioning makes us feel guilty if we don't walk around with a madonna-like expression and saintly attitude to everything. That is absurd. Being pregnant isn't all fun. Accepting the reality is the best thing you can do for yourself and your child.

Spend time daydreaming Imagining and thinking about your baby helps you to form a relationship with her even before she is born, and you shouldn't feel silly if you find that you spend a couple of hours doing nothing but thinking about the baby. Making that connection with the tiny person growing inside you is the first step in accepting your child.

The daydreams of pregnant mothers are notoriously sexist, with many having an undisguised preference for a girl or a boy. Although it isn't usually a problem if your newborn turns out to be the opposite sex from the one you wanted, it can mean readjusting, so try not to get too carried away with your plans!

Consider your parents Your parents are about to become grandparents, perhaps for the first time. They may be delighted, they may be upset, and they may feel a combination of both. In other words, it is possible that they are feeling nearly as ambiguous about their new role as you are about yours. Becoming a grandparent is often seen as being synonymous with becoming old, and can be unsettling for a person who perhaps feels only just middle-aged. Try to be understanding and loving, include them in your pregnancy, talk to them and share your feelings with them.

Confront your isolation It is quite common for a pregnant woman to feel isolated nowadays. Many women postpone having children, and some decide against it altogether. You may find that you are the first in your social circle to start a family, and that you don't know any other pregnant women or fully fledged mothers. It can be lonely. There is so much that you want to know and discuss. You may have little niggles and worries that you feel are too irrelevant or silly to talk about at your antenatal clinic, and you may wish that you knew someone who was going through the same thing or who already had a child. If so, find people to whom you can talk – join parent groups, approach other pregnant women in your childbirth classes, and ask your friends or family if they know any pregnant women, or parents with young children, whom you could get to know. These relationships may provide support long after your baby is born. Don't forget your partner either – if you are feeling isolated, he probably is too, so talk to him, include him, and expand your social circle together.

Communicate Wanting to talk and share what you are feeling and thinking during your pregnancy is natural. Your partner is the logical first choice, and will probably be anxious to talk to you. There are bound to be things that he would like to talk about: worries, things that he may have refrained from discussing with you because he thought that he might upset you, or you might think him silly, or because you were too busy, or too tired. Keep talking. You need each other more now than ever before. Denying or ignoring your fears and feelings won't make them go away. Suppressed feelings have a very nasty way of festering and then surfacing when you are least equipped to deal with them, thus becoming full-blown problems. You should be able to avoid these problems if you bring them out in the open when they first occur and then get on with your lives.

COPING WITH MATERIAL CHANGES

Everyday difficulties that you would normally deal with quite calmly can turn into dramas during pregnancy. Keep a level head, and try not to overreact if you can help it.

Finances One of the major causes of marital strife, financial problems can become especially troubling during pregnancy. You may find it difficult to cope with an inevitable reduction in income, even if you plan to return to work, but remember that you are in this together. Work out before the birth how you will cope on your income once the baby has arrived.

Housing Moving or expanding your home may be something that you are forced to consider – perhaps you need the extra space, or there may be a lack of facilities in your area. This can be stressful, and tends to be worse when you are expecting. If you must move – and it's not really recommended from a physical standpoint – do it before your pregnancy is too advanced.

GRANDPARENTS

A new baby means a new role not only for you but possibly also for your parents.

While they will, no doubt, revel in their roles as doting grandparents once the baby is born, they may feel they are still too young when you first tell them the glad tidings.

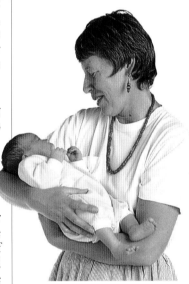

A source of help
Even before the baby is born, your parents are often invaluable sources of information, expertise, and reassurances.

MAKE-UP TIPS

Pregnancy can change the tone and colour of your skin and you may want to adjust your make-up to counteract the effects.

Fine lines or wrinkles These will become more accentuated if your skin becomes drier than usual, so stop using products that make them look more obvious. Shiny or glittering eye shadows, heavy foundations, and coloured powders will make them more prominent.

Extra greasy skin To combat this, use an astringent lotion, oil-free foundation, and dust with translucent powder.

Extra dry skin This is very rare in pregnancy, but if your skin becomes so dry that it flakes, it should be left make-up free, but make sure that you continue to moisturize it well. Otherwise, use an oil-based film of foundation and powder to help to slow water loss. Thick, creamy moisturizers will also act as a barrier to water loss on dry patches.

High colour and spider veins Stipple a thin, light coat of matt beige foundation free of any pink on to your cheeks. When dry, cover with your regular foundation and a transparent powder.

Dark circles On top of a thin layer of foundation, stipple an under-eye cover-up cream and leave to dry. Cover with another thin layer of foundation and blend carefully. Finish with a dusting of transparent powder.

Body care

Pregnancy hormones bring about changes to almost every part of your body, including your breasts, skin, hair, teeth, and gums. To keep your body in the best condition, a changed daily routine may be necessary. Moreover, your enlarging abdomen may affect your posture so pay closer attention to the way you stand or move (see p.160).

SKIN

Your skin will probably "bloom" during pregnancy because the hormones encourage it to retain moisture that plumps it out, making it more supple, less oily, and less prone to spots. The extra blood circulating round your body will also cause your skin to glow. However, the opposite can sometimes happen. Red patches may enlarge, acne may worsen, areas may become dry and scaly, and you may notice deeper pigmentation across your face.

Skin care Here are a few general tips during pregnancy. Soap removes the natural oils from the skin, so use it as infrequently as possible. Try using baby lotion, or glycerine-based soap and body wash. Always use oils in the bath to minimize the dehydrating effects of hard water, and do not lie in a bath for long periods of time because prolonged contact with water particularly dehydrates the skin. Make-up is good for your morale, and can act as a good moisturizer for the skin as it prevents the loss of water (see column, left). Aromatherapy oils can also have a wonderful effect, relaxing and invigorating you, and will leave a film of protective oil on your skin that will keep it supple, and prevent dehydration and damage due to water loss.

Deeper pigmentation This affects nearly every woman, especially on the areas of the body that are pigmented to begin with, such as freckles, moles, and the areolae of the breasts. Your genitalia, the skin of the inner sides of the thighs, underneath your eyes, and in your armpits may become darker too. A dark line, called the linea nigra, often appears down the centre of your stomach. It marks the division of your abdominal muscles, which separate slightly to accommodate your expanding uterus, and you should be very careful when getting up from a lying down position (see p.161). Even after birth the linea nigra and the areolae usually remain darker for some time, but will gradually fade and disappear.

Sunlight intensifies areas of skin that are already pigmented, and many women find that they tan more easily during pregnancy. Since ultraviolet A (UVA) rays can lead to skin cancer, and the effect they have on the unborn baby is unknown, it is best to avoid sunlamps. Keep your skin covered up in hot sunshine, or use a sun block, especially on pigmented areas such as your nipples.

Chloasma This is a special form of pigmentation, also called the mask of pregnancy, which appears as brown patches on the bridge of the nose, cheeks, and neck. The only way to handle chloasma is to camouflage it with a blemish stick or the cover-up cosmetics that are used for birthmarks. Never try to bleach out the pigment; the patches will begin to fade within three months of labour. Conversely, some black women develop patches of paler skin on their faces and necks. These will probably disappear after delivery and can be camouflaged during pregnancy.

Spider veins All the blood vessels in pregnancy become sensitive – rapidly dilating when you are hot, and constricting quickly when you are cold. Consequently, tiny broken blood vessels called spider veins may appear on your face, particularly on your cheeks. Do not worry; these will fade soon after delivery, and will probably have disappeared altogether within three months.

Pimples If your skin has a tendency to become spotty before periods, you may get pimples now, particularly in the first trimester when the pregnancy hormones stimulating the sebaceous glands in the skin have not yet reached a balanced level. Keep your skin as clean as possible, and use a cleanser two or three times a day to prevent spots altogether. If a spot appears, apply a tiny smear of antiseptic cream. Never squeeze spots as this only spreads the infection into the deeper layers of the skin.

Stretch marks About 90 percent of pregnant women get stretch marks. These usually appear across the abdomen, although they can also affect the thighs, hips, breasts, and the upper arms. Nothing you can apply to the skin (including oil), and nothing you can eat will prevent stretch marks because they are due to the breakdown of protein in the skin by the high levels of pregnancy hormones. Gradual weight gain should allow the skin to stretch without tearing, although some women are blessed with more elastic skin than others. While the reddish streaks may look prominent during pregnancy, during the weeks after delivery they will become paler, and shrink until they are nothing more than faint silvery streaks that are barely noticeable.

TEETH

During pregnancy, you will be more susceptible than normal to gum problems owing to the increased blood supply and to the high level of progesterone, which softens all of your body's tissues. The increased blood volume also puts pressure on the tiny capillaries around the gum margin, which often bleed easily. A balanced diet helps prevent teeth and gum problems. Sufficient calcium and high-quality protein, along with a good supply of vitamins B, C, and D, helps to protect you. You should see your dentist at least once during your pregnancy and have your teeth cleaned professionally to reduce the risk of gum infections, but be sure to tell him or her you are pregnant as you should avoid X-rays.

YOUR HAIR

During pregnancy, it is very common for the hair to change in quality, quantity, and manageability.

The high levels of hormones arrest the usual cycle of hair growth and loss. Usually some hair grows and some is lost every day. In pregnancy, the hair is arrested in the growth phase.

After delivery, the cycle passes into a resting phase when masses of hair can be lost. Hair loss can go on for up to two years and may be alarming, but rest assured, it will stop – pregnancy never causes baldness. The hair you will lose once your baby is born is simply the hair you would normally have lost throughout the whole of the 9 months of pregnancy.

If your hair becomes more difficult to manage this may be a good time to try a simpler hair style that is easier to care for. Use the mildest shampoo you can find and underwash by applying the shampoo only once – massage gently to a lather, leave for 30 seconds and rinse off.

Body and facial hair, also, may increase in quantity and may even darken in colour.

MAINTAINING YOUR POSTURE

Adopting and maintaining a good posture will help you to minimize the backache and fatigue that can easily arise as your pregnancy advances.

Bad posture is a common problem in pregnancy caused by the increasing weight of your baby. Your enlarging abdomen thrusts your centre of gravity forward and to balance this you tend to arch your back backwards, putting your back muscles under constant strain – hence backache.

When you are standing, sitting, or walking with the correct posture, your neck and back will be in a straight line.

Avoiding problems

The pregnancy hormones stretch and soften your ligaments, particularly in the lower back, making them more vulnerable to strain. However, with a little care you can avoid the unnecessary problems and fatigue that many women suffer during pregnancy.

Don't bend down
When you are doing household chores or working in the garden and you need to work on something at floor level, sit or kneel to bring it within easy reach. Whenever possible, avoid bending or stooping.

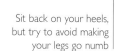

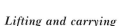

Sit back on your heels, but try to avoid making your legs go numb

Always keep your back straight, and lift by straightening your legs

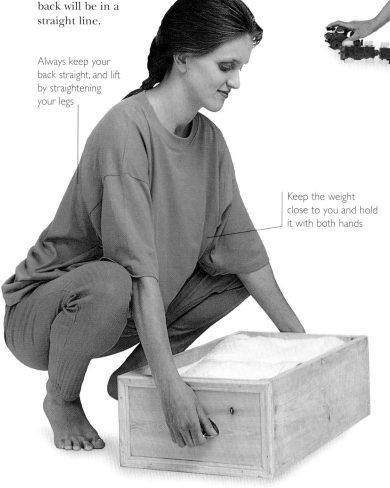

Keep the weight close to you and hold it with both hands

Lifting and carrying
To lift something from the floor, reach down to it by bending your knees, keeping your back as straight as you can. When you pick it up, hold it close in to your body, and lift it by straightening your legs, so that you use the strength of your leg and thigh muscles to do the actual lifting. Never struggle to lift objects that are too heavy – get someone to help you. Don't try lifting heavy things to or from high shelves or upwards. If you are carrying heavy bags, try to divide the weight equally between both your hands.

Getting up

When you have been lying down on the floor, for instance, if you have been exercising, get up in easy stages. First, turn on to your side (see below), then use your hands to support yourself as you move yourself into a kneeling position (see top right). From there, keeping your back straight and using the strength of your thigh muscles, push yourself up into a sitting position (see bottom right). From here you can stand up without straining your abdomen.

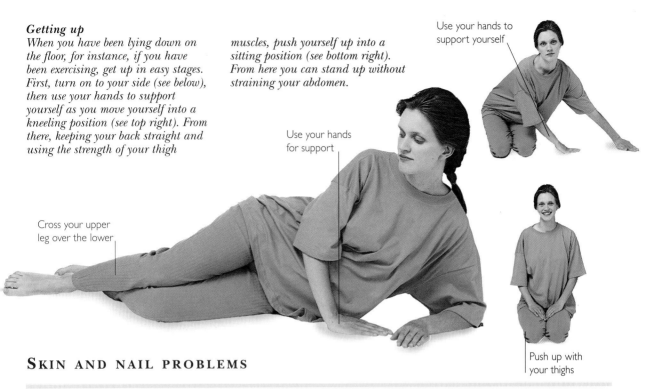

Use your hands to support yourself

Use your hands for support

Cross your upper leg over the lower

Push up with your thighs

SKIN AND NAIL PROBLEMS

POSSIBLE PROBLEMS	WHAT TO DO
Itching or chafed skin The skin of your extended abdomen may become quite itchy during pregnancy, and the area between your thighs may become chafed.	Massage your skin with baby lotion to stimulate the blood supply and ease irritation. Keep the thigh area dry; dust with powder, and wear cotton underwear.
Rashes These are not uncommon in the groin and under the breasts, and are a result of excess weight gain and sweat that accumulates in the skin folds. Poor bodily hygiene will increase the risk.	Keep your groin area and the skin under your breasts clean, and apply calamine or other drying lotion. Take care to keep your weight under control. Wear a firm, supporting bra to hold up the breasts.
Pigmentation Many women find that their skin pigmentation alters when they are pregnant; this particularly affects already-darkened areas such as moles and the areolae of the breasts.	Use a sun block to protect your skin from the ultra-violet rays in sunlight. The pigmentation effects will disappear follow-ing the birth.
Nails Your fingernails grow faster than usual in pregnancy, but may also become brittle and split, or break more easily than they did before your pregnancy.	Keep your nails short, and wear gloves for housework and gardening.

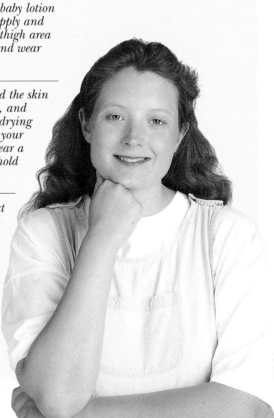

What to wear

Comfort is the watchword during pregnancy as far as clothes are concerned. As your size increases, try to stay one step ahead – there's nothing more demoralizing than feeling constricted and too big for your clothes. Because the blood is circulating round your body at a faster rate, you'll probably be warmer during pregnancy than you expect. Feet and legs tend to swell, particularly towards the end of the day, so footwear and hosiery should be chosen with care.

CLOTHES

You don't have to buy lots of expensive maternity clothes in pregnancy. A few specially bought basics, such as a pair of maternity jeans with an expandable front panel, a selection of properly fitted maternity bras, some maternity cotton or wool tights and leggings with expandable gussets, and one or two maternity dresses for special occasions, can be supplemented with inexpensive ethnic dresses, drawstring cotton trousers, leggings, and man-size tops and jumpers – all of which can be worn when you are no longer pregnant. Before you splash out on any special outfits, find out if friends or neighbours have pregnancy clothes that you could borrow. There are also shops which specialize in nearly-new maternity clothes, where you can find clothes at bargain prices. Avoid synthetic fabrics whenever you can as they're not as comfortable as natural fabrics. Stretch fabrics, for example, can become unpleasantly clingy and tight; polyester tends to trap moisture, causing discomfort in hot weather.

Work clothes Depending on where you work, you may be able to get away with wearing smarter versions of your casual wear, such as leggings with an elegant top or a loose cotton skirt with a crisp cotton blouse. However, if you work in an environment where formal clothes are worn, you may have to invest in higher-priced maternity clothes, but ordinary long-line jackets, large-size skirts and blouses, and drop-waist dresses may suffice. If you wear a uniform, make sure that you tell your employers as soon as you know you are pregnant, as they may be able to offer you financial help even if they don't provide uniforms for their staff. Make sure that you change to flat shoes if you normally wear heels to work.

SHOES

The bigger you get, the more unstable you become, so it's a good idea to wear flat or low-heeled, comfortable, easy-fitting shoes. They should give your feet good support, be sufficiently roomy, and preferably have a nonslip sole for safety. Trainers fulfil all the criteria, and you should choose a pair with a Velcro fastening because later in pregnancy it may be difficult for you to bend

Maternity underwear
A pregnancy bra and pants are invaluable for your comfort during pregnancy – and for your figure afterwards.

down to do up the laces. There are lots of smart, flat shoes available that are versatile and durable. Your feet will swell during pregnancy, so choose a size bigger than normal, and avoid anything with a heel. Best of all, go barefoot whenever you can.

UNDERWEAR

Bra This is one item that is essential in pregnancy. Your breasts may enlarge substantially, particularly during the first three months, and if you don't support them, they are likely to sag later. This is because the sling of fibrous tissue to which they are attached can never regain its former shape once it is stretched. A good, well-fitting bra will help to prevent stretching in the first place.

When you buy a bra, it is best to have it properly fitted. A store specializing in maternity clothes or lingerie, or a large department store, is the most likely to have specially trained staff. Make sure that the bra of your choice gives you good support with a deep band underneath the cups and wide shoulder straps that don't cut deep into your skin. Fastening should be adjustable for comfort, so back-fastening bras may be better than front-fastening. Only buy a couple of bras to begin with as your breasts will continue to grow, and you'll have to get larger sizes later in pregnancy. If your breasts become very big it is a good idea to wear a light bra in bed at night to give them extra support, and just before your due date buy two or three front-opening feeding bras so that you can breastfeed as well as give your breasts support when the milk comes in. They can be bought at any maternity shop or department store.

Girdles Wearing a maternity girdle during the second and third trimester will give you some much-needed support – especially if you are expecting more than one baby. By relieving your back of some of the strain, a girdle can also help prevent backache.

Socks These should be made of cotton and be loose fitting; synthetic materials don't give and can cut really deeply into swollen feet. In addition, they don't allow you to sweat, so the skin may become waterlogged and soft. Avoid knee-high socks because these can form a restricting band around the top of your calf, encouraging varicose veins (see p.212).

Tights Even sheer maternity tights give a lot of support. There are many different types available in a variety of colours. You will find them in maternity shops and most department stores.

Stockings If you find that you suffer from thrush (see p.212), you may prefer to wear stockings. Support stockings, or ones containing a high percentage of lycra, will probably be the most comfortable, although they obviously don't offer the same amount of support as maternity tights. Suspender belts will be most comfortable if they fit on your hips under your abdomen, so choose one that is big enough and shorten the straps if necessary.

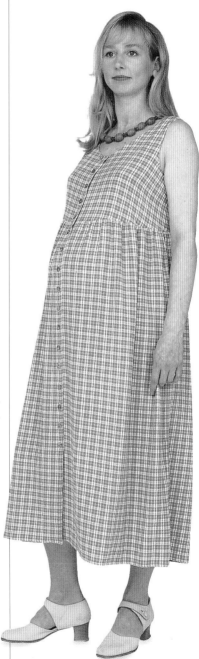

Maternity outwear
Choose clothes for comfort and practicality throughout pregnancy, bearing in mind that the seasons change as you grow bigger.

163

There are a few minor adjustments that you can make to your normal working lifestyle that will make your day more comfortable.

Put your feet up Sit down as much as possible, and put your feet up whenever you can. Convert a piece of furniture such as an overturned bin, or an extended drawer into a foot stool.

Relaxation exercises Practise a few simple neck, shoulder, pelvic, and foot exercises as often as possible when travelling, and at work. These will release any tension, and help to improve your circulation.

Practise squatting Use the squatting position whenever you have to bend down, or if there is no chair available. You will strengthen your thighs, and prepare yourself to use this position at the delivery.

Eat well Keep a supply of nutritious snacks close to hand (see p.130). Although you may still have feelings of nausea, your urge for food may strike at inconvenient moments. A wholemeal biscuit or cracker, and a glass of skimmed milk will be filling, and help relieve attacks of nausea.

Take it easy In general, you should just try to take things more slowly. Stop whenever you feel fatigued, and rest.

A working pregnancy

Whether you are working because of financial necessity, or you find your career stimulating and intend to continue after the birth, be fully aware of information that will protect both your health and your job. You may wish to carry on working well into your pregnancy, and there is no reason why you shouldn't unless your environment will pose a danger to your baby. Harmful materials or fumes, or heavy physical labour, for example, can be deleterious.

Pregnancy brings with it a variety of physical changes and discomforts but working can confer the psychological benefit of reaffirming that it is a normal state. By continuing to work, you can maintain this important and stable aspect of your life at a time when you may be feeling disorientated owing to the physical and emotional changes created by your pregnancy.

PUTTING YOUR RIGHTS INTO PLAY

Most employers will be keen to cooperate with your wish to carry on working during, and after, your pregnancy, provided you keep them well informed of your plans for stopping work before your baby is born and possibly resuming it afterwards.

Protect your job Discuss with your employer or your trade union representative your entitlements concerning maternity leave and pay (see p.64). You are allowed time off with pay for antenatal care, and this includes attending relaxation classes.

Protect your health If there is the possibility of an aspect of your work causing harm to your baby, for example, X-rays, heavy lifting, or the handling of harmful chemicals, your employer should find you an alternative job while you are pregnant, or, if this isn't possible, suspend you on full pay. This is your right no matter how many hours you work or how long you have been employed.

ADAPTING YOUR ROUTINE

Coping with fatigue while working is an ever-present situation when you are pregnant. Bouts of morning sickness can make the situation even more difficult. As your pregnancy progresses, you will lose some of your agility, so working long hours may leave you feeling very tired. Overtiredness will exacerbate your feelings of nausea, and you could also find yourself losing concentration and falling asleep. Added to this, the stress of travelling, especially if you use public transport, can prove exhausting.

Seek flexibility If aspects of your job make you uncomfortable, find out whether you can alter them until your baby is born. You may be able to change the times you start and finish work to avoid travelling in the rush hour. If you have to do a lot of standing or walking, see whether you can take up a more sedentary role.

Take it easy Don't push yourself too hard. Adopt a more lenient attitude towards household chores, letting domestic priorities slide; your health and that of your baby are far more important. Relaxation is vital and you should allow yourself enough free time to look after your body with an exercise routine, and massage.

Request support If he doesn't already help with the cooking and cleaning, ask your partner to do so. Maybe you could leave most of the chores until the weekend and do them together. If you let colleagues know you're pregnant from early on, they are more likely to understand your emotional and physical changes, such as mood swings, lack of energy, and need for comfort.

DECIDING WHEN TO STOP

Some women happily continue working until they near labour. However, most medical authorities believe that you should not continue beyond the 32nd week. It is around this time that your heart, lungs, and other vital organs will have to work harder, and when a great deal of physical stress will be placed on your spine, joints, and muscles. This is the time when you should allow your body to rest whenever possible, which may be difficult if you are working.

DECIDING WHEN TO RETURN

It is important to think carefully about when you will want to return to work after your baby is born, and what you will do when you return. You may wish to go back under different working conditions, and you will have to discuss this with your employer. There may be provision for part-time employment in your work, or a phased return that allows you to be, in effect, a part-time worker for up to one year after your baby's birth. You may also like to investigate job sharing, flexi-work, or going on your own in some freelance activity that will enable you to work from home. Try to consider these options early on in your pregnancy, as you have to inform your employer in writing whether you intend to return to your job three weeks before you stop work (see p.65).

FATHERS AND WORKING MOTHERS

If you've agreed as a couple that your baby's mother is to go back to work, then you must be accommodating. The routine at home will change and your partner will need a lot of support especially at first. Try to share the responsibility; don't always assume your partner will sort out problems or be the one to cope when, say, your baby is ill. Share chores, including collecting the baby from the childminder or getting home first to take over from the nanny. You will come to relish the time alone with your baby.

YOUR BABY'S SAFETY

Try to be aware of any chemicals in your workplace that may potentially harm your baby. If you are worried, talk to your doctor and employer about the risks, and take steps to avoid these hazards.

Many mothers working in an office environment are particularly concerned about hazards posed by exposure to radiation from copying machines and computer video display terminals. However, recent reports state that these very low levels of radiation will not harm the developing baby.

Very few workplaces now allow smoking at all, and the few that do confine it to designated areas. Try to avoid places where people smoke as passive smoking (inhaling cigarette smoke in the atmosphere) is just as bad for you and your baby as directly smoking cigarettes yourself.

Choosing single parenthood

Ros is a lawyer. She studied Politics, Philosophy, and Economics at Oxford University and went on to study law in chambers in Lincoln's Inn Fields. This involved a three-year law degree and a period of practical training. She is now a highly respected barrister, specializing in Family Law.

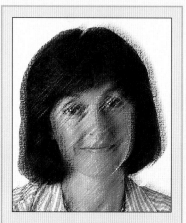

Name **Rosemary Hutchinson**

Age **38 years**

Past medical history **Appendix removed at age 15**

Obstetric history **One abortion at 11 weeks ten years ago. She is now 14 weeks pregnant.**

Ros never saw motherhood as the most pleasurable aspect of being a woman. She always felt that work would be more fulfilling and a career more satisfying. Even as a small girl, Ros was determined not to "dwindle" into marriage or adopt the role of housewife. She always takes responsibility for contraception and believes that she has the right to decide whether or not to have a baby. Indeed Ros made the decision to abort an 11-week pregnancy when she was 28 years old because she did not wish to interrupt her career.

THE CHILD'S FATHER

Ros has had two long-term relationships but in neither case felt she had found a partner with whom she could settle down. She felt she did not wish to make any form of long-term commitment to a partnership where she would have to relinquish any independence.

However, this independence has had its price. As she got older, Ros began to fear that her fertility was diminishing and she sensed that time was running out. She began to want a baby very much, but remained reluctant to commit herself to any man.

During a recent passionate and rather whirlwind affair with a younger man, Ros decided that she would be more than happy if her lover, Timothy, was to become the father of her baby, although she couldn't see the relationship lasting, and didn't particularly want it to.

She talked the idea over with Timothy, who agreed that he didn't want to make any long-term commitment to Ros either, although he was more than happy to father her baby. The affair has now ended, although they have remained firm friends, and Ros has just entered the second trimester of her pregnancy.

A HEALTHY BABY

This will be Ros's only child and she wants to do everything she can in order to ensure that the baby will be healthy. To this end, she went to a genetic counsellor before she became pregnant because a cousin on her father's side suffers from haemophilia (see p.25). However, as her father had not suffered from the disease, the counsellor was able to reassure Ros that she was not carrying the gene.

After she had discussed the possibility of pregnancy with Timothy, Ros also asked him about his family background. Happily everything seemed to be normal.

Antenatal care

On her first visit, Ros was told that her lifestyle was more important than her age in determining the smoothness of her pregnancy and her delivery. She is therefore being very careful about her diet (see p.128), exercise (see p.144), not smoking, drinking, or taking any medication.

All of her medical tests have proved normal and she is aware that she should not gain too much weight, that her blood pressure will be meticulously checked, and that she must be on the look-out for signs of water retention (tight rings, swollen ankles) as this could herald pre-eclampsia (see p.224). Ros had a scan at her last antenatal visit in order to find out amongst other things if there are any obvious abnormalities with the baby. Everything proved to be normal. Although ultrasound scanning revealed no abnormality, Ros is keen to have the added eassurance of the information about genetic or chromosomal diseases that can be revealed only by amniocentesis (see p.185). She will also have a specimen of blood examined to check her alpha-fetoprotein (AFP) levels.

PREGNANCY AND LABOUR

Ros hopes that by careful reduction and flexibility in working hours and workload, she will be able to work right up until labour begins. Despite being allowed 28 weeks maternity leave by law, she intends to return to the office part-time after only two weeks at home with her newborn baby. Given her demanding working schedule, Ros knows the importance of rest. Already she rests with her feet up for 20 minutes during her lunchbreak and at tea-time is quite likely to snatch a nap in chambers or in the car. She is rigorous about getting enough sleep, has stopped socializing except at weekends, and is in bed by 9.30 p.m. I advised her to learn deep muscle and mental relaxation and to continue with her yoga.

Ros is determined to have the very best medical care available during labour and has made the choice to enrol at a large teaching hospital that is at the forefront of technology. She has decided that she wants to have an active birth and is pleased that she will be supervised by a team of midwives as she will not have a birth partner and will therefore be relying on her carers for emotional support. She has made a birth plan (see p.122) which has been added to her hospital notes.

AFTER THE BIRTH

Being able to afford it, Ros has opted for a full-time nanny who will live in with her and the baby as soon as she returns from her hospital delivery.

The nanny will be on night duty from the end of the first two weeks so that Ros can get a full night's rest in preparation for returning to work.

Ros has decided to breastfeed her baby for as long as possible and is prepared to express her milk and store or freeze it so that her baby has the benefits of breast milk even though she herself is absent.

I warned Ros that one of the hardest things about being a single parent is that she will have no-one with whom she can share the memorable events, such as when her baby first smiles or speaks. I also warned her that although her baby would not suffer from having only one parent, it would mean that the demands on Ros herself would be very high.

While work will bring her great satisfaction I encouraged Ros to have as active a social life as her commitments will allow because it's so easy to become isolated at home with a small child. I advised her to find out about local activities where she will probably meet other mothers as well as finding hobbies or classes with creche facilities.

ROS'S BABY

Ros's baby will only have one parent right from the start, which means that her experience will be somewhat different from a child who has both parents present.

• **Feeding** She will have the advantage of having Ros's breast milk, despite the fact that Ros will be at work. However, this does mean that she will have to get used to being bottlefed by her nanny and breastfed by her mother.

• **Care** Ros will be able to provide her baby with just as much care as two parents would. Her baby will also become very attached to her nanny, who will be a very important person in her life, but there is nothing wrong in this.

• **Time** Ros's baby will not see her mother all of the time, but when she does see her, it will be quality time.

• **Relationships** Ros and her child will tend to be everything to each other, which may lead to a rather intense one-to-one relationship. However, babies also need and thrive on exposure to other people so it is important that Ros's baby is encouraged to interact with a wide range of people – both children and adults – as she will greatly benefit from this broad network of support and love.

DRUGS AND YOUR BABY

Consult your doctor before taking any drug – prescription or non-prescription – and don't consult a doctor about anything without saying you're pregnant.

It is best to avoid taking anything during pregnancy unless your doctor determines that the benefit to you outweighs any risk to the fetus. The long-term effects of many drugs on the unborn child are still largely unknown. Other drugs have been proven to be hazardous to the fetus and should be completely avoided (see below).

Avoiding hazards

Many normal activities may pose dangers in pregnancy. Cleaning out cat litter, or contact with harmful chemicals in the work environment, passive smoking while socializing, or vaccinations for travelling, may affect the development of the unborn baby, and certain precautions should be taken.

AT HOME

Very few of us can move to a perfect environment while pregnant, but you should try to avoid handling raw meat, touching other people's pets and cleaning out litter trays, breathing in exhaust gases from cars, and working with pesticides in the garden. Alcohol, coffee, and teas containing caffeine are also best avoided. Herbal teas are generally safe (although you should avoid raspberry leaf, which is said to trigger contractions), but choose organic ones, if possible, to avoid the risk of pesticides.

DRUG	USE	POSSIBLE SIDE EFFECTS
Amphetamines	Stimulant	May cause heart defects and blood diseases
Anabolic steroids	Body building	Can have a masculinizing effect on a female fetus
Tetracycline	Treats acne	Can colour both first and permanent teeth yellow
Streptomycin	Treats tuberculosis	Can cause deafness in infants
Antihistamines	Allergies/travel sickness	Some cause malformations; check with your doctor
Anti-nausea drugs	Combats nausea	May cause malformations, but can be used safely to treat morning sickness
Aspirin	Painkiller	Can cause problems with blood clotting
Diuretics	Rids body of excess fluid	Can cause fetal blood disorders
Narcotics (Codeine, etc.)	Painkillers	Addictive; baby may suffer withdrawal symptoms
Paracetamol	Reduces fever	Safe in small doses, but large doses can damage baby's kidneys and liver
LSD, cannabis	Recreational	Risk of chromosomal damage, and miscarriage
Sulphonamides	Treat infections	Can cause jaundice in the baby at birth

Harmful chemicals Limit your use of aerosol sprays in the home; there are alternatives available. Although modern aerosols contain halogenated hydrocarbons (rather than CFCs), which have not been implicated in causing harm to fetus or mother, my feeling is that we are all exposed to invisible sources of potentially harmful chemicals, and it's wise to take every possible precaution.

Avoid substances that give off vapours, such as glue and petrol, as they may be toxic and should never be inhaled, whether you are pregnant or not. Read the label of any material you use, and avoid those which are potentially harmful. Some examples are cleaning fluids, contact cement, creosote, volatile paint, lacquers, thinners, some glues, and oven cleaner. Perms are apparently safe in pregnancy, but if you have fears about their long-term effects, I would advise you to wait until after the first three months, when the most crucial organs in your baby's body have formed.

Hot baths Saunas and hot whirlpools have been implicated in fetal abnormalities, particularly those of the baby's nervous system, in exactly the same way as fever. When your body is subjected to extreme heat over a lengthy period, you can become overheated which may affect your baby. Avoid saunas and whirlpools, especially in the first trimester, and keep bath temperatures moderate.

Television rays Rays have not been shown to form ionizing radiation. It is not harmful to sit within several feet of the screen, even for long periods, but make sure you are sitting comfortably.

Immunizations Because your entire immune system is changing under the influence of your pregnancy and may be weakened, your responses to immunizations can be unpredictable. Your doctor will discuss with you any immunizations that are necessary if you have been exposed to infectious diseases or if you have to travel outside the UK. In general, vaccinations that are prepared using live viruses – including measles, rubella (German measles), mumps, and yellow fever vaccinations – are avoided. It is recommended that women do not have the flu vaccine during pregnancy, unless there is a high risk of heart or lung disease.

AT WORK

If you work outside the home, you may have many questions that have no simple answers: How safe is my workplace? Will the demands of my job put my pregnancy as risk? How long can I work? If your job is strenuous, involving a lot of standing, walking, lifting, or climbing, it may deprive you of the extra rest you need during pregnancy and aggravate fatigue. Your doctor may suggest that you reduce your work hours, transfer to less strenuous work or stop working several weeks before your EDD. In all circumstances, pregnant women must avoid activities that expose them to physical danger, including some police work, motorcycle racing, and so on.

TOXOPLASMOSIS AND YOUR BABY

This parasite normally produces only mild flu-like symptoms in an adult, but it can seriously damage the unborn child.

It can cause fetal brain damage, blindness, and is fatal in certain cases. The greatest danger is during the third trimester.

Toxoplasma is carried in the faeces of infected animals, particularly cats, but most people contract it eating undercooked meat, particularly poultry. About 80 percent of the population have had it and have developed antibodies, but the younger you are, the less likely you are to be immune. You can ask your doctor to do a blood test.

Guidelines to follow:

• don't eat raw or undercooked meat, especially pork, rare steak, or steak tartare

• don't feed raw meat to your cat or dog. Keep their food bowls away from everything else

• don't garden in soil used by cats

• do wear gloves when gardening

• don't stroke other people's pets

• don't empty your cat's box or use your dog's poop-scoop. If it is unavoidable, wear gloves and wash your hands in disinfectant immediately afterwards

• do wash your hands after gardening, or petting your animals

• do cook meat to an internal temperature of at least 54°C/140°F – at which bacteria is killed. Use a meat thermometer to be sure

• if your cat hunts, treat it regularly for worms and parasites, picked up from infected mice and birds.

YOUR RISK OF INFECTION

In the first 12 weeks of pregnancy, you must try to avoid contact with anyone, especially a young child, who has a high fever, even if the fever is not thought to be caused by German measles (see p.19).

If you contract mumps in pregnancy it will run the same course as if you were not pregnant. There is a minimal risk of increased miscarriage if you get the disease in the first 12 weeks.

The mumps vaccine will not be given during pregnancy because it is live and could therefore adversely affect the fetus.

Chickenpox is an uncommon disease in adults and is similarly uncommon in pregnancy. There is some evidence that it can cause fetal malformations.

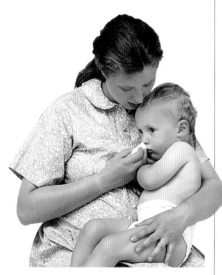

Infection
If you have small children, there is obviously not much you can do to keep away from them. If you are a school teacher, be fairly strict about sending home any feverish child.

Your doctor may also advise you to stop working if you have certain diseases, such as a heart condition, if you have a history of more than one premature baby or miscarriage, or if you're expecting more than one baby.

Be alert to jobs that could expose you to potentially harmful factors and make sure your employer transfers you to a hazard-free working place or job. Especially avoid:

• Anaesthetic gases, which are used by nurses, physicians, dentists, and anaesthetists

• Chemicals used in manufacturing and other industries – for example, lead, mercury, vinyl chloride, dry cleaning fluids, paint fumes, and solvents

• Animals, which present a risk of toxoplasmosis

• Exposure to infectious diseases, especially childhood rashes

• Exposure to toxic wastes of any kind

• Exposure to excessive levels of cigarette smoke, including passive smoking, which can happen in offices that do not have smoking restrictions

• Unacceptable levels of ionizing radiation (these are now strictly monitored by government regulation). It is generally accepted that day-to-day exposure to ultraviolet or infra-red radiation emitted by equipment such as printers, photocopiers, and computer video display terminals is not dangerous to you or your baby. But just to be extra careful, women who photocopy on a daily basis should keep the top of the photocopier closed when the machine is copying.

Otherwise, if you are a healthy woman, having a normal pregnancy and working in a job presenting hazards no greater than those encountered in daily life, you can usually work until close to the expected delivery date.

SOCIALIZING

Infections are caught from people with whom we come into contact. Although being pregnant doesn't mean that you should become a hermit, or wear a gauze mask when talking to people, it pays to be cautious – especially around children (see column, left), or adults who are running an elevated temperature.

Colds and flu will not harm your baby, but do your best to avoid running a fever. If your temperature is very high, your doctor will advise what medications are safe (aspirin is not usually recommended in pregnancy except for certain specific conditions), and using a damp sponge and a fan might help to cool the skin. Don't take cold or flu medicines that contain antihistamines. There is some evidence that virulent flu viruses can cause miscarriage.

TRAVELLING

There is absolutely no evidence that travel precipitates labour, or leads to miscarriage, or any other complication of pregnancy. You should be extra cautious if you have miscarried before, or have a history of premature labour. Ask your doctor for the name of an obstetrician in the area you are visiting and, in the last trimester, limit yourself to trips within 30 miles of home.

Trains Book a seat if possible, and make sure that it is not next to the buffet car as the smell may make you feel nauseous. Eat lightly to minimize motion sickness. Do not lean on, or stand close to, outside doors as they have been known to fly open (this obviously applies even when you are not pregnant).

Cars Travelling by car can be exhausting, so limit your journeys. Get out of the car at regular intervals and have a short walk to ensure good circulation. Always fasten your seat belt, but buckle it low, across your pelvis, and use a shoulder harness if you have one. You can do the driving as long as you are comfortable behind the wheel, but you must stop as soon as you begin to feel at all cramped. In addition, it may seem an obvious point, but don't drive yourself to the hospital if you are in labour!

Air travel After your seventh month, air travel is not a good idea because of pressure changes in the cabin. If you must fly at this time, check with the airline about whether it requires a doctor's letter to let you on the plane after your seventh month. Do not fly in small private planes that have unpressurized cabins. If you sit over the wings or towards the front of the plane you will feel less of the plane's motion.

While flying, eat lightly because pregnancy makes you more prone to motion sickness. Make sure that you empty your bladder before you board because there may be a delay in taking off, or the seat belt sign may stay on a long time. When fastening your seat belt, make sure that you buckle it low on your hips.

Foreign travel Take care when eating out that you follow the guidelines I've given to protect against listeria and other food-related diseases (see p.139). Drink bottled water when in doubt.

Check with your doctor about possible immunizations (typhoid fever vaccinations, for example, could harm the baby). Even if you have been exposed or are in an epidemic, the bad effects of the live vaccine will have to be weighed against the risk to your baby. You should refuse to have a yellow fever vaccination unless there has been direct exposure. However, you can be vaccinated against cholera, as the vaccine is probably not harmful and you may need it to satisfy travel requirements in South East Asia. Rabies and tetanus vaccinations may be necessary, particularly if there is any indication of exposure. Chloroquine may be used for malaria but only if you're going to an endemic area. The polio vaccine may be administered in pregnancy if you are not already immune.

GOOD TRAVELLING

Bearing in mind a few important points when you are travelling will make it a more comfortable experience.

• Leave more than enough time for your journey.

• Try to leave yourself a comfortable margin between any connections you have to make.

• Travel in short bursts rather than a long stretch.

• Travel safely (see main text).

• Carry a drink, such as milk or fruit juice, in a flask.

• Take adequate amounts of nutritious portable food, such as wholemeal crackers, cold hard-boiled eggs, raw fruit or vegetables, and nibbles like dried fruit, nuts, and seeds.

• Carry glucose sweets in order to help prevent nausea due to low blood sugar.

• Make use of an eye mask and ear plugs so that you can get some sleep when travelling by train or plane.

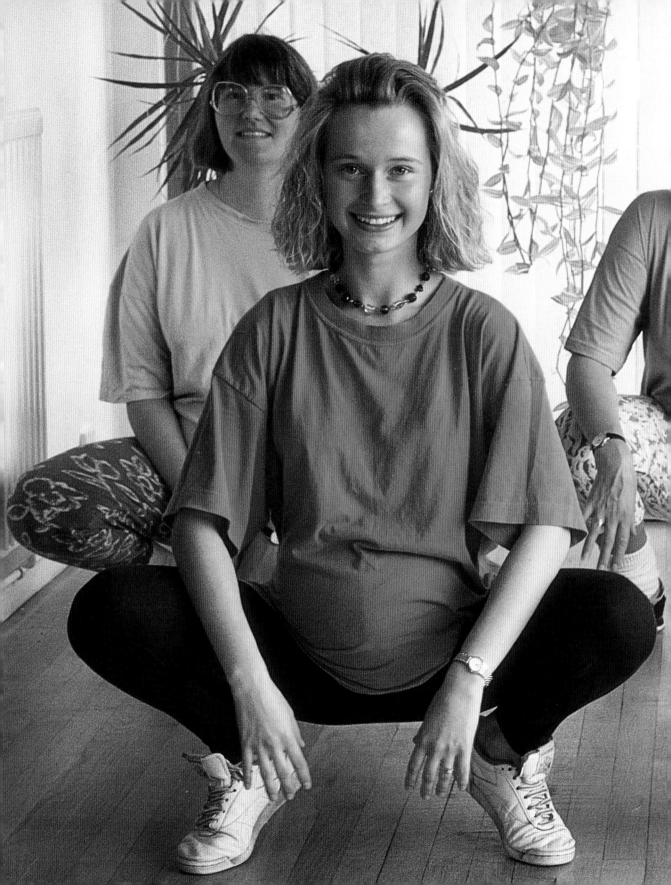

CHAPTER 7

Your ANTENATAL CARE

*Excellent antenatal care should be rewarded with
healthy mothers and babies. Routine tests will
usually spot any problems as soon as they arise,
while special tests are available for mothers
and babies with particular needs. The
antenatal clinic also provides
opportunities to ask questions and
meet other women going through
the same experience as yourself.*

Antenatal care

YOUR FIRST VISIT

On your first visit to the antenatal clinic, you will be asked various questions on the following subjects:

• your personal details and circumstances

• childhood illnesses or serious illnesses you have had

• illnesses that run in your family, or in your partner's family

• if there are twins in your family

• your menstrual history – when you started, how long your average cycle is, how many days you bleed, and the date of LMP (see p.62)

• what symptoms of pregnancy you have, and your general health

• details of previous births, pregnancies, or problems in conceiving

• if you take a prescription medicine or suffer from an allergy.

Discussing your pregnancy
Don't hesitate to request more time if you have questions that need answering.

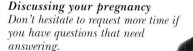

Consultations, check-ups, and tests will be carried out throughout your pregnancy to monitor your health and that of your baby. Although most pregnancies proceed normally, these visits and investigations are vital to monitor progress and spot problems early before any harm is done.

THE ANTENATAL CLINIC

You'll attend antenatal check-ups at your doctor's surgery, the local health centre, or the hospital, depending on the care in your area. You'll probably have a "booking in" appointment at around 12 weeks, and then be checked every 4–6 weeks up to about 32 weeks and every 2–3 weeks after that. If there are any complications, such as a multiple birth, a pre-existing medical condition, or you are at risk, you will attend more frequently.

Now that the majority of antenatal care is handled in the community, appointments are much less stressful than a few years ago when hospital clinics were the norm. The atmosphere is more relaxed, and if you do need to be monitored by the hospital, you'll probably find it less of a "cattle-market" than at one time.

However, there will be times when you do have to wait around, especially if you are having an ultrasound, or a blood test. Try to make the best of your time at the antenatal clinic by taking along something to read or to do, and some food just in case you don't have time to go out to the cafe during a long wait. It's a good idea for your partner to accompany you when he is able to, and you may have an opportunity to make friends with the other expectant mothers. If you have other children, try to arrange for them to be looked after so that they don't become bored.

TALKING TO YOUR CARERS

It can be hard for midwives at a hospital-based antenatal clinic to find time to talk to you in depth. However, community clinics are more relaxed and you'll be able to find out what alternatives are open to you, discuss your preferences, and be reassured about any worries and fears. If you feel that you're being hurried through, ask your midwife for extra time to discuss things. Don't be browbeaten, but do bear in mind that the emotional vulnerability that many pregnant women feel may mean that you cry very easily, even if it is the last thing you want to do. If you have strong preferences but worry that you won't be able to stand up for yourself, take along your partner for moral support. It will help to make a list of points you would like to discuss beforehand and rehearse them.

UNDERSTANDING YOUR NOTES

At your first antenatal visit you may be given your hospital notes to look after, although some units provide a "cooperation card" first, and give you your complete notes at 28 weeks. Your midwives or doctor, will record details here of routine tests and your pregnancy's progress, as well as any special tests.

The details may be difficult for you to understand as many of the medical terms are abbreviated. Compare the abbreviations on your notes with those explained below. If your notes still do not make sense, ask your midwife or doctor for an explanation.

Take your notes with you every time you go to the clinic. Ideally carry them at all times, so that if you need medical attention, all the information will be at hand. In addition, remember to take them with you to the hospital when you go into labour.

ABBREVIATIONS AND TERMS ON YOUR NOTES

NAD or nil or a tick *No abnormality detected*

Alb *Albumin in urine (a name for one of the proteins found in the urine sample)*

BP *Blood pressure*

FHH/NH *Fetal heart heard or not heard*

FH *Fetal heart*

FMF *Fetal movements felt*

Ceph. *Cephalic, baby is head down*

Vx *Vertex, baby is head down*

Br *Breech, baby is bottom down*

LMP *Last menstrual period*

EDD/EDC *Estimated date of delivery/confinement*

Hb *Haemoglobin levels to check for anaemia*

Eng/E Engaged *The baby's head has dropped down into the pelvis ready for birth*

NE *Not engaged*

Para 0 *Woman has had no other children*

Para 1 *(etc) Woman has had one or more children*

Fe *Iron has been prescribed*

TCA *To come again*

Height of fundus *The height of the top of the uterus. The baby pushes this up as it grows and often the height is used to estimate the length of the pregnancy. Some clinics measure the height of the fundus (from the top of the pubic bone to the top of the uterus) with a tape measure in centimetres*

Relation of PP to brim *This is the brim of your pelvis. The presenting part (PP) of the baby to the brim in the later stages of your pregnancy will be the part in the cervix ready to be born*

PET *Pre-eclamptic toxaemia*

Oed *Oedema*

Long L *Longitudinal lie, the baby is parallel to your spine in the uterus*

RSA *Right sacrum anterior – the most common breech presentation*

AFP *Alpha-fetoprotein*

CS *Caesarean section*

H/T *Hypertension (high blood pressure)*

MSU *Midstream urine sample*

Primigravida *First pregnancy*

Multigravida *More than one pregnancy*

VE *Vaginal examination*

1/5–5/5 *Indicates extent of head engagement*

THE LIE OF YOUR BABY

Certain abbreviations describe how the baby is lying, and refer to where the back of the baby's head (occiput) is in relation to your body – on the right or left, to the front (anterior) or back (posterior). ROA, for example, means the back of his head is to the front on your right.

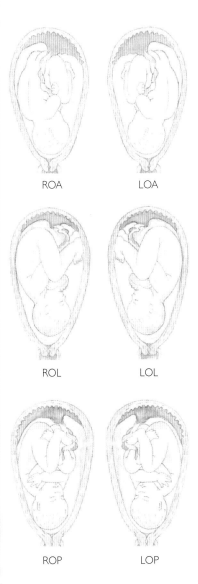

ROA   LOA

ROL   LOL

ROP   LOP

Routine checks

Every pregnant woman has routine checks to monitor her health and her baby's development. They may be performed on every visit, or at different times during her pregnancy. Some are performed only once. If the tests indicate that there is, or may be, a problem, you will be monitored closely and prompt action taken if necessary.

HEIGHT

Your height will be measured at your first visit. If you are petite, your midwife may suspect that you have a small pelvic inlet and outlet, both of which need to be assessed. (Shoe size was also once used as an initial indicator.) However, the chances are that your baby will be tailored to suit your particular physical build.

WEIGHT

Although this used to be noted at every visit, nowadays many units only weigh you at the booking clinic. In the first trimester a loss of weight usually reflects nausea and vomiting due to morning sickness and is usually nothing to worry about. Sudden weight gain may reflect fluid retention and indicate pre-eclampsia (see p.224). In the past, maternal weight gain was taken as a reliable indicator of the growth of the baby. Research now indicates, however, that maternal weight gain should not be relied upon on its own, but viewed in conjunction with external examination, blood and urinary tests, and especially ultrasound scans, which are much more accurate in measuring fetal growth.

LEGS AND HANDS

On every visit your legs will be checked for varicose veins, and your ankles and hands will be checked for swelling and puffiness (oedema). A little swelling in the final weeks of pregnancy is normal, particularly in the evening, but excessive puffiness may give an early warning of pre-eclampsia (see p.224).

BREASTS

Your breasts and nipples will be examined. A very few women have dimpled, or inverted, nipples, and these may have to be corrected by wearing a breastshield in your bra, although they do usually correct themselves in pregnancy.

YOUR BABY'S HEAD SIZE RELATIVE TO YOUR PELVIS

The shape and size of your pelvis is important because of the risk of disproportion, which could become apparent during labour and may delay the baby's delivery.

Disproportion means that your pelvis is too small for your baby's head to pass through it easily, or your baby's head is too large. To avoid delays in delivering your baby, it's important for your doctor or midwife to make an assessment of the size of your pelvic outlet. Your height is a good guide; short women tend to have small pelvises.

If difficulties are suspected, your pelvis will be examined by ultrasound (see p.180) and your baby's head size will also be determined. Severe disproportion will mean that your baby will be born by elective Caesarean section (see p.308).

Measuring your height
Potential problems may be indicated if you are very short in comparison to the average height for your racial type and build.

URINE

At your first visit you'll be asked for a sample of midstream urine to test for any underlying bladder or kidney infection. To collect a midstream sample, you'll be given a sterile pad to clean the vulva. Then you pass the first few drops of urine into the toilet bowl and then collecting a sample of the midstream urine in a sterile container. You then finish urinating into the toilet.

You'll be asked to bring a morning sample of urine to every subsequent visit which will be tested for urinary infection; for sugar, to check that you are not developing diabetes; and for ketones, which are the classic sign that diabetes is established and needs urgent treatment (see p. 140). A rare cause of ketonuria is very severe vomiting in pregnancy, called hyperemesis gravidarum, which requires urgent hospitalization. Diabetes may disappear completely after this pregnancy but return in future pregnancies. A trace of protein in your urine in late pregnancy is a strong indication of pre-eclampsia. This will be investigated promptly because of the associated risks of miscarriage, a small-for-dates baby, and premature delivery (see p.298).

BLOOD TESTS

At your first antenatal visit, a routine blood sample will be taken, usually from a vein in your arm, to find out your basic blood group (A,B,O), and also your Rhesus (Rh) blood group (positive or negative), in case a blood transfusion becomes necessary. If you are Rh negative, you will be tested for Rhesus incompatibility with your baby (see p.202).

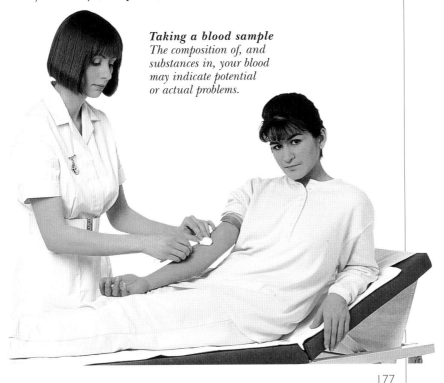

Taking a blood sample
The composition of, and substances in, your blood may indicate potential or actual problems.

177

FETAL HEARTBEAT

Your baby's heartbeat will be monitored at every visit from week 14. The baby's heartbeat is almost twice as fast as your own (approximately 140 beats per minute compared with 72 beats per minute), and sounds just like a tiny galloping horse.

Pinnard stethoscope The doctor or midwife may listen to your baby's heartbeat using a traditional ear trumpet known as a Pinnard stethoscope, although these are now rapidly falling out of use.

Sonicaid It is more likely, however, that they will use a sonicaid. This is a small portable instrument (about the size of a telephone) that is placed on your stomach and which uses ultrasound (see also p.180) to listen to the fetal heartbeat. The sonicaid magnifies the sound of your baby's heartbeat, so you can listen to it.

Electronic monitor If your baby is distressed for any reason, the heart rate dips. This occurs in labour during each contraction, and hospital staff will record the baby's progress using an electronic fetal monitor (see p.275).

Your haemoglobin level will also be measured. This is a measure of the oxygen-carrying power of your red blood cells. The normal level is between 12 and 14 grams; if it falls below 10 grams, treatment for anaemia will be given. Iron and folic acid raise the oxygen-carrying power of your blood, so it is essential that you make sure you are eating healthily (see p.128).

German measles (rubella) antibodies (see p.19) will be looked for, to see whether or not you are immune. Additionally, the presence of sexually transmitted diseases, such as syphilis, will be revealed. Certain genetic disorders such as sickle cell anaemia and thalassaemia (see pp.24 & 25) are detectable in blood. You may also have a special screening blood test to help rule out certain types of fetal abnormality.

You can ask also to have your blood tested for toxoplasmosis infection. The toxoplasma is a parasite that can be picked up from cat faeces and also from poorly cooked lamb or pork. Toxoplasmosis is harmless to adults, but it can cross the placenta and cause blindness, epilepsy, and developmental delay in the baby. You won't necessarily be offered this test unless you're thought to be at risk, so if you're worried – particularly if you have pets that hunt outside, ask for the test, as only about 20 percent of women in the UK are immune to the disease.

EXTERNAL EXAMINATION

At every visit your abdomen will be gently felt to determine the size of your growing baby. This gives a good idea of whether your baby is approximately the right size for your dates. Before the introduction of routine ultrasound scans, a series of measurements were taken over the course of your pregnancy to monitor your baby's rate of progress. Now, however, ultrasound scans at about 12 weeks and 22–24 weeks provide your doctor with an accurate picture of your baby's progress, and if there is any doubt you will be scanned more frequently (see p.180). After 26–28 weeks the doctor or midwife will also feel for your baby's "poles" (head and rump). This enables them to judge the lie of your baby (see p.175).

BLOOD PRESSURE

This reading is taken at every visit, and measures the pressure at which your heart is pumping blood through your body. The reading is made up of two numbers: the upper one is the systolic pressure – when the heart contracts it pushes out blood and "beats". This is measured when the arm band is tight. As the pressure is released, the lower, or diastolic, reading is made. This is the resting pressure between beats. The statistically average reading in pregnancy is 120 over 70, although blood pressure differs with age, and there is a range of blood pressures at one age that are considered normal. A higher reading than normal during pregnancy may indicate pre-eclampsia (see p.224) and bed rest in hospital may be advised. Constant checks ensure that changes are quickly noted.

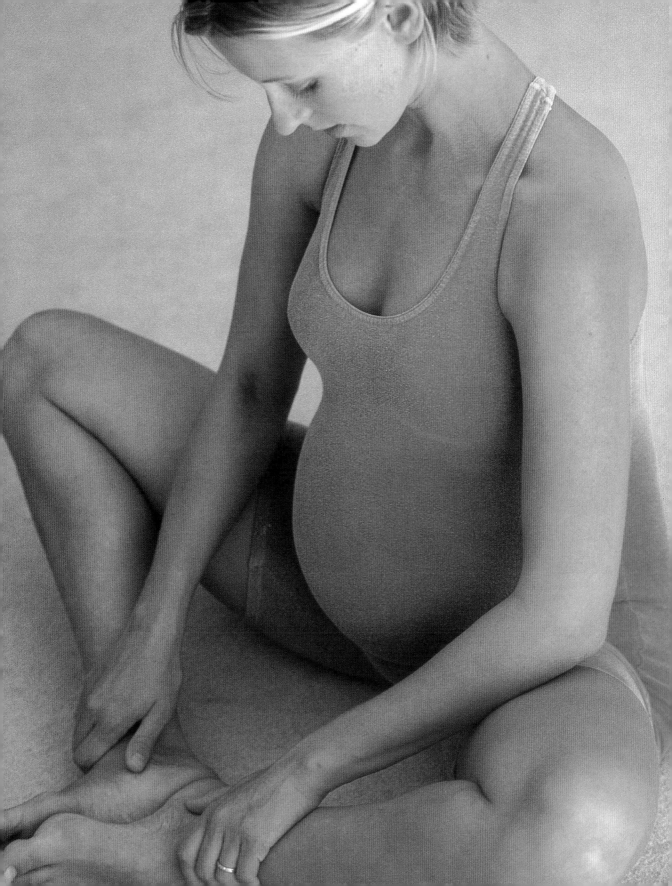

Ultrasound scan

Ultrasound is one of the most beneficial of medical technologies and is now used routinely in all antenatal care. Ultrasound scans are used to check the baby's general well-being and position, and guide doctors when performing special tests and operations. Most women will be offered two scans – the first at 11–13 weeks, to confirm dates and to screen for Down's syndrome (see p.184), and the second at 18–20 weeks. This scan (known as the anomaly scan) checks that the fetus is growing well. If any problems are detected, you may have several repeat scans up until the birth.

Ultrasound scans are done routinely to check that the fetus is developing normally, but certain situations and conditions may also necessitate extra scans. You may have extra scans:

• as part of infertility assessment

• to identify abdominal problems such as an ectopic pregnancy

• if the doctors suspect an imminent miscarriage

• to check for a multiple pregnancy.

HOW IT WORKS

The process is based on a sonar device that reveals objects in fluid, which was first used by the US Navy to detect submarines during World War II. A crystal, inside a device called a transducer, converts an electrical current into high frequency soundwaves, inaudible to the human ear. The soundwaves form a beam that penetrates the abdomen as the transducer is moved back and

HAVING A SCAN

An ultrasound scan is painless, and usually lasts for approximately 15 minutes. You will probably be asked to drink about a pint of water, and not urinate before arriving at the clinic. This may cause some discomfort, but a full bladder will provide a clearer picture of the fetus on the screen. At the clinic, you may be asked to remove your clothes and put on a hospital robe before lying on a bed beside the scanner. An oil or jelly, which acts as a conductor of the soundwaves, is rubbed on your abdomen, and the transducer is passed over this area in different directions. As the image appears on the screen you can just relax, and enjoy your first view of your baby.

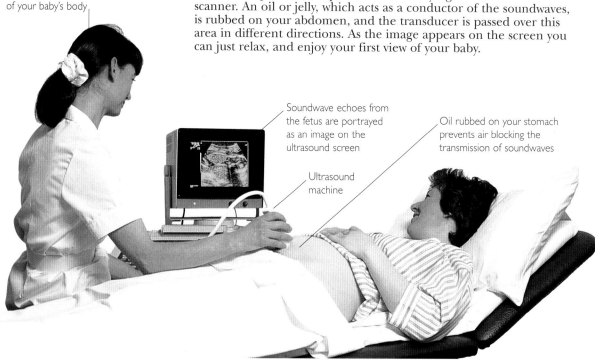

The operator will explain the image on the screen, identifying different parts of your baby's body

Soundwave echoes from the fetus are portrayed as an image on the ultrasound screen

Oil rubbed on your stomach prevents air blocking the transmission of soundwaves

Ultrasound machine

forth. The beam reflects off material in its path, and the transducer records these echoes. The echoes are converted into electrical signals, which produce an image that can be displayed on a visual monitor. The beam can only penetrate fluids and soft tissue such as the amniotic sac, kidneys, and liver. It cannot pass through bone, or register gas. An ultrasound scan is increasingly used to assess threatened miscarriage, exclude ectopic pregnancies, for infertility treatments, such as IVF, and for fetal surgery (see p.200).

YOUR FIRST SCAN

Like much else in the world of medical technology, ultrasound scanning equipment has been improved and refined over the years, and the technique is not intrusive. The scan offers an exciting opportunity for you and your partner to see your baby for the very first time.

You should be able to hear her heartbeat, and to distinguish the gentle movement of hands and feet, waving and kicking, as she floats in the amniotic fluid. Ask the ultrasound operator to explain the image on the screen as some details may be difficult to interpret. Some clinics offer you a print of the image of your baby as a memento to cherish, although there may be a charge.

IS IT SAFE?

Unlike an X-ray, ultrasound scanning poses no known risk to the fetus. Questions have been raised about long-term effects such as hearing impairment caused by the impact of soundwaves. However, recent research seems to indicate that ultrasound is not harmful to the mother or the baby, as the waves are of a very low intensity, and so it is safe for the scan to be performed repeatedly.

WHY YOUR BABY HAS IT DONE

A routine ultrasound scan will reveal if your baby is healthy, and may be used at different stages of your pregnancy for the following reasons:

• to check the baby's location and development of the placenta

• to check on growth rate of the baby, particularly when the date of conception is unknown

• to discover whether the baby is ready to be born if overdue

• to confirm your baby is in the usual head-down position, and not bottom-down, after week 38

• to detect certain fetal abnormalities, such as spina bifida

• to monitor the baby throughout special tests such as amniocentesis, and fetoscopy

• to assist in operations performed on the baby in the uterus.

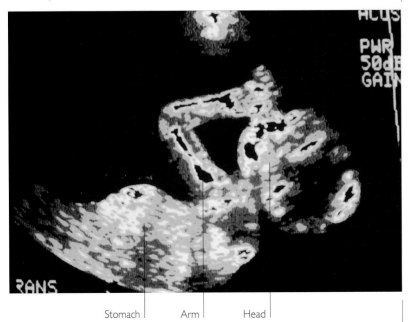

Stomach | Arm | Head

Baby at 22 weeks
An ultrasound scan will show clearly your baby's health, its position, and whether you are expecting more than one. This portrait shows the baby in its mother's uterus. The baby floats and moves about continuously in the amniotic sac performing various functions, sucking its thumb, yawning, blinking, and urinating.

Twins

Once they had got over the initial shock of finding out that they were expecting twins, Karen and Joe were delighted, if a little bit apprehensive. Their main concerns were initially for the well-being of Karen and the twins throughout the pregnancy, and how they would cope with the extra responsibilities that would follow the delivery of two babies.

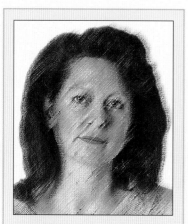

Name **Karen Phillips**

Age **36 years**

Past medical history
Nothing abnormal

Family history
No history of twins known

Obstetric history
Two previous pregnancies. Oedema in last month of both

Karen was diagnosed as expecting twins when she had an ultrasound scan at 14 weeks. She knew from the beginning that there was something different about this pregnancy as she was constantly sick in the first couple of months, which she hadn't been in her previous pregnancies. She also looked huge – at three months she looked about five! Consequently it wasn't a total surprise when her scan showed that she was carrying twins.

SUSPECTING A MULTIPLE PREGNANCY

Many women guess early on that there is something different about their pregnancies when they are carrying twins. Size is often the telling factor, as well as the shape – twins tend to push the abdomen out sideways as well as forwards. Twins can be diagnosed by week eight of the pregnancy using ultrasound scanning.

KAREN'S SPECIAL NEEDS

Some women sail through a twin pregnancy with very few or no side effects. Some do not. The stresses imposed by carrying two babies can intensify feelings of tiredness and sickness as your body adjusts. In addition, twin pregnancies need to be watched carefully for raised blood pressure, anaemia, oedema, and pre-eclampsia (see p.224). Like all expectant mothers of twins, Karen will visit her antenatal clinic more frequently than a woman expecting one baby. Her doctor will watch for the recurrence of oedema, and may hospitalize her if she seems likely to develop pre-eclampsia. A good, high-protein diet is essential.

Sheer size can be a problem in later pregnancy, and finding a comfortable position can be difficult. I told Karen that she might find that being in water helps as it reduces the effects of gravity. Gentle swimming would be fine as long as her doctor agrees. She might also consider hiring a birth pool (see **Addresses**, p.370) as an extra large bath in which she can relax. Making love is not usually prohibited, although Karen should follow her doctor's advice and consult him or her straight away if she has any discharge or bleeding or if she has contractions.

Women who are expecting twins and who do not rest, are much more likely to go into premature labour than those expecting twins who have had complete rest from the fifth month. All types of work during pregnancy, especially caring for young children, should not be too strenuous. I advised Karen to try and arrange childcare and extra help, and have at least three hours bedrest a day.

LABOUR AND TWINS

Labour is always managed in hospital because of the risks. As doctors and midwives are highly sensitive to the problems that can occur, 20 minutes is the most they will allow to elapse between births, and the second twin is always monitored closely for any signs of distress. An emergency Caesarean may be performed if a twin appears to be in danger.

WILL THEY BE IDENTICAL OR FRATERNAL?

A third of all twins are identical. They are always the same sex and usually share the placenta, although this depends on how late the egg splits. Half of fraternal twins are boy–girl pairs and half are same sex. Their placentas are separate, but may be fused together. The incidence of identical twins appears to be completely random, while fraternal twins often run in families, being inherited through the mother's side. There is no history of twins in Karen's family. However, the likelihood of having non-inherited, fraternal twins rises until a woman's mid-thirties then drops again, and seems to be higher if she is tall, well-built, and conceives easily.

The chances of having fraternal twins also appear to increase with each subsequent child.

IDENTICAL TWINS

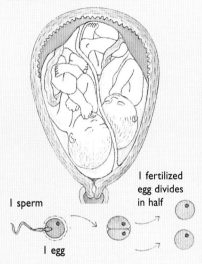

I sperm

I egg

I fertilized egg divides in half

FRATERNAL TWINS

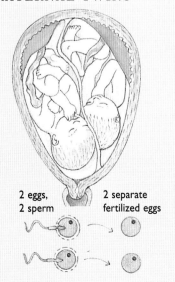

2 eggs, 2 sperm

2 separate fertilized eggs

Twins shown by ultrasound
Ultrasound scans can show if you are carrying two babies. Sometimes, however, one may be behind the other and not easily seen. If twins are still suspected despite only one being visible on the ultrasound, you will probably have another scan in 5–6 weeks' time.

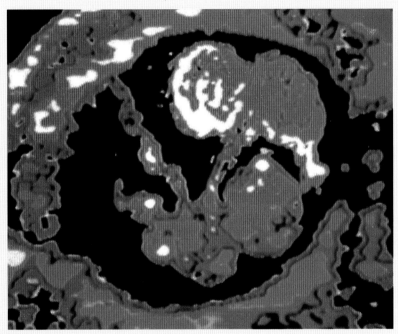

KAREN'S BABIES

A twin pregnancy and birth differs from those with a single baby (a singleton) in several important respects.

• Twins have a shorter gestation period compared with singletons – they are normally born at 37 weeks rather than 40 weeks. This is mostly due to the space restrictions in the mother's uterus, although other external factors are also important.

• Lower birthweights are caused by their shorter gestation period: twins weigh less than singletons.

• There are extra risks for the second-born: he or she has to go through the intense contractions of expulsion twice over. The second twin may also suffer from a diminished oxygen supply to the placenta because the uterus will start to contract once the first twin has been delivered.

Special tests

Antenatal care now includes a number of specialist screening and diagnostic tests that can be used to check for various complications or defects affecting the fetus. These tests can be reassuring to expectant parents if they can definitively rule out a genetic defect, such as cystic fibrosis, or they may provide you with information that makes you question whether your pregnancy should proceed. Since information like this can put enormous emotional strain on parents-to-be, it is essential that you have full discussions with your doctor about the risks of undergoing the tests and the implications of their results.

SCREENING TESTS

There are a number of tests now which are offered in most maternity units to screen mothers for a variety of possible fetal abnormalities. These tests do not tell you for certain that there is a problem. However if the test indicates that there is a high probability, you will be offered a diagnostic test to confirm or rule out the particular problem.

Nuchal scan The risk of having a Down's syndrome baby can be assessed around 11–13 weeks using a special ultrasound scan called a nuchal scan. ("Nuchal" means neck.) A shadow of a particular size and shape that is present at the back of the fetus' neck may indicate a higher risk of chromosome defects such as Down's syndrome if it is thicker than normal in relation to the age of the mother. In this case, amniocentesis will be offered to confirm the diagnosis. Many centres now only carry out amniocentesis after a nuchal scan has been done.

Serum screening (Bart's or triple test) This is a test that was developed by St. Bartholomew's Hospital in London. A sample of the pregnant mother's blood is taken at 16 weeks to measure the levels of three substances – oestriol, human chorionic gonadotrophin, and alpha-fetoprotein. The results can be assessed in relation to your age to predict the chance of your baby suffering from Down's syndrome. If the chances seem high (more than 1 in 250), amniocentesis will be offered. The Bart's triple test is not yet offered automatically at all centres, although you can request it.

AFP test Alpha-fetoprotein is found in varying amounts in your blood throughout pregnancy. Between 16 and 18 weeks the levels are usually low, so if a blood test is performed at this time and the levels are 2–3 times higher than the average of a sample group, it may indicate a neurological problem such as spina bifida or hydrocephalus. However, these problems are nearly always diagnosed with greater accuracy by ultrasound (see p.180), and the AFP test is being used less frequently. An abnormally low level of alphafetoprotein suggests that the fetus may have Down's syndrome (see p.24) and amniocentesis would be offered. However, the nuchal scan has superseded AFP testing in many units as a screening test for Down's syndrome (see opposite).

DIAGNOSTIC TESTS

These tests are used to confirm abnormalities in the fetus, and are generally only offered after screening tests or ultrasound scans have indicated that you have a high risk. The main diagnostic tests are amniocentesis and chorionic villus sampling (CVS). Amniocentesis is the most common diagnostic test; CVS is only offered in a few centres, and carries a higher risk of miscarriage. You need to think very carefully about the implications of having these tests and discuss it as a couple and with your doctor. Ask for specialist counselling if you think you may need it (see column, right).

AMNIOCENTESIS

Amniotic fluid contains cells from the baby's skin and other organs which can be used to diagnose his condition. Amniocentesis is the name given to the procedure that withdraws this fluid from the uterus.

Why it is done You will probably be offered an amniocentesis if you are over the age of 37, as the risk of chromosomal abnormalities (such as Down's syndrome) increases with age (see sidebar, right). You may also be offered it after serum screening (Bart's test), or if a nuchal scan indicated a risk of Down's syndrome (see opposite). In addition, amniocentesis can reveal other important information which may be sometimes helpful in determining the care and progress of your pregnancy.

What it can reveal Where there is cause for concern, the test may show the following:

• The sex of the baby: cells sloughed off by the fetus accumulate in the amniotic fluid. Under the microscope, male cells can be distinguished from female cells and the baby's sex ascertained. In gender-linked genetically linked disorders such as haemophilia, a male child will have a 50 percent chance of being affected

• The age of the fetus: if the lecithin/sphingomyelin (L/S) ratio in the fluid is measured, the maturity of the lungs can be assessed, which is in itself an indication of fetal age. However, this is rarely done now.

• The chemical composition of the fluid: this can reveal metabolic disorders caused by missing or defective enzymes

• The bilirubin content of the fluid: this helps to determine if a Rhesus-positive baby needs an intrauterine transfusion

THE EFFECT OF YOUR AGE

Your age is important but it's just one of several factors that can affect the outcome of your pregnancy. Your nutrition is much more important.

If your general health is good, your pregnancy will not be treated any differently from younger women. However, age is a factor in certain fetal abnormalities, and your have a higher risk of maternal diabetes and placental insufficiency, so you may be screened for these more frequently.

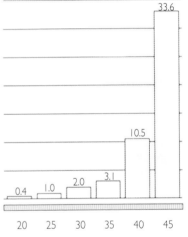

Down's syndrome and your age
Maternal age seems to be an important factor in why Down's syndrome occurs. As you can see from the graph, the risk of having a baby with this condition rises with advancing maternal age, but isn't really significant until after 35 years of age. However, as a Down's baby is born every 2,000 births, and as most babies are born to women under 35 who don't undergo screening for Down's syndrome, there are more Down's babies in the pre-35 age group than in the post-35 age group.

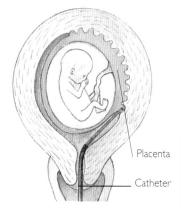

Chorionic sampling
A small amount of chorion (placental tissue) is withdrawn from the uterus through the cervix with the aid of a catheter.

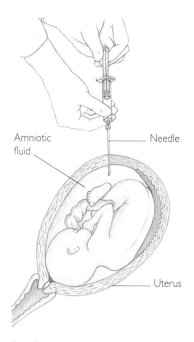

Amniocentesis
Amniotic fluid is extracted only after an ultrasound scan has determined the position of the fetus and the placenta. Using ultrasound, the doctor will pass a needle through the abdominal wall, which has been numbed with local anaesthetic, and into the uterus. A small amount of amniotic fluid is withdrawn.

• The amount of oxygen the baby is getting: gases dissolved in the amniotic fluid can be measured, revealing whether the baby is at risk from lack of oxygen

• The acidity of the fluid: this is another indication of fetal distress often caused by inadequate oxygen flow to the fetus

• The chromosome count: determined by examining discarded cells. Any deviation from the normal chromosomal structure usually means that the baby may have a disability

How is it done? Amniocentesis is usually performed at 16–18 weeks. The mother's abdomen is first numbed with a local anaesthetic. Then, guided by ultrasound, a hollow needle is inserted into the amniotic sac through the front of the abdominal wall. About 14 grams (half an ounce) of amniotic fluid is usually withdrawn and this is then spun in a centrifuge to separate the cells shed by the baby from the rest of the liquid. It takes about three weeks for the cells to be cultured and for the results to come through, which is a very stressful period for couples. Many women talk about putting their pregnancies "on hold" during this time, until the results confirm that the fetus is unaffected.

Amniocentesis is only undertaken with ultrasound monitoring to guide the needle into the amniotic sac, so that neither the placenta nor the fetus is harmed. The risk of the procedure inducing a miscarriage in early pregnancy is small – about one in 200. It has also been suggested that there may be a very small risk (less than 1 percent) of respiratory difficulties in babies after amniocentesis.

CHORIONIC VILLUS SAMPLING (CVS)

Chorionic villi, finger-like outgrowths on the edge of the chorion, are genetically identical to the fetus. They develop earlier than amniotic fluid, so examining a sample of chorionic villi provides valuable information about your baby's genes and chromosomes before amniocentesis is possible. However, CVS is only available at a few specialist centres, and is not as common as amniocentesis.

What it can reveal The most important group of mothers needing CVS are those at risk of having a Down's syndrome baby. An abnormality of haemoglobin, such as sickle-cell disease or thalassaemia, can also be diagnosed with CVS. Inborn errors of metabolism are fortunately rare, but if a family is afflicted, the incidence may be as high as one in four. The basic defect is an enzyme deficiency, and direct enzyme analysis on the chorionic tissue gives a diagnosis within two days. Single gene disorders, such as cystic fibrosis, haemophilia, Huntington's chorea, and muscular dystrophy, can be detected with the use of CVS.

How is it done? CVS is also carried out under ultrasound control, usually between 10 and 12 weeks of pregnancy, before the amniotic sac completely fills the uterine cavity. Two routes are employed, the trans-cervical route and the trans-abdominal route. For the former route, the cervix is first examined using a speculum. A plastic or metal catheter is then introduced through the cervical canal, across the uterine cavity, and then into the outside edge of the placenta. A small amount of chorionic villi tissue is then removed for analysis. The latter procedure follows that of amniocentesis, but with a sample being taken of the placental tissue rather than of the amniotic fluid. The risk of miscarriage following CVS is about 1 percent higher than the spontaneous miscarriage rate (see p.218). The advantage of CVS is that it gives an initial result within 24–48 hours, with full results in about a week.

UMBILICAL VEIN SAMPLING (CORDOCENTESIS)

This procedure is used to examine the constituents of fetal blood. and, in the case of fetal anaemia, for intrauterine blood transfusion. It is vital in four other situations.

Infection detection Rubella, toxoplasmosis, and the herpes virus may be detected by performing a specific radio analysis of certain proteins that are present in the blood of the fetus.

Rhesus iso-immunization In cases of Rhesus incompatibility (see p.202) the direct assessment of fetal haemoglobin is the best way to determine the severity of blood-cell destruction and whether an intrauterine blood transfusion (also done through the umbilical vein) needs to be carried out.

Suspected growth retardation If the fetus is considered to be growth-retarded, cordocentesis will reveal the acidity or alkalinity of the blood, the amount of oxygen, the amount of carbon dioxide, and the amount of bicarbonate in the blood. In addition, plasma levels of glucose can be estimated.

How is it done? Under ultrasonic control, a hollow needle is passed through the front wall of the abdomen and uterus into a blood vessel in the umbilical cord, about one centimetre from where it emerges from the placenta. A small quantity of blood can then be removed for testing. The risk to the fetus appears to be about 1–2 percent. In theory, cordocentesis can replace any investigation currently undertaken on a blood sample.

DOPPLER SCAN

This is a special scan, only available at a few centres. The Doppler scan looks at the flow of blood in the fetus or in the placenta. It is used when a fetus is small for dates or seems to not be growing as fast as it should. It uses a slightly different sort of soundwave from a normal ultrasound scan, which bounces off moving red blood cells, and indicates how fast they are moving through the fetus's blood vessels.

Testing for abnormalities

Modern technology has enabled doctors to investigate the health of the fetus before birth at earlier and earlier points. Like Daniella, most pregnant women are now offered routine screening tests, sometimes leading to much more invasive diagnostic tests for confirmation with little discussion of the implications.

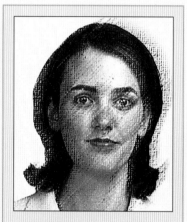

Name **Daniella Stamp**

Age **26 years**

Past medical history
Nothing abnormal

Family history
Nothing of note

Obstetric history **Dysmenorrhoea (very painful periods)**

Daniella and her partner Will had decided to try for a baby after he had secured a good promotion at work, which meant they could afford to move into a bigger house. Daniella was particularly keen to have her babies while she was young and fit. After Daniella had missed two periods and when a home pregnancy test proved positive, she and Will visited their family doctor who referred them to the antenatal clinic at the local city hospital. They both found this visit impersonal and quite off-putting.

WHEN SCREENING IS OFFERED

Without explanation, Daniella and Will were given a list of routine screening tests that would be performed as Daniella's pregnancy progressed. As a young, healthy first-time mother, Daniella hadn't expected to be screened for fetal abnormalities, and they both found the idea frightening. It set them off thinking about the implications of screening tests. They're both keen on a natural birth and resistant to the technological approach they met at the hospital. Daniella wants a minimum of medical interference at her birth. They would have preferred to have the baby at home, if at all possible, but their doctor advised them to go for a hospital delivery as this was her first pregnancy.

Routine screening tests

They were told that Daniella would start having tests to screen for abnormalities in her baby at 11–12 weeks with the first ultrasound scan. Then at 15–16 weeks, a blood test (known as the Triple test or Bart's test) would be taken to look for Down's syndrome, spina bifida, and hydrocephalus. At 16–20 weeks, she'd have her second ultrasound scan, possibly followed by an amniocentesis (a diagnostic test) if either screening test suggested a risk of abnormality in her baby.

Daniella is completely confused. She doesn't understand the difference between a screening test and a diagnostic test, and she doesn't really understand why they are necessary.

Screening and probability

I told Daniella that a screening test is by definition a blunt instrument. It doesn't give any precise information. It can do no more than pick up a tendency for something to happen. The way doctors express this tendency is in terms of probability.

So if a blood test gives a one in 150 probability (chance) of the baby having Down's syndrome, it means that if Daniella had 150 babies, one of them would have Down's. By any criteria this is a very small risk, but as Daniella says, any risk of Down's syndrome seems a big risk to her. Like all mothers, she wants the test to come back entirely negative. As I point out, on the scale of probability, one in 150 is exceedingly low. There would be little cause for concern until the risk rose to say, one in 30. But these days any result higher than one in 250 means that Daniella will be offered more tests. The next step would be a precise diagnostic test to detect a specific abnormality. This is normally only done if a screening test is positive.

Diagnostic tests

Such tests are precise enough to give the answer "yes" or "no"; "present" or "absent"; "normal" or "abnormal". Unfortunately, they are quite invasive, and the most widely used, amniocentesis (see p.185), involves a specimen of amniotic fluid containing cells from the baby being drawn out of the uterus – a delicate operation requiring skilled guidance with ultrasound. The cells are then examined for chromosomal or genetic damage in a specialist laboratory. I told Daniella that amniocentesis itself also carries a risk of miscarriage of about two in 100 (two percent).

At this point Daniella asked the right question: "How long do you wait for the result?" In most centres, even the best, it's a three week wait. Daniella was upset. She said she'd be wracked with fear in half that time. I can only agree. It's brutal and inhumane to make a pregnant mother wait three weeks to find out if she's carrying a normal baby, especially as she may be feeling her baby move by the time the result comes through, as amniocentesis is usually done at around 16–18 weeks. "And what if the amniocentesis confirms Down's?", Daniella asked. The blunt answer is: "You'd be counselled about whether to terminate the pregnancy."

Other types of tests

Daniella is feeling more and more distraught. She had never considered the possibility of

termination. Her dilemma might be eased with a nuchal scan, done as early as 11 weeks, which would alert her and Will to the possibility of a chromosome defect in her baby. This would be followed immediately with a diagnostic test, such as chorionic villus sampling or CVS (see p.186), another rather invasive test, but one which can be done much earlier in pregnancy and from which results can be obtained in as little as three days. CVS is only available in specialist centres, of which the hospital to which Daniella had been referred is one. Like amniocentesis, CVS carries a small risk of miscarriage. However, I could see Daniella was getting confused so I gave her the checklist below to help.

What happens if an abnormality is found

The thought of terminating their pregnancy is an enormous shock. Will and Daniella feel the very idea of aborting their baby is

unthinkable, whether or not tests reveal that their baby is normal. They are certain that they will continue with the pregnancy irrespective of test results. What's more, they are unshakeable in their desire to love and nurture their baby, whether or not he or she has a disability.

Their determination to take care of the baby they've created raises the question of whether they should have any screening tests at all, in that the results wouldn't change anything. They also need to weigh up the risks to the pregnancy of allowing diagnostic tests to go ahead when the chances are high that the pregnancy is perfectly healthy given Daniella's age.

Screening tests aren't compulsory, they're optional, so I suggest Will and Daniella request an interview with the obstetrician in charge of the antenatal clinic to discuss their position, before they make a final decision to forego all tests.

CHECKLIST OF SPECIALIST TESTS

Screening tests

• Nuchal scan: a fairly new non-invasive screening scan carried out at 1–13 weeks that screens for high risks of chromosomal defects (see p.184)

• Triple (or Bart's) test: A sample of the mother's blood at 15–16 weeks screens for hormone levels that indicate a higher risk of Down's syndrome (see p.184)

• AFP Test: A blood test at 15–16 weeks screens alphafetoprotein levels, which may show a risk of Down's syndrome or spina bifida

Diagnostic tests

• Chorionic villus sampling: cells from the developing placenta are examined at 11–13 weeks to check the baby for chromosomal abnormalities (see p.186)

• Amniocentesis: fetal cells from the amniotic fluid are removed at about 18 weeks and checked for chromosomal abnormalities such as Down's syndrome (see p.185)

• Cordocentesis: a test where fetal blood from the umbilical cord is tested for abnormal chromosomes or infection (see p.187)

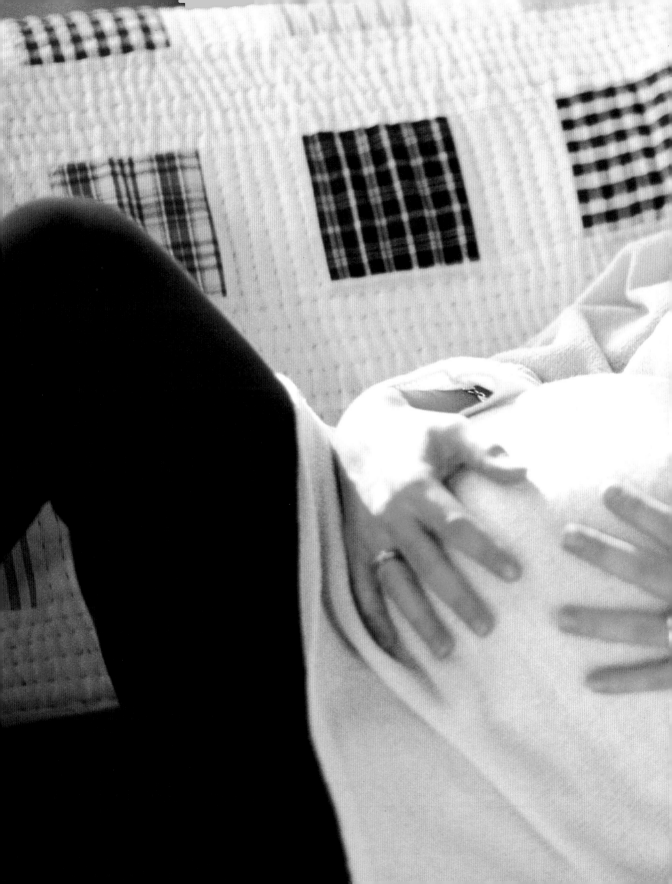

CHAPTER 8

Caring for your UNBORN BABY

By being observant and aware, you and your partner can be in touch with your unborn baby throughout pregnancy. Your baby can hear you talk and sing, and can feel you touch him through your abdominal wall. And while not all babies have the friendliest of uterine environments or develop normally, modern medical techniques mean that even these babies have the best possible chance.

Communication can begin early on. What you say, do, think, or experience, and the way you move may be transmitted to your baby.

Talk and sing Get in the habit of talking out loud to your baby, and singing to her, when possible. Some children have recognized lullabies played to them while in the uterus.

Touching Stroking your baby through your abdominal wall is another way of keeping in touch and will usually quieten her. This may continue after she is born. In the final months you may be able to distinguish her foot or hand through your skin.

Thinking Be aware of your baby. Think positive, happy thoughts about her. If you are upset about something, don't shut her out.

Moving Try to move in a relaxed manner whenever you can. The gentle movement of your uterus as you walk soothes her. Rocking and swinging will remain a favourite relaxing activity after she is born.

Feeling When you feel happy and excited, so does your baby. When you feel depressed, so does she – so reassure her that you still love her. Share feelings with her consciously.

In touch with your baby

A constant awareness of your unborn baby is a first stage in bonding with her and ensuring a good future relationship. Keeping in touch means you will be aware of what's best for your baby's physical and emotional health.

WHAT YOUR BABY EXPERIENCES

While she is still in your uterus, your baby feels, hears, sees, tastes, responds, and even learns and remembers. She is not, contrary to decades of medical opinion, an inert, unformed, blank personality. She has firm likes and dislikes. She enjoys soothing voices, simple music with a single melody line (lullabies, flute music), rhythmic movements, and feeling you stroke her through your abdomen. Her dislikes include strident voices; music with an insistent beat (hard rock); strong, flashing lights; rapid, jerky movements; and being cramped by you sitting or lying in an awkward position.

Sight Although your baby is shielded by the walls of your uterus and abdomen, light that is sufficiently strong can get through to her; for instance, she can detect sunlight if you are sunbathing. What she sees is probably just a reddish glow, but from about the fourth month, she will respond to it, usually by turning away if it is too bright. The limits of her sight at birth (she will be able to see faces within 30 centimetres of her own) may be a consequence of the parameters of her "home" before she was born.

Sound Your baby's sense of hearing develops at about the third month, and by midterm she is able to respond to sounds from the outside world (see above). The amniotic fluid in which she is suspended conducts sound well, although what she hears will be muffled in the same way that sounds are when you are under water. She is also able to distinguish the emotional tone of voices and moves her body in rhythm to your speech, so she will be soothed if you use a soft, reassuring tone.

The sound of your heartbeat is a continual presence in her world and this seems to be something that will leave a profound influence on her. One study found that when newborn babies were played a tape of maternal heart sounds, they gained more weight and slept better than a control group who did not hear the tape.

A MOTHER'S INFLUENCE

The unborn baby first experiences the world through her mother. Your baby experiences not only external stimuli (see above), but also your feelings, because our different emotions trigger the release of certain chemicals into our bloodstream – anger releases adrenalin, fear releases cholamines, elation releases endorphins. These chemicals pass across the placenta to your baby within seconds of you experiencing that particular emotion.

Babies dislike being exposed to prolonged levels of negative maternal emotions, such as anger, anxiety, or fear. However, short periods of intense anxiety or anger (caused by a child gone missing or an argument with your partner, for example), do not appear to have any long-term negative effect on your unborn child. In fact, they may even be beneficial as they may help her to begin to develop the ability to cope with future stressful situations. On the other hand, research indicates that long-term festering anger or anxiety, such as you might experience in an unsatisfactory, unsupportive relationship or poor social conditions, can have detrimental effects on your baby. These effects appear to include a problematic birth, a low birthweight, being a colicky baby, and future learning problems. However, studies have found that long-term negative maternal emotions appear to have far less effect on the baby if the mother feels generally happy and positive about being pregnant and doesn't shut out her unborn child.

A FATHER'S INFLUENCE

As the expectant father, you are the second most important factor in your unborn baby's life. Your attitude towards your partner, the pregnancy, and your child is crucial. If you are happy and looking forward to your newborn, your partner is much more likely to be happy and to enjoy her pregnancy. This, in turn, means that your baby is much more likely to be a happy, contented, healthy child. In addition, you should talk directly to your unborn baby as often as possible because research has shown that newborn babies can recognize the voices of their mothers and their fathers.

WHAT YOUR BABY DOES

There are a variety of ways in which your unborn baby interacts with her world.

Movement She moves constantly while she is awake. She will kick and wriggle her body in response to external stimuli, such as if you sit in a position that she finds uncomfortable.

Hearing From the sixth month your baby begins to respond to external sounds. She moves her body and limbs in rhythm to your voice. She may jump and kick when you raise your voice.

Seeing She dislikes bright light, especially if it flashes, and will move away, put her hands up to her face, or become agitated.

Feelings She will experience changes in mood to match yours when the chemicals your emotions release into your bloodstream cross the placenta into her body.

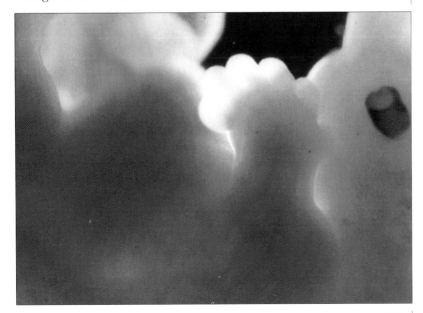

Her secure world
If she finds the world she experiences through you a reassuring place, she is likely to develop a generally trusting, positive personality. If she finds the uterus stressful she may develop a generally anxious approach to life.

SENSING THE MOVEMENTS

When you begin to feel your baby's movements, it is because they are being transmitted through the wall of the uterus to the sensitive nerve endings in your abdominal wall.

The reason you do not feel any of your baby's movements until several weeks after they actually begin is partly because they are very weak at first, and partly because the uterus does not transmit them. Only when it has grown sufficiently to touch your abdominal wall, will any movements within it be felt.

If your baby kicks or squirms more than she usually does, sit down in a comfortable, quiet place and try to calm her. Playing her gentle, relaxing music, singing her a lullaby, or humming to her are often very effective, partly because the sound will be pleasant to her and partly because you will become more relaxed and she will tend to do the same. Reading to her, or just talking, is also soothing, as is gently stroking your stomach.

Your baby's movements

For most pregnant women, the first awareness of movement within the uterus is exciting, tangible proof that the baby actually exists. Even though you may already have had an ultrasound scan which showed your baby moving about in the womb, it can seem unreal until you can actually feel it for yourself. If you are a first-time mother, you will probably begin to notice the movements of your baby within your uterus at about 18–20 weeks, but if you already have had a child, the first movements may be apparent at 16–18 weeks or even before. This is because the earliest noticeable movements of the baby – the "quickening" – produce a delicate sensation that has been likened to the fluttering of wings or the darting movements of fish. This feeling is easily mistaken for indigestion, wind, or hunger pangs, but the experienced mother knows what to expect, and is usually adept at identifying these sensations as movements of her baby.

WHY YOUR BABY MOVES

Your baby continually stretches and flexes her limbs as they develop. This activity, vital for the proper development of her muscles, starts at around the eighth week, when she begins making very tiny movements of her spine. At that stage, and for several weeks to come, her movements will go unnoticed, but by about the end of the sixteenth week, the vigorous movements of the now fully formed limbs may occasionally be felt, although you might not recognize them for what they are.

Your baby's movements – which include kicking, pushing, punching, squirming, and turning somersaults – can often be seen as well as felt. They will steadily increase as she grows, reaching their maximum between weeks 30 and 32. The typical baby averages 200 movements per day at week 20, rising to 375 per day at week 32, but the number of movements per day can range from 100 to about 700 over a period of several days. After week 32, your baby's movements become steadily more restricted as she grows to fill the uterus. Although restricted, she will still be able to give plenty of sharp kicks. When her engaged head bounces on your pelvic floor muscles, you will feel a jolt.

Changing position and emotional reactions Your baby will move about in your uterus for reasons other than the need to exercise and coordinate her growing muscles.

If you feel her moving she may, for instance, be shifting her position because she feels like a change, or because you are sitting or lying in a position that causes her discomfort. Or she may be trying to relocate the thumb that she had been happily sucking before she decided on a change of position.

However, she may also be moving about in response to your emotions. Hormones, such as adrenalin, are released into your bloodstream when you are physically or emotionally stimulated.

Pleasure, excitement, anger, stress, anxiety, or fear also stimulate the production of chemicals that will pass across the placenta and into your baby's bloodstream. These hormones make your baby react in a way that corresponds to your emotions, so if you get angry or very anxious, she may become agitated and start kicking and squirming. If you can, sit down in a quiet place and practise your relaxation techniques (see p.258). This will help to calm both you and your baby.

COUNTING THE KICKS

Just like the rest of us, your baby will feel and be more active on some days than on others, but her daily pattern of movements will become more consistent after about week 28. From then on you can monitor your baby's movements. On average, most women can feel around nine out of every ten of their baby's movements, although for some women the proportion is only six out of every ten. Whether you feel a movement or not depends on its direction and strength, and the position your baby is in when she makes it. For instance, if she is facing and kicking in towards your spine, you will not feel the sort of short, sharp jab that you will get if she kicks out towards your belly or up towards your ribs.

FETAL MOVEMENT RECORDING

There are several ways of counting fetal movements, and your antenatal clinic may give you their own "kick chart" to fill in. However, you can easily create your own "count-to-ten" kick chart like the one shown (right), which is drawn up on a piece of squared paper. You can use this to record your baby's movements during the final months of your pregnancy.

Making a kick chart Down the left of the chart, mark out a 12-hour period during which you will count the number of movements, from 9 a.m. to 9 p.m., and mark in the days and weeks across the top, with a column of squares for each day of the week. Each day, starting at 9 a.m., count the number of fetal movements until they reach ten, and then mark the time of the tenth movement on your chart. For example, if you started on the Monday of the 29th week of pregnancy, and you counted ten movements by quarter to three in the afternoon, fill in the 2.30 square. You wouldn't have to continue counting on that day, but would start again at 9 a.m. on Tuesday 17th June. However, if the number of movements is less than ten by 9 p.m., fill in the actual number in the space given at the bottom on the chart.

If you notice any significant change in your baby's movements as term approaches advise your doctor without delay. If you feel less than ten movements for two days in a row, contact your doctor or the hospital. If you don't feel any movements at all in one day, contact your doctor or the hospital immediately. Even if your baby's movements seem to have ceased altogether, don't panic. Your doctor can quickly assess your baby with ultrasound and electronic fetal monitoring and decide whether any intervention is necessary.

KICK CHART

Time	39th week							40th week						
	M	T	W	T	F	S	S	M	T	W	T	F	S	S
9am														
9.30														
10am														
10.30														
11am														
11.30														
12pm														
12.30														
1pm														
1.30														
2pm														
2.30														
3pm														
3.30														
4pm														
4.30														
5pm														
5.30														
6pm														
6.30														
7pm														
7.30														
8pm														
8.30														
9pm														

If less than ten movements by 9 p.m., record total number here.

9														
8														
7														
6														
5														
4														
3														
2														
1														

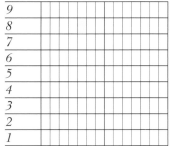

Monitoring fetal movements
This is a useful way of checking your baby's well-being, especially if you are overdue. Only you can tell if your baby is moving in a way normal for her; if there is a significant drop in the number of her movements, contact your doctor, midwife, or the hospital.

NEONATAL HEART SCANS

Congenital heart disease is diagnosed in a number of ways, such as by the use of chest X-rays or by a form of ultrasound scan called echocardiography.

A congenital heart condition, such as ventricular septal defect (hole in the heart – see main text) sometimes isn't detected until the baby is about 4 weeks old. Both chest X-rays and echocardiograms are used to confirm the diagnosis and to give an indication of the extent of the problem, so that the appropriate treatment can be given.

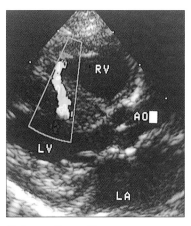

Echocardiography
The above shows a baby's heart that has a ventricular septal defect. Echocardiograms are taken by an ultrasound scan and displayed as a series of lines on the screen. By using colour-enhancement, the flow through the defect is shown up as red. The abbreviations used are: Ao = aorta (main artery); RV = right ventricle (pumping chamber that pumps blood into the lungs to be oxygenated); LA = left atrium (collecting chamber that collects reoxygenated blood from the lungs); LV = left ventricle (pumps reoxygenated blood back to the body).

Fetal problems

I am aware that this subject is an emotive one that may cause you to worry. However, I cannot stress strongly enough that fetal handicaps are extremely rare, so please try not to be too anxious. The cause of many fetal defects is still unknown. Some are genetically determined (see p.24) while others may be due to the adverse effects of drugs, radiation, fetal infections, or metabolic disturbances.

The types of malformations that may occur are numerous and varied, although most are very rare. The fetal tissues that are most actively growing at the time when the adverse factor operates are the most likely to show the defect. Some malformations are incompatible with life, and no treatment is possible. The defects that are especially important to recognize just after birth are those that endanger life but, with prompt intervention, can be treated very successfully. An increasing number of problems are now recognized before birth by ultrasound scan (see p.180) and many can be treated just after birth or later in infancy.

Imperforate anus This is when the anus is sealed, either because of a thin membrane of skin over the anal opening or because the anal canal that links the rectum with the anus has not developed. The rectal pouch may be connected to the vagina, urethra, or bladder, and so the baby must be referred for surgical treatment at once. Although rare, this condition is carefully looked for at every birth, and is treated immediately if found.

Umbilical hernia The gap in the muscle sheath in your baby's abdominal cavity, where the umbilical cord entered his or her abdomen, normally closes up in time. Sometimes, however, a soft swelling called an umbilical hernia forms when the abdominal contents bulge through this weak spot in the abdomen. In most cases the hernia eventually disappears, although a few will require surgical treatment later in childhood.

Congenital heart disease The most common form of congenital heart disease is ventricular septal defect (hole in the heart). In this disease there is a hole in the septum, the thin dividing wall between the right and left ventricles (pumping chambers) of the heart, and so the ventricles are connected instead of being divided. It does not usually produce symptoms or signs in a newborn baby, because it may take as long as four weeks for the blood vessels in the lungs to relax sufficiently to allow pressure differences to develop between the ventricles. Consequently, there may not be an appreciable left-to-right shunt of blood through the hole for a month or so, and symptoms will be absent.

Symptoms to look for are a bluish tinge to the skin especially round the mouth, floppiness, and breathlessness. One of the first signs may be breathlessness while feeding. An operation is not always required because the hole may seal spontaneously.

Congenital dislocation of the hip Dislocation of the hip happens when the ball at the head of the thighbone does not fit snugly into the socket of the hip joint. In the newborn infant this is a potential, rather than an actual, problem. It is much commoner in girls.

As part of the routine examination of newborn babies (see p.293), the hips are examined for excessive mobility, or for a characteristic "clunk" felt when the legs are spread apart and the thighs are flexed. Orthopaedic advice must be sought if there is any doubt, and early follow-up and treatment such as manipulation and splinting may prevent trouble in later infancy, although an operation may be required in severe cases.

Spina bifida This is the name given to the condition when the vertebral bones of the spine do not fuse so that the meninges (the coverings of the brain and spinal cord) bulge through at some level in the spinal column. The area may be covered with skin, or only by a bluish membrane. It may contain nerve roots, or the spinal cord itself may be exposed. In many cases, the place where the bones of the vertebrae are not fused is covered with skin and is only marked by a small, dark, hairy mole. The incidence of spina bifida is fortunately decreasing, probably due to careful monitoring of those more at risk and better knowledge of the importance of folic acid in preconception and the early weeks of pregnancy (see p.20).

The absence of the various coverings that normally protect the cord means that meningeal infection can occur very easily, but this can be prevented by immediate surgery to cover the defect. Spina bifida can be detected by ultrasound and babies with a good prognosis can be sent to a special centre where appropriate surgery can be performed without delay. However, the overall prognosis is poor for babies with severe defects. Problems may include complete paralysis of the legs, incontinence of urine and faeces, mental retardation, and the appearance of hydrocephalus (see below).

Hydrocephalus (water on the brain) In hydrocephalus there is an excessive amount of cerebrospinal fluid within the skull. It often occurs with other neurological defects such as spina bifida and it is caused by restricted circulation of cerebrospinal fluid in the brain. It is most common following brain haemorrhage in the preterm baby. The head swells, and soft tissues between the skull bones and the fontanelles become wide and bulging. The condition may be present before birth owing to congenital malformations, and will obstruct labour, or the baby's head may enlarge excessively after birth. If hydrocephalus is suspected before birth, frequent ultrasound checks are performed, and the head circumference is measured every two or three days. If the rate of growth is much faster than normal, a neurosurgical

CLEFT LIP AND CLEFT PALATE

These conditions are due to the incomplete development of the upper lip or of the palate or, in some cases, both.

A cleft lip, sometimes known as a harelip, occurs when the halves of the upper lip fail to join properly during fetal development. Similarly, a cleft palate is the result of the halves of the fetal palate failing to join.

These defects can cause surprisingly little difficulty in feeding – breastfeeding can often be successfully achieved but bottlefeeding may be more difficult, and it may be necessary to resort to cup and spoon. Care is necessary when feeding a baby who has a cleft palate, because the cleft may permit milk to enter the nose and cause him to gag.

Early consultation with a plastic surgeon is advisable so that treatment can be planned. Some hospitals are now performing immediate closure of the cleft lip at birth. However, if a cleft palate is closed too early, it may mean a major operation during early adulthood, as the palate may be unable to develop fully.

TRISOMIES

Trisomy is a chromosomal disorder in which there are three chromosomes where normally there would only be a pair. This defect would exist in all the cells of the body of the affected person.

The most common trisomy is Down's syndrome (see p.24), also known as trisomy 21, in which there are three number 21 chromosomes.

The infant is born with small features, a tongue that tends to protrude, and slanting eyes that have folds of skin at their inner corners. The head is flat at the back, and the ears are unusual. He or she is rather floppy, and the hands and feet are usually short and wide, with a single transverse crease across the palms and soles. In addition congenital heart disease may be detected.

Down's syndrome sufferers are usually mentally handicapped, although the degree of handicap varies, and many Down's syndrome children are near normal.

Children with Down's syndrome are very rewarding. They're affectionate, outgoing, and have a great sense of humour. With careful attention and early education they often do very well. Some manage to live independently.

Other trisomies include trisomy 13 (Patau's syndrome) and trisomy 18 (Edwards' syndrome), both of which produce a number of severe physical and mental abnormalities but which are much rarer than Down's syndrome.

opinion is sought as it is possible to prevent progression of the hydrocephalus by repeated lumbar punctures or by inserting a drainage tube and valve into a tiny hole made in the skull.

Neural tube defects such as spina bifida and hydrocephalus may be diagnosed by ultrasound (see p.180) or amniocentesis (see p.185) well before the child is born. High alpha-fetoprotein (AFP) levels can indicate a need for more investigation.

Cerebral palsy This is muscular paralysis, stiffness, or incoordination that occurs because of damage to the brain before, during, or after birth, for instance, because of a poor supply of oxygen to the brain in late pregnancy or a difficult labour. Premature babies are particularly vulnerable. An infection of the mother's uterus may also cause cerebral palsy, as may meningitis or a severe injury to the baby's head after birth. It is not possible to detect cerebral palsy before birth. The symptoms are usually not obvious until the baby is several months old and his development appears to be delayed. He may not be walking, sitting, or making progress as expected; there may be a stiffness in the arms or legs, or a persistent abnormal posture. The degree of disability ranges from slight – where the child may just be very clumsy or unsteady – to severe, where at the very worst the child is totally immobile.

If there are muscular spasms and the limbs are abnormally stiff, the baby is termed spastic. Rigidity may affect the arm and leg on one side (hemiplegia), the legs only (paraplegia), or all four limbs and trunk (quadriplegia). A child may display unintentional writhing movements, which is termed athetosis, or a loss of coordination and balance, known as ataxia. Very often, a child's other abilities – speech, vision, or hearing – may be affected. Unfortunately, a number of children may suffer severe mental handicap, particularly quadriplegics, but a significant number do have normal intelligence. Cerebral palsy is incurable but it is not progressive – it does not get worse as the child grows older. Physiotherapy will help to prevent deformities caused by stiffness and spasms, and develop muscular balance and control; speech therapy will help to ease communication problems.

Respiratory distress syndrome In this condition, the baby's lungs are deficient in surfactant, a substance that keeps open the minute air sacs in the lungs through which oxygen is absorbed into the blood. This is due to immaturity of the lungs, or because the function of crucial lung cells is temporarily depressed because of a lack of oxygen. Respiratory distress syndrome is most commonly found in small preterm babies, but also occurs in the infants of diabetic mothers whose diabetes is not sufficiently well controlled. A low fetal oxygen level just prior to birth is a predisposing factor and it is very rare in full-term infants.

With increasing skill in detecting immaturity of the baby's lungs before birth and in the management of preterm deliveries and early and effective resuscitation, the incidence of the disorder has fallen in recent years. Infants that are born with the established disease require full support in an intensive care unit and are given surfactant to mature their lungs.

Pyloric stenosis The narrowing of the pylorus, the passage from the stomach to the small intestine, because of thickening of the pyloric muscle, is more common in males. The cause is unknown, but symptoms typically first appear at two to four weeks.

Food builds up in the stomach, which contracts powerfully in an attempt to force the food through the narrow pylorus. As this is impossible, milk is vomited up violently after feeding, known as projectile vomiting, when the vomit may be propelled a couple of metres. The baby may suffer constipation and dehydration. A simple operation widens the pylorus, giving a complete cure.

Epispadias and hypospadias About one in 1,000 male babies has an abnormality of the penile opening of the urethra. In epispadias, the opening is on the upper surface of the penis; the penis may curve upwards. In hypospadias, the opening is on the underside of the glans (head) and the penis may curve down. In extreme, but rare forms of hypospadias, the urethral opening lies between genitals and anus, and the genitals may appear female. Surgery is straightforward and usually successful, enabling normal passage of urine and, later, sexual intercourse. Neither epispadias nor hypospadias cause infertility.

CLUB FOOT (TALIPES)

This is when a child is born with the sole of one foot, or both feet, facing down and inwards or up and outwards.

The exact causes of the many varieties of club foot are not fully understood, but it is known that the condition can be inherited, and on rare occasions may spontaneously recover.

In most cases, though, treatment is necessary if the defect is to be corrected. The most common remedy is repeated manipulation of the child's foot over a period of many months. In the intervals between manipulations, the foot is held in the required position by some form of bracing such as a splint or a plaster cast. In some cases surgery may be required.

FETAL DEFECTS PER 10,000 BIRTHS

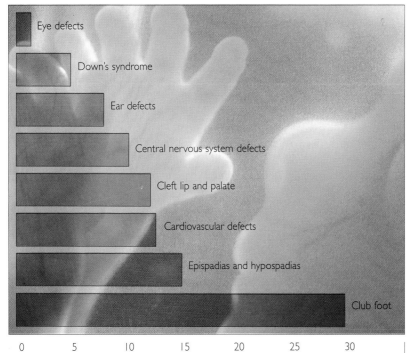

Eye defects

Down's syndrome

Ear defects

Central nervous system defects

Cleft lip and palate

Cardiovascular defects

Epispadias and hypospadias

Club foot

0   5   10   15   20   25   30

Incidence of fetal defects
This chart summarizes typical incidences of birth defects found in babies born in England and Wales. The most common is club foot, which affects both boys and girls. Epispadias and hypospadias, together the second most common, are defects of the urethra and affect only boys. Cardiovascular defects are those of the heart and circulatory system, including congenital heart disease, and the defects of the central nervous system include spina bifida and hydrocephalus.

Despite the physical and emotional stresses involved in fetal surgery, most parents cope extremely well.

When an unborn baby is diagnosed as having a serious illness or defect, and the doctors contemplate fetal surgery, the parents are given extensive counselling to help them decide whether or not to agree to it. Fetal surgery, although advancing rapidly, is still very much at the experimental stage. The most complicated techniques are only attempted if there is nothing to lose. In some experienced centres, however, simple procedures like exchange transfusions are performed routinely.

If the surgery succeeds, the rewards are immense, and there appears to be little effect on the mother's fertility. Many women subsequently become pregnant again, and their pregnancies are normal. With less successful surgery, there is the possibility of subsequent miscarriage, premature birth, and the necessity of a Caesarean section. There may also be complications for the mother after the operation, which can be extremely stressful for all concerned.

Fetal surgery

Thanks to the development of specialized surgical techniques, it is possible to correct some defects before birth. Although some procedures are still experimental, they may offer the only chance for the baby, and many parents see this as a risk worth taking.

Only a small number of pioneering surgeons are involved in fetal surgery, and the number of defects they can help is limited, but research continues. New methods are constantly being tried and evaluated, and advances in the diagnosis of fetal defects make it easier for doctors to decide if surgery is appropriate.

ULTRASOUND-GUIDED SURGERY

More straightforward types of fetal surgery are carried out by thin needles inserted through the mother's abdomen and uterus and into the amniotic sac. Ultrasound gives the surgeon a view of the fetus, and enables him to manipulate the needles (only one at a time is used), with which blood or tissue samples are taken from the fetus and with which drugs or blood transfusions are given.

Using ultrasound-guided techniques, surgeons are able to treat a growing number of life-threatening conditions. Rhesus and other incompatibilities between the immune systems of mother and baby may be corrected through intrauterine blood transfusions. Drugs that will correct fetal heartbeat irregularities and destroy tumours may be injected into the fetus; minute drainage tubes (shunts) that prevent further build-up of fluids may be inserted to drain excess fluids from the baby – for instance from the brain in cases of hydrocephalus – and to clear urinary tract blockages. Ultrasound is also used to guide the tiny forceps and scalpels with which surgery can be carried out.

Intrauterine blood transfusions In some cases of Rhesus incompatibility (see p.202), where a mother's blood is Rhesus (Rh) negative and her baby's is Rh positive, the baby may become dangerously anaemic. In this case he will be given one or more blood transfusions into one of the blood vessels in the umbilical cord to sustain him until he can be delivered safely. Fresh Rhesus negative blood will be injected slowly, in volumes related to the estimated weight of the fetus and the degree of anaemia.

Fetal blood transfusions have a good success rate, but in some severe cases, Rh incompatibility results in miscarriage or stillbirth, despite numerous transfusions. Until recently, if transfusions were unsuccessful there was nothing more that could be done, but now research is underway to investigate whether injecting the baby with donated Rh-negative bone marrow will stimulate him to become Rh negative and so remove the incompatibility.

A more uncommon type of incompatibility between mother and child results in the mother producing antibodies that destroy the baby's blood platelets. These platelets help blood to clot, and without them the baby could be in danger of suffering a haemorrhage and die. This can now be prevented by giving the fetus transfusions of platelets and, in severe cases, donor antibodies that counteract those of his mother.

Shunts for urinary tract problems   Hydronephrosis, which is when a kidney becomes swollen with urine because the ureter that drains it is narrow or blocked, sometimes occurs in unborn babies. If it is left untreated, it can lead to severe kidney damage; if it affects both kidneys, it can cause kidney failure. Hydronephrosis can sometimes be corrected by the insertion of shunts.

OPEN FETAL SURGERY

Some fetal defects that cannot be treated by ultrasound-guided techniques can be corrected by open fetal surgery. This involves opening up the uterus and partially removing the baby so that he can be operated on. Open fetal surgery has been used to repair diaphragmatic hernias, where a hole in the baby's diaphragm allows his intestines to protrude into his chest cavity and damage his lungs, and to remove certain types of tumour.

The operation   Unlike ultrasound-guided techniques, which are always carried out under local anaesthetic, open fetal surgery requires a general anaesthetic for both mother and baby. When the anaesthetic has taken effect, an incision is made in the mother's abdomen to expose the uterus, and an ultrasound scan is used to locate the exact position of the placenta. The amniotic fluid is then drawn off and kept warm, and an incision about 12 centimetres (five inches) long is made in the uterus and amniotic membranes, well away from the placenta to avoid damaging it. The baby is eased gently out of the uterus through this opening just far enough for the surgeon to be able to repair the defect.

After the operation   Once the surgeon has finished, the baby is carefully replaced in the uterus along with the amniotic fluid (to which is added a small amount of antibiotic in order to prevent infection). The incisions in the amniotic membranes and the uterus are closed with absorbable stitches and surgical glue, and the incision in the abdomen is stitched together.

The mother rests in bed for at least three days after the operation, during which time both she and her baby are intensively monitored, and she usually leaves hospital within ten days. Contractions of her uterus, caused by irritation following the operation, must be suppressed by drugs to prevent her going into labour at this early stage. These drugs are given intravenously while she is in hospital, and she is switched to oral medication when she leaves. Although generally fit, most babies who undergo open fetal surgery are born before term, usually by Caesarean section.

PROSPECTS FOR THE BABY

Fetal surgery is used to help babies who have defects that are easier to correct before they are born than afterwards, or who will die without it.

In general, the earlier in pregnancy that fetal surgery is performed, the better the baby's prospects of survival. This is partly because wounds will heal relatively quickly in a developing baby, and partly because organs unable to grow until the defect is repaired can complete their normal development. For instance, if a baby's lungs cannot grow properly because of a diaphragmatic hernia, they will need time to mature so that he will be able to use them when he is born.

The exact time when a baby can be operated on depends upon a number of factors, one of the most important being the point at which the defect can be diagnosed. Blood and antibody problems are usually diagnosable in the earliest weeks of pregnancy, and often, as in many cases of Rh incompatibility, they are predictable. One baby who was given 25 transfusions of antibodies received the first at 11 weeks, when she was only about 5cm (2in) long. Most physical malformations, however, are not diagnosable until the organ or organs they affect have grown enough for the defect to be apparent. As a result, surgery to correct defects of this type is typically carried out after about week 18.

Rh-negative Mother

About 85 percent of people have the Rhesus factor in their red blood cells and they are Rhesus positive. The other 15 percent who lack the factor are Rhesus negative. A Rhesus positive mother who's carrying a Rhesus positive baby may develop antibodies to her Rhesus baby's Rhesus positive blood cells and injure them.

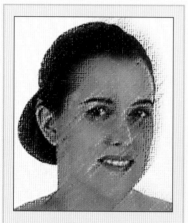

Name **Elizabeth Duncan**

Age **27 years**

Past medical history
Nothing abnormal

Obstetric history **One daughter aged two years; normal birth, no postnatal complications; child's blood group Rhesus positive**

Elizabeth's blood group is Rhesus negative and her partner's, Chris, is Rhesus positive. Their second baby has a 50:50 chance of being Rhesus-negative however if Chris passes on a recessive Rhesus-negative gene. Their first baby was Rhesus positive so Elizabeth may have developed anti-Rhesus-positive antibodies. If this second baby is Rhesus positive, the baby's red blood cells may be damaged by the antibodies. To prevent any damage, Elizabeth will have special care throughout pregnancy.

AN INCOMPATIBLE MOTHER AND BABY

Elizabeth's first pregnancy went without a hitch. This is usual with first pregnancies where the mother has Rhesus-negative blood and the baby Rhesus-positive (an incompatible pregnancy).

However, when fetal blood cells mix with maternal cells, for example during delivery, the mother's blood becomes sensitized. When the Rh factor from the baby's blood enters the mother's bloodstream, it acts as an antigen and stimulates production of anti-Rhesus-positive antibodies. These will attack and destroy the blood cells of her next Rhesus-positive (incompatible) baby. This causes haemolytic disease of the newborn (see p.342) and infants affected with blood conditions ranging from mild jaundice to serious, possibly fatal, anaemia. Fetuses who develop the disease can often be saved by intrauterine blood transfusion (see p.200).

DO ALL WOMEN BECOME SENSITIZED?

Not all Rh-negative women with Rh-positive babies become sensitized, but there is no way of predicting which women will. All of these women, therefore, should have an Anti-D injection.

Women who are Rhesus negative are also given an Anti-D injection after the follwoing:
• an abortion
• chorionic villus sampling
• an amniocentesis or cordocentesis, especially if there is blood on the needle after it has been withdrawn from the uterus

DESENSITIZING ELIZABETH

Within 48 hours of delivering her first baby, Elizabeth was injected intra-muscularly with Anti-D (Rh immune-globulin) to help prevent the destructive antibodies from forming. Had this pregnancy miscarried, she would have also needed the injection, because her blood and that of the baby's would have mixed.

CAREFUL MONITORING

Elizabeth is hoping that she will be only mildly affected by Rhesus incompatibility. However, if antibodies have already formed, the Rhogham injection will be ineffective. Therefore, Elizabeth's blood will be monitored throughout her pregnancy. At each visit, Elizabeth will have a special specimen of blood taken to examine for increasing levels of antibodies. Only if they increase beyond a certain point is her developing baby in any danger.

ELIZABETH'S BABY

Elizabeth's baby is likely to be fit and healthy, owing to the Anti-D injections and the special care she receives during her pregnancy.

• Immediately after the birth Elizabeth's baby will have a Coomb's test to look for the presence of maternal anti-Rhesus-positive antibodies.

• If the baby is affected by Rh incompatibility, his bilirubin levels will rise quickly after birth because his liver can't get rid of it.

• He may need a transfusion – blood is withdrawn from the baby via the umbilical vein and replaced with donor blood compatible with his mother's blood. If severe

haemolytic disease had been predicted before he was born, he may have been successfully treated by a transfusion while in the womb.

• A high level of bilirubin will make him look yellow. This can be treated by placing him under ultraviolet "bili" light which converts bilirubin into a harmless substance.

If increasing antibodies are noted, she will have an ultrasound scan at 18 weeks. This can check for the presence of fetal bilirubin (a by-product of red blood cell destruction) in the amniotic fluid.

In the third trimester, a direct test for the presence of bilirubin can be done by a process called cordocentesis (see p.187). This will enable the doctors to assess the severity of the condition and determine whether blood transfusions are necessary.

ELIZABETH'S BIRTH EXPECTATIONS

If her antibody count remains low, Elizabeth will not require further special care during her pregnancy. However, if the count rises moderately, her baby may be induced early to prevent serious consequences. In this case, home birth is out of the question and she will need to deliver in a hospital with an experienced obstetric department. She will probably have a Caesarean section. In a very few cases the baby has to be given a blood transfusion to replace its own blood cells which have become damaged during pregnancy.

RHESUS DISEASE IN PREGNANCY

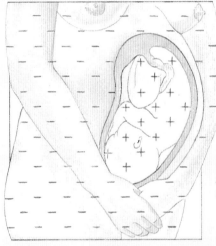

Rhesus disease only occurs when a woman who has Rhesus-negative blood (symbolized by red minus signs in the picture) is pregnant with a Rhesus-positive (symbolized by blue plus signs) baby. Most Rhesus-negative mothers carry their first babies without any problems – just as Elizabeth did. However, if they subsequently develop antibodies to Rhesus-positive blood (symbolized by green triangles in the pictures below) any babies that they have later could be at risk.

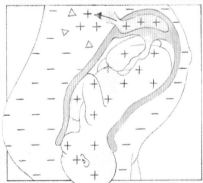

Mother is sensitized
If the mother is not given an Anti-D injection within 48 hours of delivery, she may develop anti-bodies to Rhesus-positive blood.

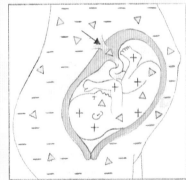

A future pregnancy
If she becomes pregnant with another Rhesus-positive baby, her antibodies may attack this baby's red blood cells.

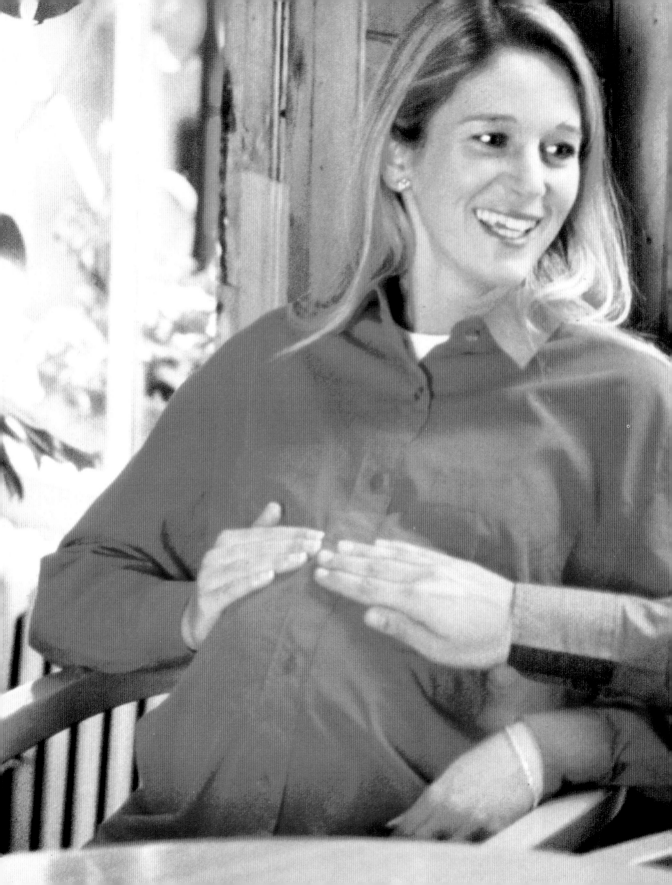

CHAPTER 9

Common
COMPLAINTS

Very few women go through pregnancy without suffering a few complaints that are, in the main, uncomfortable rather than serious. Being prepared for them is half the battle and also enables you to differentiate between those that are just uncomfortable and those that are potentially serious.

Common Complaints

COMPLAINT	WHY IT HAPPENS
Backache is usually a general discomfort across the lower part of the back, often with pain across the buttocks and down the legs. It can occur when you have been standing for too long with bad posture or after lifting a heavy weight, especially during the third trimester.	High progesterone levels cause softening and stretching of the ligaments of the pelvic bones, allowing the baby to be born. The ligaments of the spine also relax, putting extra strain on the joints of the back and hips.
Intensely painful low backache may also occur when you rotate your spine and pelvis in opposite directions, such as when you turn over sideways in bed.	The baby is resting against your sacroiliac joint, which is located some 7½cm (3in) in from the top of your buttocks. Rotary movements of the spine and pelvis open and close the sacroiliac joint, causing pain.
Carpal tunnel syndrome is a sensation of pins and needles, mainly in the thumb and first finger, with numbness and sometimes weakness. Occasionally the whole hand and forearm are affected. It can occur from conception onwards.	Pressure on the nerve that passes from the arm to the hand along the front of the wrist. The pressure is caused by swelling of the carpal tunnel (a ring of fibres around the wrist under which the nerve passes) owing to water retention.
Constipation is when you have dry, hard stools that are difficult to pass. It can occur from conception onwards.	Progesterone relaxes the muscles in the intestinal walls, so there are fewer contractions to push the food along. Consequently much more water than usual is absorbed from the stool in the colon, making it hard and dry. Stools may be less frequent, too.
Cramps are a sudden pain in the thigh, calf, and/or foot, followed by a general ache that lasts for some time. They tend to be more common in the third trimester, and usually waken you from sleep.	Cramps are thought to be caused by low calcium levels in the blood, or they may be due to salt deficiency. Check with your doctor.

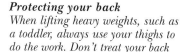

Protecting your back
When lifting heavy weights, such as a toddler, always use your thighs to do the work. Don't treat your back as a crane.

During pregnancy you may experience a number of discomforts that are often no more than irritating. Most are caused by a combination of hormonal changes and the extra strain that your body is experiencing, can be treated very simply, and are nothing to worry about. A few, however, can be serious, so be aware of the symptoms and be prepared to act promptly if you suspect all may not be well.

WHAT CAN BE DONE	RISK TO BABY
Massage may help (see p.152). Do exercises to strengthen your spine. Make sure your mattress is firm. Lift heavy weights correctly (see bottom left, opposite). Try to improve your posture (see p.160), and avoid high-heeled shoes. If the pain runs down your leg towards your foot, consult your doctor in case it's a slipped disc.	*None.*
Osteopathic manipulation can help you in even the most severe cases. Backache usually eases by itself in the fifth month when the fetus tips forward – although you may not be able to wait that long!	
Diuretics prescribed by your doctor may alleviate the symptoms. A splint on the wrist at night may help, as may holding your hand above your head and wiggling your fingers. Acupuncture may help. Sleep with your arm on a pillow. Symptoms usually disappear soon after delivery.	*None.*
Drink lots of water. Eat as much roughage in the form of fruit, vegetables, and fibre as you can. Walk briskly for 20 minutes once a day or more. Don't take a laxative without consulting your doctor. Natural fibre laxatives are best as they simply increase the amount of water in the stool, making it soft. Figs and prunes will also do the job.	*None.*
Massage the area very firmly. Flex your foot up and push into the heel. You may be prescribed calcium or salt tablets if your levels are low, but don't self-prescribe without first consulting your doctor.	*None.*

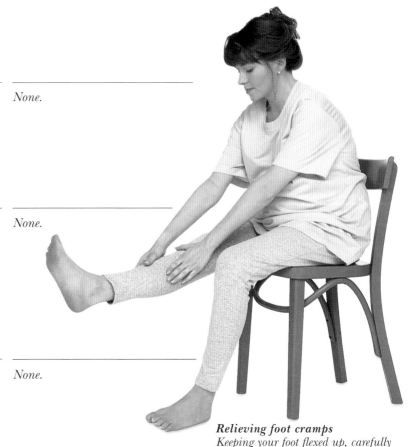

Relieving foot cramps
Keeping your foot flexed up, carefully make circling movements with your lower leg.

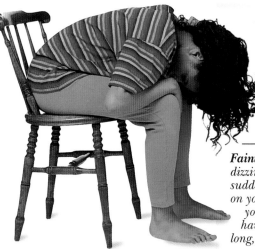

COMPLAINT	WHY IT HAPPENS
Diarrhoea *is when you have soft, watery stools, requiring frequent visits to the toilet. It can occur at any time.*	*Usually because an infection by bacteria or a virus is present.*
Faintness *is a feeling of dizziness or vertigo that occurs suddenly, making you unsteady on your feet. It can come on if you stand up too quickly, or have been on your feet for too long, especially in hot weather.*	*A lack of blood supply to the brain, often caused by pooling of the blood in the legs and feet when standing, together with the demands of the uterus for an increased blood supply.*
Heartburn *is a burning sensation just behind the breastbone, sometimes with regurgitation of stomach acid into the mouth. It happens most commonly on lying down, coughing, straining when passing a stool, and when you are lifting heavy weights.*	*Early in pregnancy, the muscular valve at the entrance to the stomach relaxes under the influence of progesterone. This allows stomach acid to flow up into the oesophagus, causing a burning sensation. Later in pregnancy, the baby can press up on the stomach, forcing the contents back into the oesophagus.*
High blood pressure **(hypertension)** *is an increase in blood pressure. It can be mild or severe, and there may be no, few, or many symptoms including frontal headaches, visual disturbances, and vomiting. Water retention (see p.212) with swelling of the feet, hands, and ankles may also occur. It can happen at any time, but it is more likely to occur near term. It is more common in women having their first baby, especially if they are over 35, and also in women having more than one baby. It is always looked for because it may herald pre-eclamptic toxaemia (PET or **Pre-eclampsia**, see p.224).*	*The cause is not fully understood. In some women, cells from the placenta produce chemicals called vasoconstrictors that may cause the blood vessels to constrict. This may cause the blood pressure to rise, and the kidneys to retain sodium, leading to water retention.*

Coping with faintness
If you do feel faint, put your head as far down as you can – between your knees if you can still manage it! Get up slowly.

Avoiding heartburn
To prevent your stomach overfilling, eat smaller meals. Learn to snack on nutritious food and split meals if they fill you up.

WHAT CAN BE DONE	RISK TO BABY
Increase your water intake to 12–14 glasses a day to replace lost fluid. This will ensure that your blood pressure remains normal. Consult your doctor, who will test your stools for infection and give you the appropriate treatment.	*Diarrhoea can cause dehydration and loss of calories that can put your baby at risk if it goes untreated for a long time. If it is profuse and protracted, you will need to be hospitalized for intravenous feeding.*
Avoid standing for long periods. Always sit or lie down when you feel dizzy. Don't get up suddenly from sitting or get out of a hot bath too quickly. Keep cool in hot weather. If dizzy, sit with head between knees – if you still can – or lie down with your feet higher than your head.	*None, unless you fall very heavily on to your stomach.*
Keep meals small so that the stomach is never overfilled. Sleep propped up with several pillows. A glass of milk at bedtime will help to neutralize stomach acid. Your doctor may prescribe antacids, but only in the later stages of pregnancy.	*None.*
If you suffered from high blood pressure before you were pregnant, tell your doctor. Keep an eye on your weight. Always report persistent headaches and nausea. *Your doctor will test your blood pressure and urine, and look for any swelling (oedema – see **Water retention**, p.212) of your hands, face, and ankles at each antenatal visit. He or she will almost certainly increase the frequency of your antenatal visits.* *If your blood pressure goes up at any stage of your pregnancy, you will be advised to stay in bed and rest, and your doctor will suggest home visits.* *If the rise is severe, you will be admitted to hospital, where you can be monitored continuously. If the baby appears to be suffering, labour may be induced or you may have a Caesarean section. Your blood pressure will return to normal once your baby has been born.*	*Pregnancy-induced hypertension (see **Pre-eclampsia**, p.224) can slow the baby's growth rate, owing to a reduced blood flow to the uterus. The baby may also be short of oxygen. Both these factors may lead to low birthweight. There is a severe form called eclampsia (see p.224), which can be life threatening. Fortunately this is now very rare in the West, owing to excellent antenatal care that spots the signs very early.*

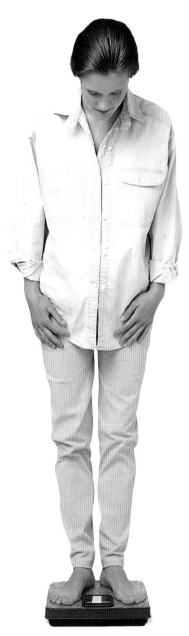

Monitor your weight
Gaining a lot of weight suddenly may indicate the onset of pre-eclampsia.

Self massage
Massaging your face, especially your temples and neck, is a wonderful and effective way of relieving tension and will help to dispel insomnia.

COMPLAINT	WHY IT HAPPENS
Insomnia *is the inability to sleep at night, making you tired and irritable during the day. It can happen at any time from conception onwards.*	*Your baby lives on a 24-hour clock, and his or her metabolism keeps going even when you want to sleep. This can affect your body's responses. Other causes include night sweats and a desire to empty your bladder more frequently, particularly during the third trimester.*
Mood swings *describes rapid, uncharacteristic changes in mood, often with unexplained crying and anxiety attacks. They are common from conception onwards, but are especially likely to occur in the third trimester.*	*Changes in your hormone balance during pregnancy have a depressant effect on the nervous system, causing symptoms similar to those that can occur pre-menstrually. Body image changes and identity crises may have a profound effect on you as your pregnancy progresses, and mixed feelings about pregnancy and parenthood can cause sudden shifts in your moods.*
Morning sickness *is a feeling of sickness and nausea, sometimes with vomiting. Contrary to its name, it can occur at any time of the day, but generally happens when you haven't eaten, or after a long night's sleep. These symptoms usually occur in the first trimester, then abate.*	*The main cause is low blood sugar, but pregnancy hormones may irritate the stomach directly.*
Piles *are dilated rectal veins (varicose veins – see p.212) that may protrude through the anus. Usually they do not occur until the second trimester.*	*Your increasingly larger baby presses down on your rectum and impedes venous flow to the heart. The blood therefore pools, causing the veins to dilate to accommodate the dammed-up blood.*

WHAT CAN BE DONE	RISK TO BABY
A warm bath and a hot milky drink may help, as may a relaxing massage (see p.152). Watch television or read until you feel tired and sleepy. Find a comfortable position, and try to stay cool. Your doctor will not prescribe sleeping pills until the third trimester, and then only if you are exhausted by lack of sleep, because they can cross the placenta and affect the baby (see also p.258).	*None.*
*You should consider these feelings as natural. Depression, anxiety, and confusion can occur even in the easiest of pregnancies. Analysing such feelings may only serve to prolong them. (See also **Emotional Changes**, p.154.)*	*None.*
Food will provide relief from nausea, so eat little and often. Eat high-carbohydrate foods such as wholemeal bread, potatoes, rice, and cereals, and avoid fried food and coffee, which trigger nausea. *Keep glucose sweets in your car, desk, or handbag. To prevent sickness in the morning, put a glass of water and a plain biscuit by your bed before sleeping, and have them as a snack 15 minutes before you get out of bed.* *Cigarette smoke and other strong smells may also trigger nausea. Drink extra fluids such as fruit juice or skimmed milk – if you can keep them down.*	*In its severe form (called hyperemesis gravidarum), vomiting can deplete you of fluid and minerals, leading to low blood pressure. This is always harmful to your baby. Inform your doctor if you vomit more than three times a day for three days. In very severe cases, hospitalization may be necessary to replace the fluids that you have lost.*
Keep your bowels regular and the stools soft by eating sufficient fibre – this will help you avoid straining down. Don't lift weights, as this increases intra-abdominal pressure and back pressure in the rectal veins. Have coughs treated promptly for the same reasons. Aromatherapy may be able to relieve symptoms.	*None.*

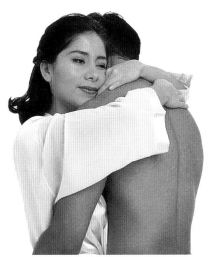

Coping with mood swings
A reassuring cuddle is probably just what you need when you're feeling anxious and upset.

COMPLAINT	WHY IT HAPPENS
Rib pain can be felt as extreme soreness and tenderness of the ribs, usually on the right side, just below the breasts. The pain is more severe on sitting down. It tends to occur mainly during the third trimester.	It is caused by compression of the ribs as the uterus rises in the abdomen. In addition, the baby can bruise your lower ribs with his or her head, or by excessive punching and kicking.
Tender, painful breasts, with a feeling of heaviness and discomfort, and a tingling sensation in the nipples, can be one of the first signs of pregnancy. Tenderness is present throughout, but may increase towards term.	Hormones are preparing your breasts for lactation. The milk ducts are growing and being stretched as they fill with milk.
Thrush is a yeast infection, characterized by a thick, white, curdy discharge from the vagina, accompanied by dryness and intense itching around your vagina, vulva, perineum, and, sometimes, your anus. You may also have pain when passing urine. Thrush can happen at any time.	It is an infection by the yeast Candida albicans, which occurs normally in the bowel. Infection occurs when the yeast grows uncontrolled by other bacteria, perhaps following a course of antibiotics. It is more common in pregnancy, probably because of the leakage of sugar into body fluids due to increased vaginal blood flow. Excess sugar intake often aggravates it.
Varicose veins are swollen veins just below the skin. Although most common in the legs or anus, they can also occur in the vulva.	See **Piles** p.210.
Water retention happens when there is an increase in the amount of fluid present in the tissues. This causes swelling (oedema), especially of the feet, face, and hands. Your rings may become tight.	Standing all day, especially in hot weather, can cause fluid to pool in the ankles. High blood pressure (see p.208), which is often associated with pregnancy, can force fluid from the bloodstream into the tissues, causing oedema. Pregnancy hormones can cause retention of sodium by the kidneys, which in turn causes the body to retain fluid.

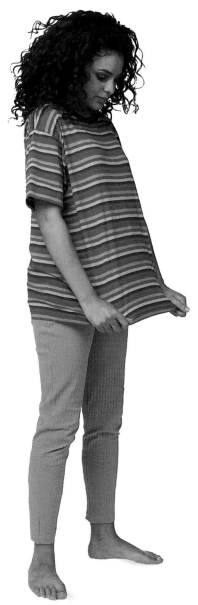

Wear comfortable clothes
Loose fitting, comfortable outerwear is essential during pregnancy. Tight fitting tops will constrict you.

WHAT CAN BE DONE

RISK TO BABY

Wear loose clothes that won't compress your ribs. Improve your posture. Prop yourself up on cushions when you lie down. The pain ceases when the baby's head drops into the pelvic cavity prior to birth.

None.

Wear a good supportive bra from early in pregnancy. If your breasts are large, wear a bra at night as well (see p.163). Wash your breasts gently once a day with a mild soap and pat dry. Apply baby lotion or oil if your nipples are sore.

None.

Avoid wearing tight pants and trousers, as this encourages infection. Choose cotton instead of man-made fibres. The doctor will prescribe pessaries that you should place in your vagina at night, as directed. You will also be prescribed a cream that should be gently rubbed into the skin surrounding the vaginal opening, the anus, and on the thighs. This will stop the itching.

The baby can become infected as it passes down the birth canal on delivery. If this happens, white clumps like curds of milk will appear in the baby's mouth. The baby must be treated promptly with a course of antifungal agents, which will quickly clear up the infection.

Avoid standing for too long. Put your feet up. Wear pregnancy support tights. Gentle massage may help to prevent varicose veins, but do not massage the area if you develop them.

None.

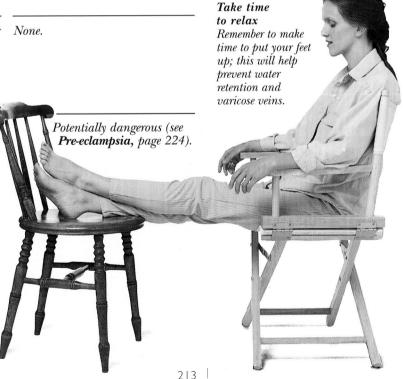

Take time to relax
Remember to make time to put your feet up; this will help prevent water retention and varicose veins.

Avoid standing for prolonged periods. Put your feet up. Avoid salty foods. Your doctor will check your hands, face, and ankles for any swelling at each antenatal visit, and occasionally diuretics may be prescribed.

Potentially dangerous (see **Pre-eclampsia,** *page 224).*

213

Mother who has MS

Kathy has always longed to have children, but because of her multiple sclerosis (MS), she and Tom believed that their chances of having a family were nil. They talked matters over with their elderly family doctor who continued to advise them against pregnancy. However, they were recently recommended to see a new obstetrician.

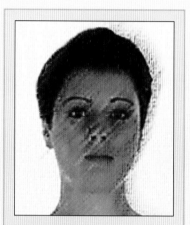

Name **Kathy Dixon**

Age **29 years**

Past medical history
Developed multiple sclerosis at the age of 23 years

Obstetric history
14 weeks pregnant

When Kathy developed multiple sclerosis a year after her marriage to Tom, both were devastated. Each had dreamed of having children. Kathy and Tom came to believe that Kathy's MS reduced the possibility of her conceiving, even rendering her infertile, and that pregnancy was not advisable for women suffering from MS because it caused a deterioration of the condition with serious relapses and increased disability.

A NEW PICTURE

As Kathy's walking was steady, her eyesight was hardly affected, and she had no troublesome urinary symptoms or vertigo, she and Tom eventually decided to press for a second opinion. They saw a modern obstetrician who had monitored several MS patients through successful pregnancies, and who enlisted the help of a neurologist throughout antenatal care. This way, both the baby and the mother received the best care.

To their delight, Kathy and Tom were given an entirely new and encouraging picture by the obstetrician. He told them that their general practitioner's advice was now out of date. MS, he told them, does not affect a woman's fertility in any way and has no effect on the course of pregnancy, labour, or delivery. Women with MS have very few complications during pregnancy. In a study of 36 pregnant women with MS, the only complications noted were two cases of mild vomiting. There is no increase in spontaneous abortions, complications in pregnancy or delivery, malformations, or stillbirths.

A GOOD PROGNOSIS

Kathy wondered whether pregnancy would make her MS worse. I told her that many research studies suggest that pregnancy is a protection for women with MS. This is probably because the natural state of immuno-suppression that occurs in pregnancy to prevent a woman from rejecting her baby also suppresses the inflammation that causes nerve and brain damage in MS. On the other hand, there is a slightly increased risk of a flare-up for three to six months after the birth. Between 40 and 60 percent of women have a relapse during this time – 20 percent of these suffer from permanent side effects while 80 percent go back to their pre-pregnant state of MS. Pregnancy does not appear to affect the long-term course of MS.

I reassured Kathy that the management of her labour and delivery would follow normal medical routine. She could be given analgesics – gas, injection, or epidural anaesthetic – and these would have no effect on her MS. A Caesarean would not affect her MS, nor would forceps if they proved necessary.

MS AND THE BABY

Tom was concerned that Kathy's MS might be passed on to their child. I explained that in an area with a high prevalence of MS, one person in 1000 out of the normal population would be likely to develop the disease. One study has shown that among children of people with MS, the figure could rise to one in 100. Dietary and genetic factors appear to be involved, although nothing has as yet been proved conclusively. However, most people feel that the risk of their child having MS is not great enough to stop them from choosing to conceive.

MS MEDICATION AND THE DEVELOPING BABY

Kathy was worried that the drugs she is given for MS might harm the baby in the uterus. I told her that in the first 12 weeks of pregnancy a woman is never given drugs, even if she does have MS, unless her life or the life of the baby is in danger. Drugs to stop painful muscle spasms would be discontinued before conception, as would long-term anti-inflammatory therapies. Drugs that help to control urinary frequency or incontinence would also be stopped. Very powerful drugs like steroids, which are only given if either the mother or the baby's life is in danger, are hardly ever needed during pregnancy.

AFTER THE BIRTH

Kathy wanted to know whether MS would affect her ability to feed and care for her baby. I told her that there are no medical reasons for her not to breastfeed and that she should insist on doing so. Rest, however, is extremely important, so she should make arrangements to have nursery help and express enough milk for the night feeds so that they can be given by others. Also, if she was already feeling insecure because of her MS, having a baby to look

after might increase her sense of insecurity. I told Tom that he would be the best person to calm Kathy's fears in that situation.

HAPPILY PREGNANT

Kathy and Tom thought about what they'd been told, and read the ARMS (Action for Research into Multiple Sclerosis) booklet 'MS and Pregnancy', which they found very helpful (see **Addresses**, p.370). They were a little stunned that after all the years that they had spent hoping for a miracle, there didn't appear to be much of a risk for Kathy after all. They decided to try for a baby, and Kathy is now 14 weeks pregnant. She is attending routine antenatal clinics and seeing her neurologist once a month. Kathy's doctors have told her that there is no need for special testing or monitoring of her pregnancy. She is being given iron to avoid anaemia and her doctors are on the look-out for warning signs of a urinary tract

infection, which must be treated promptly if it occurs. So far her pregnancy is proceeding normally and her MS remains unchanged.

PREGNANCY ADVICE

One of the most prominent symptoms of MS is fatigue. Tiredness is also a feature of pregnancy so an MS mother can easily become profoundly fatigued. Any MS mother should acknowledge that she needs to pay special attention to having rest periods throughout the day. She should also make sure that everyone around her, especially her partner, understands her needs and, if necessary, saves her from herself by insisting that she rests. Here are some guidelines I gave to Kathy:
• stop activity if you get breathless
• put your feet up when you can
• learn to catnap in spare time
• take two sleeps a day of at least 30 minutes each
• go to bed early, say, not later than 9.30pm.

KATHY'S BABY

There is every expectation that she will develop normally and be born in a straightforward way without the need for special medical intervention.

• She cannot inherit MS from her mother by transmission across the placenta, and the risk of transmission through genes appears to be very small.

• While she is in the uterus, she will not be at risk from the drugs given for MS because her mother will cease taking medication.

• After she is born, Kathy should be able to breastfeed, or to express milk for bottlefeeding.

• If Kathy consults the doctor before resuming drug treatment, the baby won't be at risk from drugs in the breast milk.

• Kathy should rest while feeding to conserve her energy so I advised her to practise breast-feeding a doll before the birth while lying on her bed or sofa. She would place a pillow or a cushion under each arm on which to rest the doll.

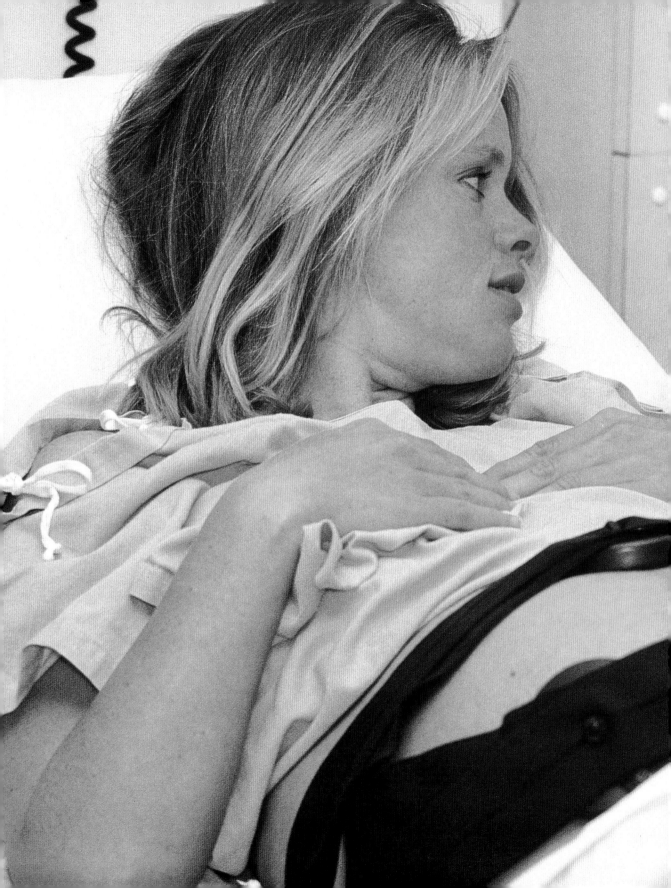

CHAPTER 10

Medical EMERGENCIES

Medical emergencies in pregnancy tend to be concentrated in the first and third trimesters. In the first trimester, most emergencies are associated with the loss of the fetus (miscarriage), or with it being misplaced, as in an ectopic pregnancy. In the third trimester, there may be complications such as pre-eclampsia, or associated problems with the placenta. Nonetheless, the vast majority of babies are delivered safely.

VAGINAL BLEEDING

Vaginal bleeding at any stage of pregnancy should be taken seriously. It may indicate an abnormally placed placenta, placenta praevia (see p.222), or it may be a warning of imminent miscarriage. Both of these conditions require prompt medical treatment.

• Vaginal bleeding occurs in the first trimester in about a quarter of all pregnancies. Over half of these pregnancies continue, with delivery of a healthy baby at term. If you experience any bleeding, call your doctor. He or she will probably refer you to the Early Pregnancy Unit at your local hospital. These are walk-in clinics, where you can be scanned quickly to check whether there is a heartbeat in the baby. If so, there is a very good chance (more than 80 percent) that all will be well. EPUs are used by women with a history of repeated miscarriage as weekly or bi-weekly reassurance boosts. Studies have shown that reassurance alone can positively affect outcome.

• If you start to bleed at any time during the second or third trimester, go straight to the maternity unit at hospital. The reasons are likely to be serious problems with the placenta, or premature labour (see pp.298 and 299) and will be treated as an emergency.

Medical emergencies

Most pregnancies continue to term with no problems or emergencies. However, it is wise to be aware of the danger signs so that medical care can be sought if necessary.

MISCARRIAGE

Medically known as spontaneous abortion, miscarriage is when the fetus aborts before the 24th week. After the 24th week, it is called a stillbirth. In the first few weeks about a third of all pregnancies end in miscarriage, but a quarter of these occur before pregnancy has been diagnosed or even suspected, so women are often unaware that they have miscarried.

Miscarriages increase in frequency with age and the number of previous pregnancies. They usually happen in the first trimester, the most common symptom being bleeding, which occurs in 95 percent of cases. If bleeding occurs at any time in your pregnancy consult your doctor. Most early miscarriages are due to a seriously abnormal fetus failing to implant in the uterine wall. Maternal causes of miscarriage include uterine abnormalities such as large fibroids and hormonal imbalances. Some bacterial and viral infections can also cause miscarriage. Cervical incompetence (see p.223) accounts for only 1 percent of spontaneous abortions. Paternal factors include abnormal sperm, or incompatible blood type, which causes the mother to produce antibodies to her partner's blood. These antibodies then attack and kill her fetus. Doctors divide spontaneous abortion into:

Threatened abortion Miscarriage is possible but not inevitable. There is vaginal bleeding and sometimes pain. This occurs in about 10 percent of all pregnancies and may be confused with the slight bleeding that can occur at the time of the first missed period.

Inevitable abortion Vaginal bleeding is accompanied by pain owing to the uterus contracting. If there is dilatation of the cervix, the loss of the embryo, unfortunately, is bound to occur.

Complete abortion The fetus and placenta are expelled from the uterus, sometimes without any symptoms. This can be confirmed by ultrasound examination.

Missed abortion The fetus and placenta die, but remain in the uterus for some time, even months, before being expelled. The symptoms of pregnancy disappear but there is no other indication of fetal death until much later.

Incomplete abortion This is when abortion has occurred but some of the products of conception, such as the amniotic sac or placenta, remain within the uterus.

Habitual abortion Three or more miscarriages have occurred at the same stage of pregnancy, possibly for the same reason.

Recurrent abortion Miscarriage has occurred on three or more occasions, but each one is for a different reason and occurs at a different stage of the pregnancy.

Treatment If you are bleeding in the second or third trimester, you should go to bed and stay there until the bleeding has stopped. However, there's no need to go to bed in the first trimester, but do call the doctor. You should stop any physical activities, such as strenuous exercise and sexual intercourse. If the bleeding and pain subside, you are quite likely to go on to deliver a healthy baby.

If a miscarriage appears to be inevitable there is little that doctors can do to prevent it. Complete and incomplete abortions should always be treated in hospital. If incomplete abortion occurs, the uterus will be cleaned out by a procedure called dilatation and curettage (D and C) carried out under anaesthetic. Painkillers are given, along with drugs to stop the bleeding. If a lot of blood has been lost (at least 500 millilitres/a pint), a transfusion may be necessary.

There is no urgency in treating a missed abortion, but if, after a time, a spontaneous abortion hasn't occurred, a D and C procedure will be carried out. If fetal death occurs later in pregnancy, prostaglandin pessaries or an oxytocin injection will be given to stimulate delivery (see also p.312).

Habitual abortion that has occurred because of cervical incompetence (see p.223) can be treated by stitching the cervix shut at the beginning of the next pregnancy.

Other possible reasons for habitual abortion are genetic or hormonal disorders, which often can be pinpointed (see pp.42–47); long-term infections, such as listeria, may sometimes cause repeated miscarriages, however, these can be difficult to diagnose and treat; poor nutrition can be a contributing factor; chronic disease, such as renal disease; tumours in the uterus (particularly fibroids) or abnormalities such as partial or complete septums (see column, right) that can usually be corrected by surgery; and immune disorders.

This last happens when the mother's immune system identifies the fetus as foreign, and therefore attacks it – Rhesus blood incompatibility (see p.202) is one example of such a situation. Other immune problems can sometimes be treated by using medication, which acts to suppress the mother's immune reaction, or the fetus itself can occasionally be injected with antibodies, either via the umbilical cord or directly into the fetus if the cord is underdeveloped.

UTERINE SEPTUMS

In all mammals, the uterus develops from two separate tubes in the embryo.

In some, such as monkeys, horses, and human beings, the tubes fuse to form a single uterus. In others, such as cats and dogs, the tubes develop into two separate uteri.

Problems arise in women when the tubes have not fused completely, thus leaving a partition in the uterus. A birth complicated by a uterine septum usually requires a Caesarean section.

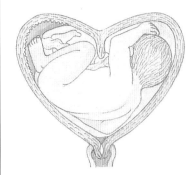

Bicornuate (horn-shaped) uterus
The baby is forced to lie in a transverse position from the second trimester.

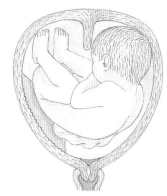

Subseptate uterus
The septum restricts the baby's movements, which can hinder birth.

Mother who has miscarried

Liz was deeply distressed by her miscarriage. What made the situation even harder to bear was that there didn't seem to be a cause, and nobody seemed to understand her intense feelings of grief, despair, and anger. Liz is now pregnant again and is naturally concerned about what will happen this time.

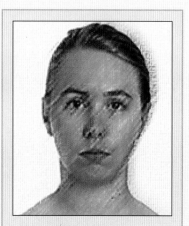

Name **Liz Turner**

Age **34 years**

Past medical history
Nothing abnormal

Obstetric history **Became pregnant for the first time a year ago; pregnancy miscarried in 11th week. She is now eight weeks pregnant**

Liz and her partner, Alan, desperately wanted their first baby and were both deeply upset by her miscarriage nine months ago. Alan buried himself in work while Liz struggled with her feelings of bereavement. Liz is now eight weeks into her second pregnancy and is determined to keep this baby. Her pleasure at being pregnant again is marred by fears that the same thing might happen again.

FIRST REACTIONS

When she miscarried nine months ago, Liz found herself fighting back guilt, despair, and anger in seeming isolation. Her doctor couldn't look her in the eye or talk openly about her lost baby. Her family and friends were sympathetic but their attempts to console her were rather clumsy. Some suggested that it was all for the best, because there must have been something wrong with the baby. Others reassured her that she could soon have another one. The unborn baby was not real to them as it had been to Liz, and they did not understand her intense sense of loss.

She began to wonder if her reactions were normal – perhaps she was not justified in grieving for a baby who had never really existed? I reassured Liz that it is natural for a mother to mourn the loss of a child, even if the child has not been born. Her emotions as well as her body needed time to readjust. I also encouraged her to share her feelings with Alan, so that they could grieve together.

ACCEPTING THEIR LOSS

At first Alan was reluctant to share his feelings with Liz, and she felt she had to force him to talk to her. She knew that it would be impossible to care for another baby until she had given up this one, and this was something that they had to do together. I encouraged them to share their anxieties and frustration, talk through their feelings and cry together. It was important that they did not deny their grief. I also suggested that it might help if they had a private memorial ceremony – perhaps something as simple as planting a tree in memory of their miscarried baby.

WAS SOMETHING WRONG WITH THE BABY?

After her miscarriage, Liz was taken to hospital and examined to make sure that no fragments of the placenta were left in her uterus, where they could create a site for infection. Following her doctor's advice, she collected up everything her body had expelled and took it with her so that the fetus could be tested for chromosomal abnormalities. None were found. Liz was reassured by this but then began to blame herself – perhaps the miscarriage was her fault? I explained that a first pregnancy is more likely to abort than any other – in fact one in three do. There are thought to be two reasons for this: an immature uterus needs to mature by having a trial run before it is fit to carry a pregnancy to term, and defects in the sperm or ova can produce an abnormal fetus.

ARE THERE CHANCES OF ANOTHER MISCARRIAGE?

Recent studies of early pregnancy loss show that a woman who has had one miscarriage is more likely to miscarry again. The risk seems to increase if conception occurs too soon after the miscarriage. Fortunately I had warned Liz and Alan about this, so they had waited for four months before trying to conceive again.

PREDICTIVE TESTING

A simple predictive test, carried out before pregnancy, can help to identify women who are more likely to miscarry again. During the menstrual cycle, too high a level of LH (luteinizing hormone) before ovulation increases the risk of miscarriage – LH controls other hormones involved in pregnancy, including oestrogen. Liz's LH levels were tested and proved to be normal.

REPEATED INSTANCES OF MISCARRIAGE

Some women do, however, miscarry repeatedly, but even for them the chance of a successful pregnancy after three previous miscarriages is about 60 percent. Women who have miscarried repeatedly are tested for uterine abnormalities, hormone imbalances, and disorders of the immunological system. Recently, scientific investigations have focused on a woman's immunological system and on hormone imbalances as causes of recurrent miscarriage.

IMMUNOLOGICALLY INDUCED MISCARRIAGES

The immune system is designed to repel foreign bodies because they are potentially harmful. Pregnancy normally overrides this, so that the woman's body protects the baby rather than rejecting it. In some mothers, for unknown reasons, the override fails, the immune system reasserts itself, and the baby is aborted. One treatment, still experimental, is to immunize women so that they do not produce antibodies hostile to their babies.

HORMONALLY INDUCED MISCARRIAGES

It has been found that 80 percent of repeat miscarriers suffer from polycystic ovary syndrome; a condition usually characterized by multiple ovarian cysts. This syndrome is caused by a hormone imbalance that results in over-production of testosterone and excessive stimulation of the ovaries resulting in immature ova (eggs).

Women with this condition who are considering pregnancy will be tested for hormone imbalances, abnormal ovulation and helped with fertility drugs such as clomiphene (see p.46).

PREGNANT AGAIN

Now that Liz is pregnant again, she's being extremely careful in every aspect of her life. She goes to relaxation classes to reduce her levels of stress and Alan has learnt how to give her a relaxing massage (see p.152).

Most importantly, she has given up blaming herself for the miscarriage and is taking a positive attitude towards her new pregnancy. I told Liz that although she can't be certain what the outcome will be, she can relax in the knowledge that her body is better prepared for pregnancy than it was last time. Alan is "sure it's going to be all right this time" but is reluctant to make plans for its future as he did with the first one.

LIZ'S BABY

Liz is fit and healthy and doesn't appear to have any condition that predisposes her to miscarry again. Liz's baby has every chance of developing perfectly in the uterus.

In several ways, Liz's baby will actually benefit both before and after birth – because of her mother's history of miscarriage.

• Liz's baby will be well nourished because her mother is paying such careful attention to diet, nutrition, and to relaxation and exercise routines.

• The baby should be comforted by the positive feelings that Liz is directing towards her.

• When she is born, Liz's baby will be greeted with relief and delight because she is making up for a previous disappointment. She represents success.

• Because of her previous history, Liz will be given extra care during her pregnancy and the health of her baby will be closely monitored for any signs of distress so that any problems can be averted.

ABNORMAL POSITION OF THE PLACENTA

If the placenta has implanted incorrectly, it can obstruct the baby's birth.

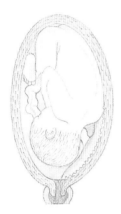

Side position
The placenta implants on the side and extends to the cervix, but does not cover it.

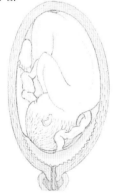

Blocking the cervix
The placenta implants centrally, completely covering the cervix – even when it is fully dilated.

PLACENTAL SEPARATION

Bleeding can occur from the placental bed owing to partial or complete separation of the placenta from the uterus. Blood builds up in the spaces, and eventually escapes around the membranes and through the cervix into the vagina. Known as placental abruption (*abruptio placentae*), it occurs in about one in 200 pregnancies. The cause is unknown, but tends to be more common in women who have had two or more children. Obstetricians divide placental separation into three types according to its severity.

In mild separation, blood loss can be slight. Bed rest is the best treatment, with ultrasound examination to monitor the situation. If it occurs late in pregnancy, labour may be induced.

In moderate separation, a quarter of the placenta separates and 500 millilitres to one litre (between one and two pints) of blood is lost. This requires a blood transfusion and, if the pregnancy is at or nearing term, a Caesarean section is usually performed.

Severe separation is an acute emergency, when at least two-thirds of the placenta shears off the uterine wall, and up to two litres (four pints) of blood are lost. This causes severe shock, disturbance of blood coagulation, and full kidney shutdown. A rapid blood transfusion will be given, and if the pregnancy is approaching term, a Caesarean may be performed to try to save the baby. If placental abruption occurs before the third trimester, fetal death is inevitable.

PLACENTA PRAEVIA

This occurs when the placenta is implanted in the lower segment of the uterus instead of the upper part (see column, left). It therefore lies in front of the baby as she comes to descend the birth canal at the onset of labour. The baby cannot pass down the canal without dislodging the placenta, thereby interrupting her own blood supply. Placenta praevia is a major cause of bleeding after the 20th week and of haemorrhage in the final two months of pregnancy. It is more common in women who have had several children, although the cause is unknown.

The greater the proportion of the placenta lying in the lower uterine segment, the greater the likelihood of complications during delivery. Even though the growth of the placenta in both size and weight slows down after the 30th week of pregnancy, the lower segment of the uterus is increasing in length quite rapidly. Therefore, shearing stresses between the placenta and the uterine wall may occur, leading to episodes of bleeding.

This extremely dangerous condition can be diagnosed well ahead of delivery by ultrasound (see p.180). Early symptoms include episodes of bleeding, with bright red blood, which may occur after sexual intercourse. If this happens, the doctor will advise hospital admission for ultrasound examination and bed rest, with blood transfusion if necessary. Bed rest should continue, if possible, until the 37th week, at which time the baby will be delivered by Caesarean section (see p.308).

Postpartum haemorrhage may occur after the delivery of the baby and is usually anticipated. Drugs to prevent it will be given as soon as the baby is born. In a very few cases, haemorrhage will continue despite treatment and then a hysterectomy may have to be considered. For these reasons, placenta praevia should only be treated by obstetricians qualified to cope with these complications. Delivery in a well-equipped hospital is vital, where a blood transfusion service is on hand.

PLACENTAL INSUFFICIENCY

During pregnancy the fetus receives oxygen and nourishment, and excretes carbon dioxide and waste products, via the placenta and the umbilical blood vessels. A healthy placenta, one that is able to act as an effective organ of transfer, is therefore crucial in maintaining the health of the fetus.

Assessment and treatment There is no reliable test for placental function. However, insufficiency may be signalled if you show less than normal weight gain, if your uterus is growing too slowly, or if your baby's development is below normal.

Ultrasound is the most reliable way to measure the growth of the fetus. If it shows that the baby is not growing adequately, your doctor will carry out tests that measure placental hormone and enzyme levels in the blood. A bio-physical profile that takes account of fetal breathing, body movement, tone and quantity of amniotic fluid, and a non-stress test may also be compiled. As the most useful sign in the last months, however, is the baby's activity level, you may be asked to keep a kick count (see p.195). Placental insufficiency may warrant the induction of labour, and even Caesarean section.

INCOMPETENT CERVIX

Fortunately, this condition is rare, unless the cervix has been damaged during previous surgery or pregnancy. During pregnancy, the cervix normally remains tightly shut and is sealed with a plug of mucus. This means that the fetus is safely held in the uterus until labour begins, when the cervix begins to dilate.

Occasionally, however, the cervical canal is incompetent and begins to open before term, usually in the third or fourth month. This allows the amniotic sac containing the fetus to sag through into the vagina, and rupture, with a sudden loss of amniotic fluid followed by miscarriage. Unfortunately, an incompetent cervix is usually diagnosed only after a first miscarriage has occurred. If cervical incompetence is thought to be the cause of previous miscarriage, a soft non-absorbable thread will be inserted around your cervix to tighten it (see column, right).

After bed rest in hospital, you will be able to return home, but you should ensure that you rest adequately throughout the remainder of your pregnancy. The thread will be cut approximately seven days before term and your baby will be delivered vaginally in the normal way.

REASONS FOR PLACENTAL INSUFFICIENCY

The placenta may be unable to support the fetus sufficiently for a number of reasons:

• the placenta may have developed abnormally

• blood flow through the placenta may be restricted, or placental tissue lost because of a blood clot

• the placenta may separate, or may partly separate, from the uterine wall

• the placenta may be too small

• the placenta may be poorly developed

• the pregnancy may go beyond dates, so that the placenta becomes relatively inadequate for the fetus (see p.260)

• if maternal diabetes (see also p.140) is present, this can affect the placenta adversely.

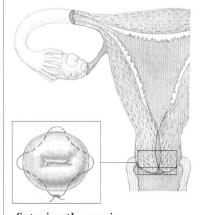

Suturing the cervix
The cervix is kept closed by passing a suture right around it – like the strings of a purse. The thread is normally cut approximately seven days before the expected delivery date.

223

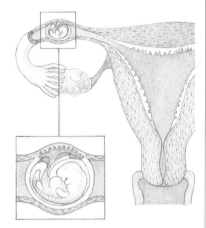

Tubal implantation
Ectopic pregnancy occurs in about 1 in every 300 pregnancies. The blastocyst (see p.32) usually implants in the fallopian tube (this happens in 99 percent of ectopic pregnancies). Very rarely, it may implant in the abdominal cavity, the cervix, or on one of the ovaries.

PRE-ECLAMPSIA

Pre-eclampsia is a potentially serious condition that can affect as many as one in 10 women, especially first-time mothers and women carrying more than one baby. It is unique to pregnancy, arising in the placenta, so the baby may grow more slowly than normal. The cause is not fully understood, but it does tend to run in families.

Symptoms Pre-eclampsia itself is in fact symptomless, but your midwife or doctor may be alerted to its presence if you are found to have significantly raised blood pressure and protein in your urine, both of which will be detected at an antenatal check, which is why it is very important to have your blood pressure checked regularly at each antenatal visit. You may also have oedema – swelling of the ankles and wrists.

Pre-eclampsia itself rarely occurs before the 20th week, but your blood pressure may start to rise progressively before this. The pregnancy can't be restored to normal, but delivery of the baby and placenta ends the disease.

Treatment You will be admitted to hospital or asked to go to a special day unit, so that delivery can be arranged before serious complications arise. Blood pressure, kidney and liver function, and blood clotting, are all monitored closely as all may be affected by the condition. Very rarely pre-eclampsia can develop into eclampsia, one of the most dangerous complications of pregnancy, which causes coma and convulsions. However, this condition is nearly always preceded by pre-eclampsia, which acts as an early warning signal, and can be prevented by delivery of the baby.

ECLAMPSIA

The word eclampsia derives from the Greek words meaning "like a flash of lightening" because the condition seemed to strike from out of the blue with fits and, eventually, coma. Eclampsia is a potentially life-threatening condition for both mother and baby and it used to be quite common. However, it is now extremely rare in the Western world owing to the ability of doctors to diagnose the condition in its earliest phase (**Pre-eclampsia,** see above) and because doctors and midwives are constantly alert for the warning signs. When eclampsia does occur, it is a full-blown medical emergency.

Symptoms Eclampsia is an emergency because the blood vessels in the uterus go into spasm (vasospasm), thereby cutting down the blood flow to the fetus with dangerous tissue hypoxia (low oxygen).

Your own life is threatened because vasospasm leads to kidney failure. Brain oxygen is also lowered, causing heightened brain sensitivity, which shows as fits. Tissues become waterlogged because of fluid retention and haemorrhages can occur in tissues such as the liver. The earliest signs are drowsiness, headache, dimness of vision, all of which are superimposed on rising blood pressure, oedema (see p.212), and protein in the urine (see **Urine,** p.177).

Treatment Where eclampsia does develop, treatment is aimed at increasing the blood flow to the brain, sedating the brain, reducing high blood pressure, and delivering the baby, which is usually by Caesarean section. As soon as the baby is born, the condition subsides, although fits may continue for five days or more after the birth.

Ectopic pregnancy

In ectopic pregnancy, the fertilized ovum implants somewhere other than in the cavity of the uterus, usually in a fallopian tube. The rapidly growing embryo causes the tube to distend, and the invading placenta weakens its walls, causing bleeding. Eventually the tube bursts under the strain.

However, before a fallopian tube bursts, certain symptoms that signal all is not well usually occur around the sixth week of pregnancy. They must be reported to your doctor immediately. Doctors define two forms of ectopic pregnancy:

Subacute form After a positive pregnancy test, the ectopic pregnancy may be signalled by pain in the abdomen, usually only on one side, sometimes accompanied by vaginal bleeding, fainting, and pain in the shoulder (on the same side as any pain in the abdomen). Sometimes an ectopic pregnancy is detected by an ultrasound scan after a small vaginal bleed early in the pregnancy. Although there is some leakage, there is no rupture as yet, and it may not be detected until eight to ten weeks gestation. This form can sometimes be treated by injecting a drug into the embryo, causing it to die and then be reabsorbed, which can save the fallopian tube.

Acute form This happens when the tube bursts, leading to severe pain and shock, with extreme paleness, weak but rapid pulse, and falling blood pressure. This acute form requires immediate hospital admission and treatment is by emergency surgical removal of the pregnancy from the fallopian tube. This may be done by laparoscopy if the tube is unruptured. The tube itself may also have to be removed, depending on the extent of the damage and a blood transfusion is sometimes necessary.

Ectopic pregnancy is becoming more common in developed countries. The reasons for this are still unknown, although some doctors think there could be a link with the increases in pelvic inflammatory disease, which causes scarring and blockage of the fallopian tubes. However, the apparent increase in ectopic pregnancies may be due to improved diagnosis made possible by the advent of ultrasound.

Outlook Almost 60 percent of women who have had an ectopic pregnancy become pregnant again, 30 percent avoid further pregnancy voluntarily; the rest are infertile. If you have had a previous ectopic pregnancy, tell your doctor as you will need special care during your current pregnancy.

POSTNATAL INFECTION

Postnatal infection, which used to be known as childbed fever, is now very rare indeed, although before the advent of antibiotics it was a primary cause of maternal mortality.

Postnatal infection is normally caused by remnants of the placenta remaining in the uterus. If one should occur, the first symptoms are a high temperature, acute stomach pains, and unpleasant-smelling lochia (see p.354).

If any of these symptoms develop, it is important to notify the doctor immediately; medical staff will promptly remove any remaining tissue and give you antibiotics to treat the infection.

A mother with pre-eclampsia

This condition, which is unique to pregnancy, is identified by the presence of the following symptoms: a rise in blood pressure, swollen ankles, feet, and hands, and protein in the urine. Although nothing can be done to prevent its onset, good antenatal care can ensure that the condition does not escalate.

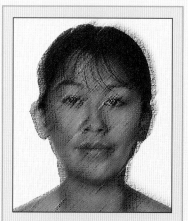

Name **Amie Lloyd**

Age **29 years**

Family history
Mother had high blood pressure

Obstetric history
This is Amie's second child

During Amie's first pregnancy three years ago she had very mild pre-eclamptic toxaemia in the last trimester of her pregnancy. Although Amie in the end had a normal delivery and her baby Isobel was perfectly normal, Amie is worried lest she has a recurrence of her PET during this her second pregnancy, possibly worse than last time. She knows that both mother and baby could be affected by the condition and naturally wants to be as well prepared as possible should any signs of PET arise during this pregnancy.

AMIE'S HISTORY OF PRE-ECLAMPSIA

There are quite a few statistics I can draw on to reassure Amie. Pre-eclamptic toxaemia (PET) is commonest in first pregnancies, so in a way she's been exposed to the highest risk already. Secondly her PET was very mild and took the form of slight oedema: swelling of the hands, fingers, feet and face with a marginally raised blood pressure requiring no treatment. But the other important sign of PET, the appearance of protein in the urine, was totally absent. And best of all, the PET came on only four weeks prior to term. In the end, Amie had a perfectly normal vaginal delivery and the baby was completely healthy and normal.

Statistics show that the later PET starts in pregnancy the lower the risk of it recurring in a second pregnancy. However, it's impossible to predict who will get pre-eclampsia again.

SOME FACTS ABOUT DIET AND PET

Amie's very keen to know if she can do anything to reduce the risk of recurrence but we know of no self-help measures that are guaranteed to work. What we do know is that PET is neither caused nor prevented by diet; by how you

feel about your pregnancy; by whether or not you exercise; by how hard you work; or by how much rest you take.

Amie eats a healthy diet and has heard that high protein diets might have a protective effect, but I had to tell her that this theory is entirely unproven.

Even the anecdotal evidence that calcium and fish oil supplements may help is not firm enough for me to recommend that she add any supplements to her diet.

WHAT IS PET?

Pre-eclampsia is an illness which arises only in pregnancy, possibly affecting mother and baby, and commonest towards the end of pregnancy. We don't really know what causes PET though it seems to run in families because the daughters of women who have had pre-eclampsia are slightly more likely to get it themselves.

PET AND THE PLACENTA

What's known for certain is that pre-eclampsia originates in the placenta. Towards the end of pregnancy the placenta gets as large as a dinner plate, about two inches (five centimetres) thick and needs a large and efficient blood supply from the mother to keep her baby growing healthily. In pre-eclampsia the placenta seems to run short of an adequate blood supply, and this has potentially serious consequences for mother and baby.

WARNING SIGNS ON THE MOTHER'S SIDE ARE:
• her blood pressure starts to rise
• valuable protein leaks out into the urine as her kidneys can't function as efficiently as before
• fluid starts to accumulate in the extremities – the hands, the feet, and the face
• the blood clotting mechanism may be affected.

It's likely that if PET did recur in her second pregnancy it would be milder than before. Nonetheless I advised Amie to take an active interest in everything that goes on at her antenatal clinic and in the results of her antenatal tests. I also suggested that she got her partner, Ed, involved because there might be moments when she's confused or alarmed and she would need to talk to him. She'd also need him for moral support at her antenatal visits.

GOOD ANTENATAL CARE
I told Amie that by far the most important preventative measure is for her to make sure she has excellent antenatal care throughout the term of her pregnancy. Monthly checks to 28 weeks, fortnightly to 36 weeks then weekly to term are the minimum she requires, and probably more often if any signs of PET are detected. I reassured her that because of her past history she'll be checked meticulously and frequently.

BASELINE TESTS
While there are no screening tests that can predict Amie's risk of developing pre-eclampsia during her pregnancy, there are some baseline tests that she could have done in the first half of her pregnancy and have repeated at regular intervals to give early warning of the onset of PET. So apart from the normal checks on blood pressure, urine, and her weight she should make sure she has tests for:
• kidney and blood-clotting function
• ultrasound scans to track the baby's growth
• doppler scans to measure the efficiency of blood flow to the placenta.

HOSPITAL ADMISSION
I reassured Amie that at the first sign of PET, in even its mildest form, she would be admitted to hospital to enable doctors and midwives to monitor her progress as well as that of her baby, enabling the delivery to be carried out before complications set in. Pre-eclampsia is progressive. It doesn't get better so once admitted Amie shouldn't expect to be allowed home until after the delivery.

DRUGS
Drugs are often prescribed to bring down a mother's blood pressure if it is found to be high. Though these drugs don't affect the underlying disease they can reduce the risk of some of the associated complications.

It's also possible that Amie may be given small daily doses of aspirin during her pregnancy which could prevent or delay the onset of PET. Aspirin works directly on the clotting blood cells, known as platelets, which are involved in PET.

CONSEQUENCES OF PET
If PET is worsening, if the baby shows signs of distress, or if the mother's condition is deteriorating there's only one treatment: urgent termination of the pregnancy – sometimes by Caesarean if the situation warrants it. However, last time Amie had a perfectly normal delivery and the chances are she'll have the same this time. Furthermore, I reassured her that if she was delivered by Caesarean section subsequent deliveries didn't necessarily have to be in the same way. Women who have had one Caesarean section can be allowed to try for a normal delivery next time. I suggested to Amie that if she should opt for an epidural rather than general anaesthesia, then she and Ed could take part in the delivery.

INVOLVEMENT OF EXPERTS
At their first antenatal visit I suggested that she and Ed discuss the need to be cared for by a PET specialist. Not all obstetricians are expert in the subject and I felt sure Amie and Ed would find it reassuring to see an expert early on. Research shows that the most important factor in a happy outcome to a PET birth is the involvement of specialized consultants who take action and treat the condition at once. I advised Amie to get in touch with Action on Pre-Eclampsia (APEC): 31–33 College Road, Harrow, Middlesex, HA1 1EJ. 24-hour helpline: 01923 266778

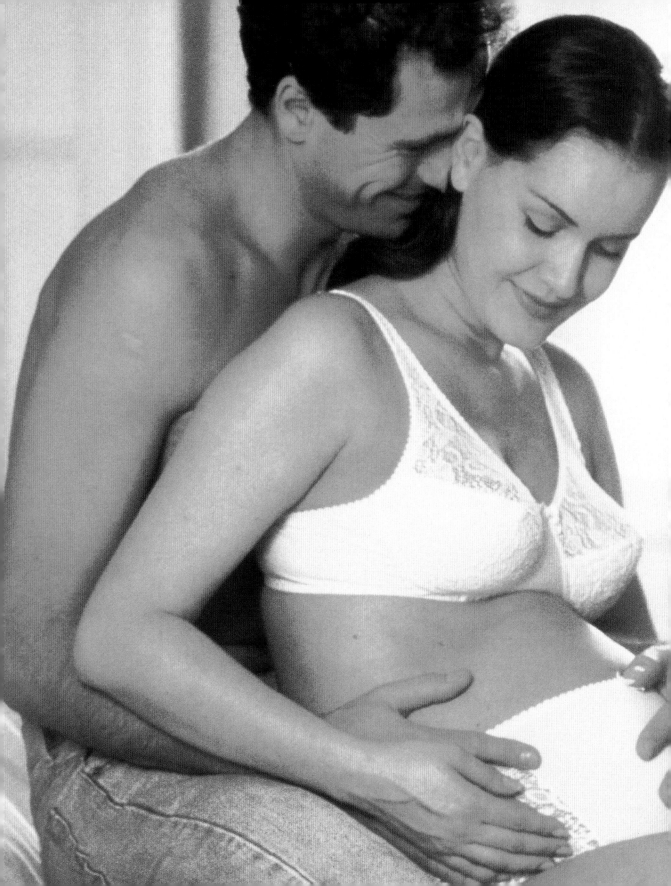

CHAPTER 11

A sensual PREGNANCY

The very high levels of female hormones present in your body during pregnancy mean that you have the potential to enjoy all aspects of sex, from massage to sexual intercourse, far more than ever before. However, you may experience sexual problems and these can easily wash over into other aspects of your lives, but the majority can be averted or resolved with open communication.

YOUR HORMONES

A woman undergoes many physical, emotional, and psychological changes during pregnancy, which will influence her attitude to sex and her enjoyment of it. These changes are due mainly to the vastly increased levels of hormones circulating in her body.

The most important hormones involved in maintaining pregnancy are progesterone and oestrogen. In the early days of a pregnancy these are produced by the corpus luteum in the ovary. However, once the embryo has implanted in the uterine lining, it and the developing placenta take over as the primary sources of progesterone and oestrogen.

The increase in the amounts of progesterone and oestrogen circulating in the body is swift and dramatic. The level of progesterone rises to 10 times what it was before conception, while the amount of oestrogen produced in a single day is equivalent to that generated by a non-pregnant woman's ovaries in three years. In fact, during the course of a single pregnancy, a woman will produce as much oestrogen as a non-pregnant woman could over 150 years.

Progesterone and oestrogen induce a sense of well-being and also lead to shining hair, supple and glowing skin, and an aura of tranquillity and contentment.

A sensual pregnancy

Unless there are medical reasons for abstaining from it, sexual intercourse is safe and permissible in pregnancy. Moreover, every pregnant woman has the potential to enjoy sex – perhaps more than she ever has before.

The desire for sex and the enjoyment of it varies widely, not only from one woman to another during pregnancy, but also in the same woman at different times throughout its duration. Typically, though, there is a decline in interest in sex during the first trimester (especially if you are suffering from tiredness and nausea), followed by an increase in the second trimester, and then another decline in the third trimester.

When a pregnant woman does have sex, she may find it far more exciting and satisfying than it was before she conceived. In fact, a woman will sometimes achieve orgasm or multiple orgasms for the first time when she is pregnant. This enhanced sexuality is principally because of the high levels of female hormones and pregnancy hormones that circulate throughout her body when she is pregnant (see column, left). These cause a number of important changes to her breasts and sexual organs, making them more sensitive and responsive. In addition, as being pregnant is such an affirmation of being female, a woman may find her condition leads to enhanced sensuality.

EROTICISM DURING PREGNANCY

One of the effects of the rise in oestrogen levels during pregnancy is an increase in blood flow, especially in the pelvic area. Because of this, the vagina and its folds, the labia, become slightly stretched and swollen. This stretching and swelling, which normally occur only during sexual excitement, make the sensory nerve endings hypersensitive, resulting in rapid arousal.

The breasts start to enlarge almost as soon as pregnancy occurs and one of the classic signs of pregnancy is sensitive, enlarged breasts with nipples that may tingle or even feel painful. The increased sensitivity of the breasts makes them a focus of sensory arousal, and a woman can feel the most exquisite sensations when her nipples and breasts are caressed and kissed by her partner. This sexual foreplay can result also in the arousal of the clitoris and the vagina, which will swell very readily.

Because of the increased blood flow the vaginal secretions are quite profuse, so a pregnant woman usually becomes ready for penetration much earlier than usual. Penetration is particularly easy because of the plenitude of vaginal fluid, and a climax can be achieved quite quickly if the clitoris is stimulated simultaneously. The intensity of orgasm may reach new heights and the time taken to "come down" from an orgasm can be greatly extended. This is evident in the labia minora and the lower end of the vagina, which can remain swollen for anything up to two hours after orgasm, particularly in the last trimester.

Incidental to stimulating the whole of the genital tract, the pregnancy hormones stimulate the production of a hormone within the brain called melanocyte-stimulating hormone (or MSH), which results in deeper skin pigmentation – as in the darkening of the nipple area. Darkening of the nipples can act as a sexual signal to a man, making his partner's breasts very attractive to him.

WHEN TO MAKE LOVE

You can make love whenever you want to, given that it's not too athletic and that there are no medical reasons for you to forego it (see p.236). Good sex in pregnancy is very enjoyable, and it helps to prepare you for childbirth by keeping your pelvic muscles strong and supple. It also bonds you closer to your partner, which will help you cope much better with the stresses of parenthood.

There is absolutely no physical reason why a woman having a normal pregnancy should not enjoy sexual relations with her partner to the full, and sex need not stop any earlier than the onset of labour, both partners being willing. In a low-risk pregnancy, the uterine spasms that accompany orgasms are perfectly safe, and in late pregnancy may be beneficial because they help prepare the uterus for the rigours of labour.

It is a fallacy that sex can cause an infection during pregnancy and may harm the baby – infection is virtually impossible because the cervix is plugged with a tough mucus that prevents the ascent of bacteria into the uterus. In addition, the baby is completely enclosed within the amniotic sac, which resists rupture even when under great pressure and cushions him against all external forces (including the weight of a partner during intercourse). There is no question, however, that extremely athletic sex is not a good idea, because it may cause soreness and abrasions and a pregnant woman should be free of these unnecessary discomforts.

Lovemaking positions There are several sexual positions that you can use to enhance your enjoyment – without in any way diminishing that of your partner – once the missionary position becomes too awkward and uncomfortable. Side-by-side positions are often pleasurable, as are rear-entry positions, because in these positions your abdomen is not under any pressure from the weight of your partner. Sitting positions are particularly enjoyable in the later months of pregnancy, and enable you to adjust your position but still see your partner's face and feel close to him.

If you are feeling sexy, but you don't really want intercourse, you and your partner could explore other forms of sensual and sexual pleasuring, such as erotically stroking and kissing each other, massage (see p.232), mutual masturbation, and oral sex.

BUILDING YOUR RELATIONSHIP

The physical and emotional changes that take place during pregnancy will inevitably have an impact on your sexual relationship with your partner. Love and understanding will help you to minimize any problems that may arise.

As pregnancy advances you may find that you have to change your sexual habits, and the best way to approach this change is to realize that it is a chance to build on and enhance the physical side of your relationship. For instance, it might prompt you to explore (perhaps for the first time) the pleasures of new lovemaking positions and of other forms of sexual activity such as mutual masturbation and oral sex.

Try to understand any changes in your own and your partner's sexual desires, and be open with each other when discussing your needs, but never allow your sex life to become the dominant feature of your overall relationship. Concentrate on loving rather than lovemaking, and if at any time you or your partner don't feel like sex, rediscover the intimacy and joy of simply being with the one you love.

GOOD FOR YOU

Use sensual massage as a source of pleasure in itself, or use it as a form of foreplay.

Sensual massage is a highly enjoyable way of maintaining a close physical relationship with your partner during your pregnancy, especially if intercourse is not possible for medical reasons, or if you find it uncomfortable or undesirable. If you make the massage as sexy as you can, and masturbate each other while you do it, both of you will probably be able to reach orgasm without penetration. Alternatively, if you are still having intercourse, use sensual massage as a loving, prolonged, and highly effective method of foreplay.

Sensual massage

When you and your partner give each other a loving, sensual massage you will find it both relaxing and highly erotic, and it will reinforce the feelings of love you have for each other. Begin with tender hugs, cuddles, and stroking, and then take it in turns to massage each other all over, from head to toe, using slow, sensuous hand movements and plenty of massage oil.

A SHARED PLEASURE

Massage is a way of discovering what gives you pleasure, and you should approach it with a completely open mind. You may both be surprised at how sexy it feels to have certain parts of your bodies caressed that you had never thought of as erotic.

Preparing for massage Choose a time when you are not likely to be disturbed (switch on the answering machine and put your mobile on to voice mail), and prepare your bedroom beforehand, making sure it is warm and comfortable. If your bed is too soft for giving a massage, put a mattress, duvet, or folded blankets on the floor, covered by a large, clean towel or sheet. Dim the lighting if necessary, and play some soft music to create a soothing atmosphere.

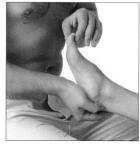

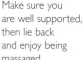

Make sure you are well supported, then lie back and enjoy being massaged

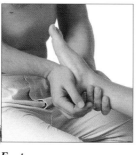

Foot massage
Press upwards into her foot with the heel of your hand and work downwards. Avoid massaging her heel and ankles, as this can cause uterine contractions.

Toe massage
Keeping the arch of her foot supported with one hand, clasp all her toes. Gently bend them back and forth. Rotate each toe in both directions.

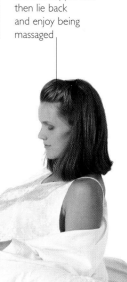

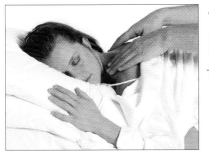

Shoulder and back massage
Gently knead the back of her neck, and then her shoulder muscles, between your palms, thumbs, and fingers. Massage her lower back with the heel of your hand.

GOOD FOR YOUR BABY

Your baby may also respond with pleasure as your body is stroked and caressed, and can share some of the benefits you receive through massage.

• From about the fifth month onwards your baby may feel stroking movements through your abdomen, which she will find very comforting and soothing.

• Learning to massage your own and your partner's body during pregnancy will help you to soothe your baby through touch after her birth.

• Continue to massage your baby after she's born: babies find massage soothing too.

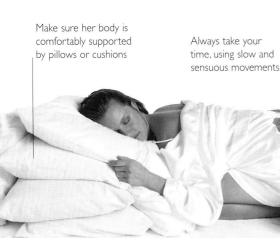

Make sure her body is comfortably supported by pillows or cushions

Always take your time, using slow and sensuous movements

Lubricating the skin Use a proper massage oil or lotion, because substitutes such as hand cream or body lotion will be absorbed into the skin too quickly, while baby oil will leave an oily film on the skin. Warm the oil before you use it (by putting the bottle in a bowl of warm water, for instance) and make sure your hands are warm and your fingernails are short and smooth. When you are giving the massage, put the oil on your hands and then smooth it on to your partner's skin (never just pour the oil directly on to your partner because that can be distracting as well as wasteful and messy).

Touching intimately Lightly coat your fingertips with massage oil and delicately trace the outlines of each other's lips, cheeks, jaws, ears, and neck. Then, using plenty of oil, work your fingers and the palm of your hands sensuously over breasts, chest, sides, and abdomen, and across the shoulders and down the arms. Stroke firmly up the inside of each thigh in turn, using the lightest of finger pressure on the return stroke. Always handle her breasts carefully as they will be tender.

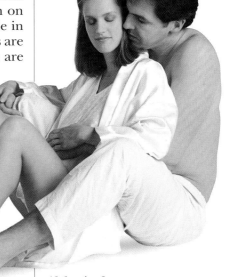

Abdominal massage
Make light, circular movements with your fingertips all over her abdomen as she leans back.

By making a few adjustments to your lovemaking you can make the experience happier for the mother-to-be.

Do:

• be tender, romantic, patient, and understanding

• use different kinds of stroking, such as using a firm hand over her abdomen if the baby kicks

• keep your weight off her stomach and breasts when making love

• use lots of pillows for greater comfort and to get the right angles around the curves of her body

• take your time when lovemaking, and don't be afraid to experiment.

Don't:

• force her to make love if she doesn't feel like it

• expect her to have simultaneous orgasms – or even one orgasm.

Making love

You can make love as late into pregnancy as you wish, as long as there are no medical reasons for abstaining (see p.236). Your baby, safe in your uterus, is not harmed by normal sexual activity (see column, left), and probably enjoys sex as much as you do as your hormones reach him via the placenta (see also p.192).

In the early months you can use any position you choose, but as your abdomen swells you may find some lovemaking positions uncomfortable. After about 24 weeks it's not advisable to lie on your back for any length of time so avoid the missionary position, with your partner on top – there are plenty of other exciting positions. Also, these alternatives are often the best positions to use when you resume lovemaking after the birth (see p.364).

WOMAN-ON-TOP POSITIONS

You will probably find these most comfortable from the second trimester onwards. As your abdomen grows, you can lift yourself further off his stomach by supporting yourself on your bent legs. This also prevents too much pressure on your abdomen and breasts. In these positions, too, you can better control the depth of penetration and the speed and rhythm of lovemaking.

These positions allow a great deal of intimacy. You and your partner have your hands free to caress and stroke each other and he can easily reach your breasts with his mouth. Alternatively, you can brush his chest with your breasts to stimulate him further.

KNEELING AND SIDE-BY-SIDE POSITIONS

Many of these involve entering from behind, and are useful in pregnancy, particularly if you don't feel comfortable on your back, or you do not want to take too active a part in lovemaking.

Kneeling positions allow your partner freedom of movement and let him vary the amount of penetration. Side-by-side positions are comfortable and permit plenty of kissing and caressing. The "spoons" position, so called because the partners nestle together like a pair of spoons, will also be useful if you experience any soreness or discomfort when you resume lovemaking after you have given birth, especially if you have an episiotomy.

SITTING POSITIONS

Most useful in the middle and late months, these don't allow a lot of movement but are comfortable for both partners and alleviate pressure on the abdomen. Also, the depth of penetration can be controlled. Your partner sits on a sturdy, comfortable chair or the edge of the bed and you sit on his lap, either facing him (if your abdomen is not too big), facing to one side, or facing away.

When you are facing to one side or away from your partner, he can use his hands to caress your body and breasts and to stimulate your clitoris. In addition, because his range of movement is limited, you have control of the sexual tempo.

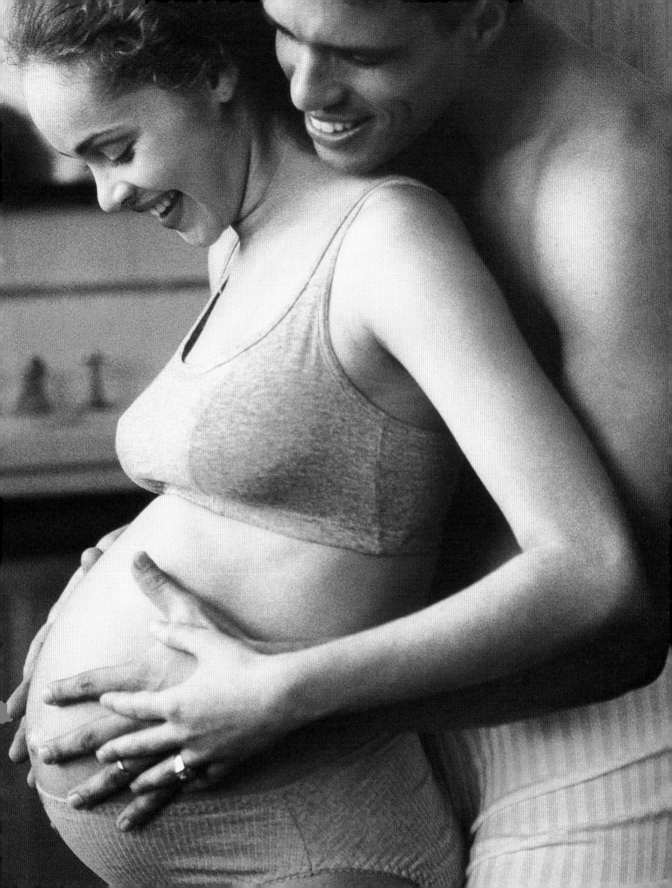

WHEN SEX MAY BE DANGEROUS

In some high-risk pregnancies, intercourse must be avoided at certain times or sometimes completely.

Your doctor will warn you if there is any risk of sexual activity being a danger to your pregnancy, and advise you on what (and when) is safe. You should always make sure that he or she explains the problem fully, and that you are completely clear about what you can and cannot safely do.

The most common reasons and times for restricting intercourse during pregnancy are:

• at any time if there is any sign of bleeding. The bleeding may well be quite harmless, but you should consult your doctor without delay

• if placenta praevia is suspected or confirmed (see p.222)

• in the last trimester if you have a multiple pregnancy

• in the last 12 weeks if you have a history of premature labour or if you are showing signs that you might go into premature labour

• if your waters have broken.

Sexual problems

During pregnancy, there are numerous physical and emotional factors that can diminish your enjoyment of sex. Fortunately, the few that actually prevent you from having intercourse are relatively uncommon.

Probably the most common reason for a drop in sexual enjoyment is that you believe your body is becoming less and less attractive to your partner as your pregnancy proceeds. In addition to a swelling abdomen with its growing baby, you may view with some alarm the loss of your waistline, your spreading hips, your swelling breasts, and your widening thighs and upper arms. When heavily pregnant, women sometimes become shy and defensive about their appearance and believe that all their femininity has gone. This, too, can lead to an increased reticence about being seen naked.

The best thing to do if this happens is to seek reassurance from your partner, who will allay your fears and probably be astonished that you feel unsure of your attractiveness.

LOSS OF LIBIDO

While you may experience an increased libido (sex drive) during pregnancy, it has to be said that some women feel a loss of sex drive during the first trimester. This is largely the result of morning sickness, which can make you feel thoroughly wretched and unattractive in every way. Fatigue is another enemy of the libido, and because pregnancy can be exhausting, you may sometimes have little energy left over to devote to enjoying sex with your partner. Like morning sickness, fatigue is a common problem of the first trimester and usually diminishes or disappears in the second.

In the second trimester, once free of the distractions of morning sickness and fatigue, most women find that their interest and pleasure in sex increase. Towards the latter end of pregnancy, though, libido may wane again, largely due once more to fatigue. It is sad that so many women feel like beached whales at this time and do not enjoy their rounded beauty. In addition, some may feel too embarrassed to want to strip bare and make love.

Hormone levels can swing quite violently during pregnancy and a woman may find that she's emotionally volatile, switching from contentment to sadness and tearfulness, and then to great elation. This is perfectly normal but, of course, it can have an adverse effect on your sexual relationship with your partner. In situations like this, you must be open with your partner and honest about your feelings. If you don't want to make love because you feel physically ill or excessively tired, tell him so, otherwise he may feel rejected.

DISCOMFORT

The hormone-controlled changes in your breasts and genitals make them more sensitive and responsive to touch. This usually has the effect of heightening your sexuality, but sometimes the increased sensitivity causes discomfort. This is especially true of the breasts in early pregnancy, and you may find that for the first couple of months they are very tender. Tell your partner about this discomfort, so that he will avoid touching them during love play.

The engorgement of your genitals may also cause some slight discomfort, particularly later in pregnancy, as they remain swollen and aching after orgasm. This can create a feeling of unrelieved fullness, which may make sex less satisfying. Some women find they can overcome this lack of satisfaction by masturbation, especially if they often have better orgasms through masturbation (by themselves or by their partners) than via intercourse.

A common source of discomfort comes when the baby enlarges. Eventually, your abdomen is so swollen that it is increasingly difficult for you to engage in sex in the usual missionary position. When you reach that stage you could try one or more of the alternative lovemaking positions discussed on page 234.

WHEN TO STOP

Refrain from sex if bleeding occurs at any time, and consult your doctor as soon as possible as to the possible cause. The likelihood is that the bleeding is not serious at all, and is the result of changes in the cervix that make it soft and easily damaged by deep penetration, but medical advice is essential. If the bleeding is confirmed as being due to the sensitivity of the cervix, you should avoid deep penetration when you subsequently have intercourse.

It is inadvisable to have sex if the mucus plug that seals the cervix has become dislodged (a show, see p.271), and you should also abstain after the waters have broken. Both of these are signs that labour is about to begin, although a show can occur as much as 7–10 days before contractions start. They usually happen near term, although they can happen earlier and could be a sign that you're going into premature labour (see p.298)

ANXIETIES

In any relationship, relaxed and happy lovemaking can be difficult to achieve if either or both of the partners are feeling anxious, tense, or nervous. During pregnancy there are many potential sources of anxiety, including fears about the safety of having sex, and the difficulty some couples or individuals have in adjusting to the idea of imminent parenthood.

Worries about the safety of sex during pregnancy are usually unfounded, and you and your partner should openly and fully discuss your feelings about the growth and extension of your relationship from partnership into parenthood.

If your sex life is causing you concern, and you and your partner cannot resolve it between you, do not hesitate to seek professional advice and counselling.

SEX WITHOUT INTERCOURSE

When intercourse is unwanted or unwise, there are alternative routes to sexual pleasure.

Extended foreplay Sensual massage and passionate kissing and caressing can stop short of or lead to orgasm, as desired.

Mutual masturbation This enables you and your partner to give each other sexual pleasure, and bring each other to orgasm, without having intercourse. To make the experience more sensual and also to avoid harming the delicate skin of your genitals, have your partner smear his hands and fingers with a suitable lubricant such as saliva.

Oral sex Fellatio and cunnilingus, as well as or instead of mutual masturbation, are perfectly safe throughout pregnancy. However, the vaginal secretions generally have a much stronger odour during pregnancy than at other times, and some men find this off-putting.

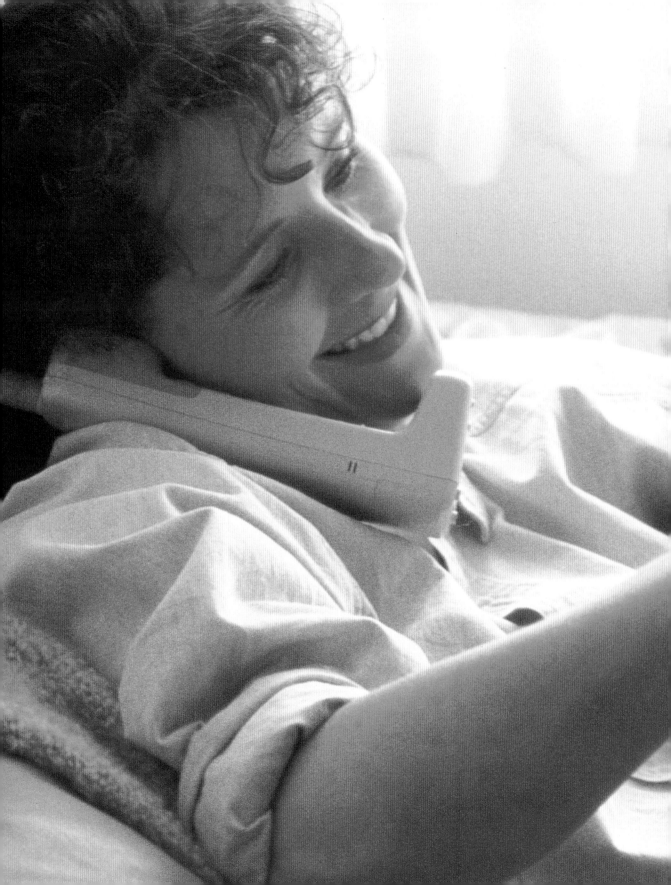

CHAPTER 12

Getting ready for
YOUR
BABY

From the 36th week, nesting begins in earnest. There's plenty to do in terms of getting the baby's room ready, choosing nursery equipment and baby clothes, finalizing your choice of names, deciding on the kind of care, if any, you will seek for your child, and making preparations for the sort of birth you are going to have.

When arranging the nursery, remember to think of your own needs; equipment and accessories should be easy and convenient to reach without creating hazards.

• Put up shelves so that you are able to see everything at a glance and withdraw items with ease.

• Keep powders and creams on shelves close to the changing mat but out of your baby's reach.

• Make sure there are no obstructions between the changing table, bath, your chair, and her cot.

• There should be no cords running across the floor. Set the lamp close to the wall socket.

• Put a comfortable, low chair in the nursery for night feeds – make sure it is easy to get out of and will support your back effectively.

Preparing for your baby

Getting ready for your baby can be one of the most enjoyable aspects of your pregnancy – there is something indefinably thrilling about a finished nursery and tiny baby clothes. To avoid fatigue, try to make preparations in small bursts, rather than all at once, and get your partner to help you – it helps you both to bond with your unborn child.

YOUR BABY'S ROOM

Over the past few months you may have had many ideas concerning the layout of your baby's room. It is a good idea to prepare the room before she arrives as once she is here your time and energy will be mainly taken up by her care. Safety and comfort for you both should be uppermost in your mind.

SLEEPING

During the first few weeks after delivery you may wish to have your baby sleeping in your own room. However, try to make sure there is a special place that can also be designated as your baby's nursery. This may be either a whole room, or an area in another child's room. Make sure you have enough space for sleeping, feeding, bathing, nappy changing, and dressing. The room doesn't have to be expensively decorated; a less elaborate treatment means fewer changes as she grows up. Much of the equipment can be obtained secondhand, or sometimes existing furniture can be easily adapted to your needs (see below).

Whether your baby has her own room or shares yours at first, the room needs to be kept warm. Try to maintain a constant temperature of around 16–20°C (60–70°F) and, if possible, install a thermostatically controlled heater.

FURNITURE AND STORAGE

A chest of drawers with a sturdy frame and legs is ideal both for storage and as a table for nappy changing. It should be high enough (about hip-height) to allow you or your partner to bend over without discomfort. Make sure the surface can be cleaned easily and, if wooden, that there are no cracks or splinters. A plastic-covered changing mat with raised sides is hygienic and comfortable. Choose a chest with at least three spacious drawers or one that allows shelves to be inserted underneath. You can then store baby-changing supplies in the top drawer or along the back edge where they are easily at hand. A small pedal-bin, lined with a plastic bag, should be placed nearby for the disposing of dirty nappies. Wall shelf units allow baby equipment to be stored neatly, and can be used later for books and toys. A straight-backed chair allows you or your partner to feed your baby in comfort. If possible, keep a small, sturdy table nearby for placing items on.

LIGHTING

You may want to check your baby while she is sleeping during the night. It is best to have lighting that will allow you to enter the room safely without disturbing her sleep. A dimmer switch fitted to the overhead lighting system will allow you to adjust the level of brightness so she is not suddenly woken. A night light or shaded lamp may be used, but be very careful to avoid extended wires.

FLOORS AND WALLS

Your nursery floor needs to be non-slippery, warm, and easily cleaned. Don't use small rugs or mats as you may trip or slip on them. If possible, lay down hardwearing and easy to clean linoleum or vinyl floor covering. Cork tiles provide warmth and damaged ones can be replaced. Walls should be painted with a non-toxic, washable emulsion paint, or if you are using wallpaper, make sure it can be wiped clean and doesn't stain.

WINDOWS AND CURTAINS

The nursery must be well ventilated, but make sure windows are draught proof, and above your baby's reach. Well-lined curtains, or blinds plus curtains, will block out daylight when your baby is sleeping; take care to choose nonflammable materials.

SAFETY PRECAUTIONS

- A safety lock should be fitted on each window in the nursery, along with bars if the window is close to the floor.

- Flameproof fabric must be used for bedding, upholstery, and curtains.

- Place childproof covers over all power point sockets.

- Screen electric bar and gas fires with a fire guard.

- Coat walls and furniture in non-toxic, lead-free paint or varnish.

- Put child-proof safety catches on all cupboards and drawers, especially in the kitchen.

- Instal smoke alarms.

- Ensure that all electrical flexes are well out of your baby's reach.

- Use non-slip mats in the bath and on the bathroom floor.

WHAT'S GOOD FOR BABY

A very young baby will be stimulated by a brightly coloured and noisy environment.

A bright musical cot mobile provides her with much pleasure if placed low down; hang another mobile above the changing table. Hang plastic-coated photographs or a small mirror in the cot; she likes looking at faces close up. Offer her rattles, and toys that make a noise when thrown, batted, sucked, or shaken. Moulded soft toys are good for sucking.

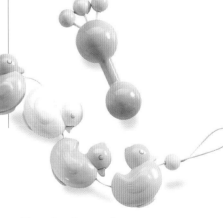

Toys for the newborn
Choose highly coloured light-weight toys that can't be swallowed or trap your baby's fingers.

Choosing equipment

Initially you need only a few pieces of equipment – something in which to transport your baby, somewhere for him to sleep, and something in which to bathe him.

A baby grows quickly and certain items of equipment may prove to be poor investments. Try to choose equipment that has a long life – a cot that becomes a child's bed, for example. Baby equipment is rarely worn out, simply outgrown, and there is no need to splash out on expensive items – check for secondhand items in your local paper or on your baby clinic notice board. Seek advice from friends and family; they may also be willing to loan or give you items.

TRAVEL

You will need some form of transportation for your baby as soon as he arrives. Before you buy, think carefully about how much space you have for storage, and the kind of lifestyle you lead. You can take your baby anywhere if you use a baby sling.

Carry cots Your newborn should be transported in a carry cot or pram, where he can lie flat. A pushchair in which he can lie flat may also be suitable. Although a carriage pram is comfortable and sturdy, you may have difficulty when storing or transporting it, or if you have to use steps.

You may find a carry cot easier to store as the stand folds flat; you can also use it for the baby's bed, and the frame can support his bath. Later, once your baby is able to sit upright, a pushchair may be more manageable. Most of these have a reclining seat that can face backwards or forwards.

Convertible transport
Buying a pram that will later convert to a pushchair will save you money, and mean that you get the full use from your equipment.

Opt for a pram or lie-back buggy that is easy to push with the handles at a comfortable height; you may strain your back if not. Good brakes are essential: you must be able to apply them without letting go of the handle.

A baby will quickly outgrow a cradle, so it is better to choose a cot that later converts into a bed. Make sure its height can be adjusted so you don't have to bend low to lift out your baby.

Car seats The law demands your child be safely restrained in a car, so buy an appropriate safety seat before taking your baby home from the hospital and check that it is securely anchored.

The seat should not be bought secondhand, and it must meet British safety regulations.

Baby sling
Your baby will enjoy the warmth of your body and the sound of your heartbeat when carried next to your chest.

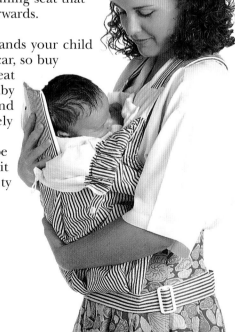

Portable baby chair This will allow your baby to see what's happening around him. A bouncing chair will provide enjoyment when he kicks his feet. While these are easy to carry, always check that the base is wide and sturdy to prevent his tipping over, and always strap him in securely.

SLEEPING AND BATHING

At first your baby will fit snugly in a baby basket, carry cot, or even a drawer! The important thing is that it is the right size and is comfortable. Choose a thin, close-fitting, waterproof mattress and cotton sheets. He must not have a pillow. Cot bumpers are not recommended as they impede air circulation and may make your baby too hot. It is much more important to make the baby's room draft-free and of an even temperature. Warm, light cotton cellular blankets are probably the best for bedding. Bear in mind that if your sleeping baby appears to be chilly, don't just add an extra covering as this will trap cold air inside, making him colder. Pick him up and cuddle him until he is warm, then add an extra blanket to his bedding.

His first bed
A baby (Moses) basket will make a snug first bed for your newborn baby

His cot Once your baby outgrows his first bed, choose a new or secondhand cot. Make sure it is sturdy and has non-toxic paint or varnish. The bars should be no wider than six centimetres (two and a half inches) so he can't push his head through. Cot sides should be high enough to stop him from climbing over, and have safety catches on the drop side to stop it being accidentally released. The mattress should be close-fitting and waterproof, with no gaps between the edges of the mattress and the frame. Cot bumpers are not recommended as an adventurous baby may try to use one as a step to help him climb over the bars of the cot.

Changing There is no need for a changing table if you have a sturdy table top or chest of drawers and a plastic changing mat. But if you do want a special changing area, opt for a stable changing unit with storage. Your baby can be bathed in a sink, but if you choose a special bath with a stand, ensure it is stable and the right height.

Bathtime
Choose sturdy, practical equipment for bathing. Yellow ducks are fun and are visually stimulating for your baby!

MEETING YOUR BABY'S NEEDS

Safety should be the most important consideration when choosing equipment, as any number of items can take care of his basic needs.

• Blankets, and quilts once your baby is six months or over, should not have a fringe or any loose ends that he can choke on.

• Blankets must be closely woven to avoid trapping fingers and toes.

• A sling should have a neck support, and wide straps that will support your baby's weight.

• Cots, prams, and pushchairs must not have any sharp edges or sharp screws.

• If you buy a pushchair make sure there is adequate protection for his head.

• There must be nothing on the pushchair that will trap his fingers or toes.

• Covers should be brightly coloured with vivid patterns to stimulate your baby.

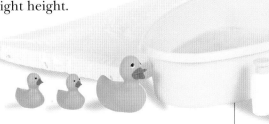

Don't wait until the last minute to purchase your layette; shop while you still feel comfortable enough to enjoy it.

• Shop on more than one occasion, and ask your partner or a friend to help you carry any heavy bags.

• Colour and style are irrelevant to your baby, so choose machine-washable garments with colours that will not run.

• Don't buy too many clothes in advance as you can't predict how fast your baby's going to grow or what the weather will be like.

• Opt for medium-priced items from well-known stores. Cheap baby clothes fall apart at the seams, fabrics become rough and irritating, and they may have to be discarded after only a few washes.

• However, don't skimp on the number of essential items. You always need more than you think.

Assembling a layette

Most of us over-prepare for a new baby, especially if it's our first. Babies, however, grow extremely fast, and very small garments will soon be outgrown. On the whole, it is always better to buy bigger, rather than smaller, as too close-fitting clothes will cause soreness and overheating. As babies have no idea what they are wearing, the golden rule is to keep all clothing simple and comfortable, causing fewer problems for both of you.

Choosing clothes and accessories Infant clothing is improving all the time in terms of fabric, design, and washability, so do shop around to get a feel for what's available before making a final choice. You will probably never use many of the items sold, so don't waste your money. A friend or relative with a baby will be able to give advice, and maybe clothes and accessories their baby has outgrown. Don't be reluctant to accept such gifts.

You will need several sheets, stretch suits, vests, and shawls so that you can have a few in the wash without running out. In order to prevent every stain showing, opt for patterned fabrics when choosing sheets and clothing, rather than solid pastels. Natural fibres are best as they allow sweat to evaporate but do bear in mind that bedding or clothes with a high percentage of cotton may shrink once they are washed, so buy at least a size bigger than you think you will need. Choose vests with wide necks, as babies hate having tight things pulled over their heads. Avoid any clothing with buttons or zippers that are close to the neck. Also, think what's convenient for you. Even if you prefer terry nappies, keep a supply of disposable nappies on hand; they can be used when a quick change with minimum fuss is desired.

ESSENTIAL BABY ITEMS

1 bonnet: the type will depend on the season

6 cotton vests with wide or envelope neck

2 plain knitted cardigans or loose jumpers

2 pairs cotton socks or slip on bootees

2 shawls

6 stretch suits

gloves or scratch mittens

6 pairs of plastic pants

1 box smallest-size disposable nappies or 2 dozen reusable nappies and 1 packet nappy liners

2 nappy buckets

2 soft new towels

8 muslin squares

1 packet cotton wool

baby lotion

1 packet safe nappy pins or plastic fasteners

blunt-edged scissors

nappy rash cream

CHOOSING YOUR BABY'S CLOTHING

Choosing clothes for your baby can seem like a daunting task when entering a shop for the first time as there are so many items to choose from. Just remember to be practical in your choice, taking into consideration some of the points that I have outlined below.

Cardigan should not have ribbons or lacy patterns that will catch fingers

Outdoor wear
When choosing clothing for outdoors your first priority is warmth. Don't be distracted by colour or fashion. Be aware that his head, feet, and hands are vulnerable to the cold, and keep them covered.

Stretchsuits are ideal for keeping baby warm all over; fastenings in crotch and inside leg will make nappy changing easy

Nightie should be long enough for warmth, with a wide opening

Going to bed
Babies move around during their sleep – not as much as adults but it's something to consider. Choose clothing that will allow free movement and not entangle his limbs.

YOUR BABY'S NEEDS

Comfort and safety, rather than style, should be the main priorities when you choose your baby's clothing.

• Fabrics should be soft and machine-washable. Cotton is ideal. Synthetics don't always absorb sweat, and wool can irritate a newborn's skin.

• In warm weather two layers are usually ample. In winter add more layers but do not overwrap him with tight clothes.

• A baby's gestures are jerky and expansive so make sure garments are loose, and easily stretched.

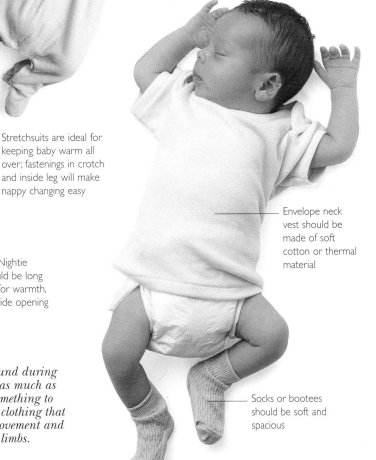

Envelope neck vest should be made of soft cotton or thermal material

Socks or bootees should be soft and spacious

MOTHER'S EXPERIENCE

Unless there are good reasons, breastfeeding is always preferable to bottlefeeding.

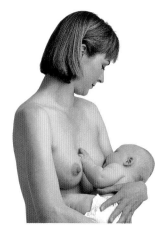

Breastfeeding This ensures that your baby is getting the ideal food; breast milk is always available, and doesn't require special equipment or preparation. It is also physically beneficial for you: for instance, it helps your uterus to return quickly to its normal size and – like many women – you may find it hugely enjoyable.

Breastfeeding has a few drawbacks, but these can be easily overcome. The quantity and quality of your milk depend on your overall health, so eat well and stay in good condition. Breastfeeding can lead to sore nipples or breast infections (see p.356), which need prompt treatment. Also it can be tiring so you must get sufficient rest.

Bottlefeeding Infant formulas are very nourishing, but they are still only second-best to breast milk, they can prove expensive and, if you take your baby out for any length of time, you have to carry equipment and a supply of formula with you.

Breast or bottle?

Breastfeeding is better for your baby than bottlefeeding. However, if you cannot breastfeed your baby, modern milk formulas ensure that she will be adequately nourished.

The best possible preparation for breastfeeding your baby is to acquaint yourself with the very real benefits that it offers (see below). Then, make sure that you are aware of what is involved, and that you are physically and mentally ready for it. The physical preparations that you can make are quite simple and straightforward, and consist mainly of being well-nourished, avoiding hazards that could affect your milk supply, and making sure your breasts are properly looked after. Your midwife, doctor, obstetrician, or childbirth teacher can answer any questions you might have.

If you decide on bottlefeeding (see pp.332 & 334), you will have to buy adequate supplies of formula, bottles and teats, and sterilizing equipment in advance of the birth.

BREASTFEEDING

Breast milk is the perfect food for a baby. It contains all the essential nutrients (fat, protein, carbohydrate, vitamins, and iron) that the baby needs; it is never too rich or too watery; it is clean, readily available, and always at the right temperature; and, like the colostrum produced by your breasts before your milk comes in (see **Producing milk**, p.326), it contains antibodies that help protect the baby from common infections such as gastro-enteritis.

Breastfeeding is a fulfilling and enjoyable experience that will enhance the loving relationship between you and your baby. Despite occasional snags, such as sore nipples or engorged breasts, it is physically beneficial. The extra calories you use up in producing breast milk help to deplete the fat reserves you accumulated during pregnancy, and it is therefore easier and quicker for you to get back to your pre-pregnant weight. When you breastfeed, the hormone oxytocin that makes your milk glands contract when your baby suckles (see p.326) also causes contractions in your uterus, enabling it to return to its normal size more quickly.

There is also some evidence that women who have breastfed are less prone to breast cancer and to osteoporosis (brittle bones). From a purely practical point of view, breastfeeding is quick, easy, and convenient, virtually free, and needs no special equipment.

However, breastfeeding does have some drawbacks. Until you have a well-established milk supply that enables you to collect and store some for later feeding by bottle (see p.327), you are the only person who can feed your baby. If you prefer privacy when breastfeeding, it may not be easy to find away from home.

246

Breastfeeding can lead to sore or cracked nipples and other breast problems (see p.356); illness, tiredness, worry, and menstruation can reduce your milk supply; if you are taking any medication or drugs while breastfeeding, these can pass into your milk and possibly cause harm to your baby, while some foods that you eat, such as oranges, may upset your baby's stomach.

Most problems and difficulties you may have in getting your baby to breastfeed tend to occur in the first couple of weeks. So if you find breastfeeding trying at first, stick with it for a while – once the initial difficulties have passed, you will probably find that it is easy, immensely rewarding, and enjoyable.

BOTTLEFEEDING

Although modern infant formula provides adequate nourishment for the baby (as you can see from the chart below), it contains none of the protective antibodies found in colostrum and breast milk. It is also harder to digest than breast milk (but because of this, your baby will need feeding less frequently); gives more formed bowel movements with a stronger smell than those of a breastfed baby; may lay the foundation for a milk allergy later on; preparing it is time-consuming; and you may find it harder to lose weight because you are not using up calories in producing milk. You have to buy the equipment and the formula, and if you go out you need to take a supply of made-up formula with you.

COMPARISON OF MILKS AND FORMULAS

Nutrient (per 100 millilitres)	Human milk	Cow's milk formula	Soya-based formula
Energy (kcal)	68	66	65
Fat (g)	3.8	3.7	3.6
Protein (g)	1.25	1.45	1.8
Carbohydrate (g)	7.2	7.22	6.9
Vitamin A (mg)	60	80	60
Vitamin D (mg)	0.025	1.0	1.0
Vitamin C (mg)	3.7	6.8	5.5
Iron (mg)	0.07	0.58	0.67

BABY'S EXPERIENCE

Your baby will derive great pleasure from being breastfed and breast milk is specifically designed to give her the best start in life.

Breast milk Nutritionally superior to formula, breast milk is easy to digest, and, like colostrum, protects against many common infections, particularly those of the gastro-intestinal and respiratory tracts. Even if you only breastfeed for the first few weeks, the antibodies in your colostrum and milk will be of great benefit to your baby, and the close contact between you will enhance your relationship.

Formula Should you be unable to breastfeed, your baby will, of course, thrive and grow on formula. Whenever you bottlefeed, give your baby lots of skin and eye contact, and talk, or sing to her to help to intensify the bonding between you.

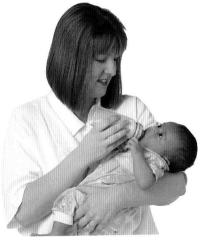

Creating intimacy
As you bottlefeed your baby, keep your attention focused on her. Maintain eye contact, and smile and talk to her.

Here are a few points that you should bear in mind when choosing a first name for your newborn baby.

• Will the name be suitable for your child at all stages throughout his or her life?

• Is it obvious how the name is spelt and pronounced?

• Does the name sound right when put together with the middle name(s) and your surname?

• Will the initials of the full name make a word when they are put together?

• Are you happy with any associations that may be apparent?

• Is there any way in which your child may be teased as a result of the name that you have chosen?

Choosing a name

Naming your baby can be surprisingly difficult. There are so many things to consider – will the chosen name go with the family name, will the name you have chosen go out of fashion? Many different associations and considerations may influence you, but you should always bear in mind that the name you choose is for your baby, and hopefully it will please him throughout the whole of his life.

FASHION

This is something that influences a great many parents, either consciously or unconsciously. For example, some names can suddenly become highly popular, such as Tracy or Jason in recent times, and are then in danger of falling out of fashion equally suddenly, thus dating the child who bears it.

It is very difficult to predict which names will become the "in" names in any given year, although some remain perennial favourites and many parents define what is fashionable or unfashionable by their own social set. The annual publication, *The Top Ten of Everything*, lists the most popular names for boys and girls in any given year.

You may be influenced by whether a name is traditional or modern. Some people prefer old, familiar names and shrink from new, invented, or imported names; others see no reason to use fossilized names from the past, and choose names that are meaningful to them and part of the age in which they live. Both points of view are equally valid, although traditional names are often easier for people to spell and pronounce.

ASSOCIATIONS

Given names are often the result of association, rather than being chosen because of their particular meaning. Meaning tends to play a much smaller role in the Western world than it does in other parts of the world.

Personal associations can have a positive or negative influence. Family, friends, or someone you respect, may provide a name; someone you dislike, a badly behaved child, or someone whose name is very much theirs is a name to reject. Godparents are sometimes honoured, and public personal associations might include royalty personalities (Charles, Diana), pop singers (Robbie, Melanie), or film stars (Kevin). Place-names, too, have begun to be used if they have a particular resonance for parents (Brooklyn, Phoenix), but take care when combining these with surnames (Brooklyn Bridge) to avoid opportunities for teasing.

Characters in books and films can also inspire parents. The 1956 film *High Society* starred Grace Kelly as Tracy Samantha Lord, which led to a surge of popularity for Grace, and the use of Tracy,

Samantha, and Kelly as first names for girls. In 1970, the name Jennifer became the second-most popular girl's name in America, following the film success of *Love Story* earlier the same year. Hit songs, such as "Michelle" and "Sweet Caroline", have also led to surges in popularity for these particular names.

For many people, a name can conjure up a particular image or character and they may expect children to fit or suit a name. As this can influence the way a child is treated, and consequently how the child responds, children may well grow into their names.

Other names, such as Patience or Faith, can reflect a desire for the child (usually female in the Western world) to manifest a particular virtue, and were first introduced by the Puritans (see column, right).

Some first names are inspired by incidents that happen at conception, during pregnancy, or around the time of birth. These can include the place of conception or birth; the time of birth – Noël or Natalie for a Christmas baby; month names such as May, June, or occasionally Octavia for an October birth; or a favourite record played during pregnancy, at or after birth; Dawn or Eve for the actual time of birth.

FAMILY TRADITIONS

Names that have passed down through a family from generation to generation have long been the automatic choice, especially for a first-born. If the traditional name was masculine, it was sometimes feminized for a girl (Thomas, Thomasina), especially if there was no male heir. In recent times, however, these customs have lapsed, with many traditional family names being dropped, although they are sometimes used as the middle name.

Some families, particularly in the aristocracy, in Scotland, and the American South, used the mother's maiden name as the firstborn son's given name. This appears to be dying out, although the maiden name is still given as a middle name. This tradition has resulted in the transferral of surnames (Russell, Howard, Cameron) to first-name usage, particularly for boys.

Many parents choose names for their children that work together, although few go as far as the Victorians (see column, right). Some parents like all their children's names to start with the same initial, although this can cause confusion with letters and official documents.

NATIONALITY

Many parents choose names that reflect their own nationality, as separate from their country of residence. This can lead to problems of spelling and pronunciation, so the spelling may be simplified – from Gaelic to English, for example (Síle – Sheila; Aodán – Aidan). In other cases, first names that are perceived as being "national" may not be used in their country of origin. Colleen, for example, comes from the Celtic word *caitlín*, meaning "girl" or "wench", and is popular for girls of Irish origin in America and Australia although it is not actually used as a given name in Ireland.

NAMING FASHIONS

There are trends in name-giving just as there are in other things. Many of today's first names have been used for centuries.

Norman After their British conquest in 1066, the Normans introduced a fixed name system. Norman names included Alan, Henry, Hugh, Ralph, Richard, Oliver, William, Alice, Emma, Rosamund, and Yvonne. These were names given to the aristocracy and later copied by those lower on the social scale, so Norman names rapidly replaced most Old English names. Of the latter, some, such as Edward and Edith, survived.

Biblical In the 16th century many names were used primarily by Catholics. These included Mary, and saints' names such as Sebastian, Benedict, and Agnes. The Protestants turned to the Bible for inspiration and Adam, Benjamin, David, Joshua, Michael, Samuel, Abigail, Dinah, Hannah, Rachel, Ruth, and Sarah became popular. The Puritans in the 17th century produced the "virtue" names – Faith, Charity, Grace, Hope, Patience, and Prudence.

Victorian At the end of the 19th century, there was a vogue for using gemstones or flowers as first names for girls. Thus Amber, Pearl, Ruby, Lily, Ivy, and Rose, became popular. Sometimes, all the girls in a family would bear the name of a flower or gem.

Contemporary This century saw the rise of exotic spellings, such as Jayne, Nikki, Debra, and of combinations, such as Raelene and Charlene. Since the 1960s many descriptive words, such as Sky, Free, Rainbow, and River, have been given as first names.

NAMING TWINS

There is a tradition of giving twins names that are related. The names may reflect an association; begin with the same initial (Paul, Patricia); sound alike (Suzanna, Hannah); or have a similar rhythm (Benjamin, Jonathan).

However, there are lots of reasons why your twins will not thank you if their names are too closely associated for comfort.

First, and most important, people will be much more likely to get them confused if there is a strong link between their names. Names are used as labels and twins, perhaps more than other children, need individual labels that belong solely to them.

Second, official forms, examination papers, and letters can easily become confused, especially if initials are shared.

Third, if the names are closely linked by association, they are likely to come in for a lot of name teasing or punning.

MEANINGS

The meaning or origin of a name tends to be a secondary factor for most modern Western parents. Many Western first names have had a more convoluted history than those of other cultures. This is because these names, along with other traditions and customs, have been transferred from one society to another, often by invasion followed by integration, migration, or intercultural contact. Consequently, many names, particularly those of dead or obscure languages, have become divorced from their original meanings. However, some Western parents do still choose names primarily because of their meanings.

FORM OF A NAME

The way our names are pronounced and spelt, and the shortened forms we prefer, are very important to us. It is extremely irritating if your name is constantly misspelt or mispronounced, and it can be very annoying if someone uses a short version you don't like, or the formal version that wasn't actually bestowed.

Diminutives The pet forms of names (Megan, Kate, Jamie) are often used, and sometimes given, in preference to the full versions (Margaret, Katherine, James). However, even if you intend always to use the diminutive, it is worth considering bestowing the formal name since there are likely to be occasions when the more dignified version is appropriate. On the other hand, if you intend always to use the full version of a name (Patricia, Edward) it is as well to consider the pet forms (Pat, Patty, Patsy, Trish, Tricia; Ed, Eddie, Ted, Ned) as your child's name will almost certainly be shortened by his or her friends.

Sound You may be particularly attracted to a name because of its sound – it could be that the name is naturally harmonious or perhaps it sounds good alongside the middle and surnames. Most parents take particular care to select a happy partnership, with surnames balanced by given names. Indeed, some parents bestow names in the order they feel sounds best (Elizabeth Anne, Arthur James), but use the middle name (Anne, James) as the primary form of address.

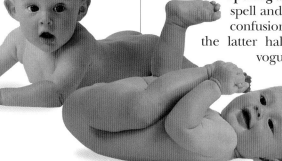

Spelling and pronunciation A name that everyone can spell and pronounce is a good idea in order to avoid confusion and irritation for your child in later life. In the latter half of the 20th century, there has been a vogue for exotic spellings of ordinary first names (Jayne, Kathryn, Jonothon), which may confer no discernible advantage. Some names have more than one pronunciation (Helena), while others are confusing (Phoebe), and still others have more than one spelling (Clare, Clair, Claire).

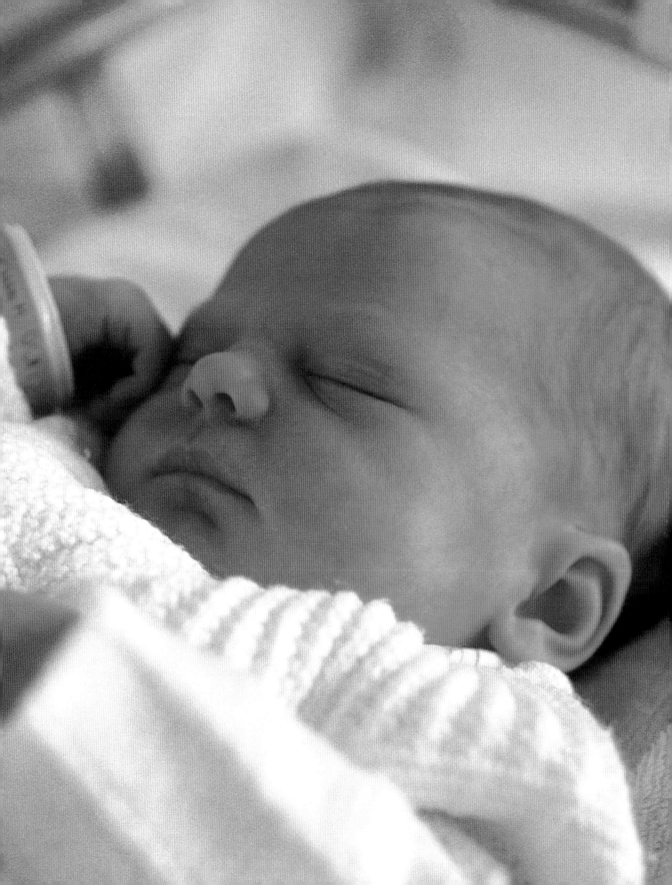

Preparing siblings for a new baby

Any child who's enjoyed the undivided attention of both parents for any length of time, say 12 months or longer, will suffer what child psychologists call dethronement when a new baby arrives. This is not simply having to take second place with mum and dad nor putting up with less attention than before. It's about feeling displaced and rejected. Nearly all toddlers suffer a deep sense of loss of parental love when a new sibling arrives. It's not surprising that their psychological disturbance shows in their behaviour.

Involving your older child
Talking to your older child about the arrival of the new baby and encouraging her to take an interest in the baby's development, will help her feel involved and avoid feelings of neglect.

To a small child, the arrival of a new baby topples him from pride of place, from being first in his mother's considerations, from being the apple of her eye, and the focus of her love, nurture, and attention. A child feels this displacement very dramatically and of course responds as only a small child knows how by using all the tactics at his disposal to regain his parents' love and attention.

The result can be "regression", which is a toddler's reversion to earlier, happier times when he couldn't feed himself perhaps, or when he wet and soiled his nappies, or when before he had learned to talk. Though this appears to adults like some sort of rebellion, a toddler can't help this kind of behaviour. So it would be absolutely wrong for you or your partner to chastise or punish him for it. In fact, the opposite is essential – extra special time alone with

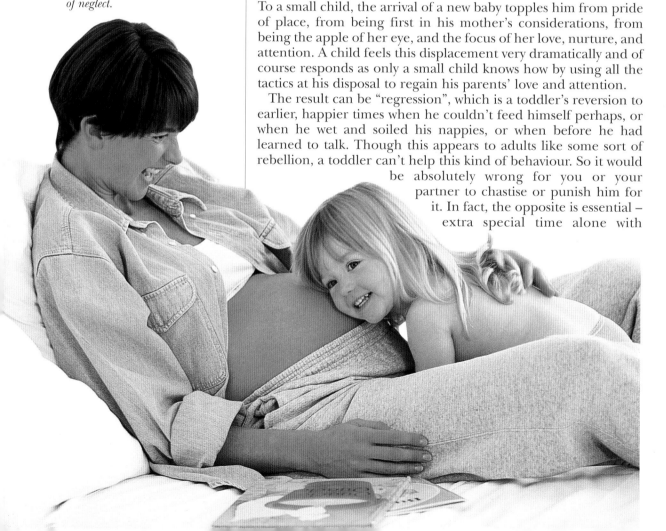

mum and dad, extra special loving care, plenty of rewards, praise and lots of physical affection with games, kisses, cuddles, lots of jokes and laughter.

Armed with this knowledge of how your toddler is likely to react to the advent of a brother or sister, with some preparation and planning you can ease him through this painful time.

Involving your older child in the pregnancy   You should be honest with your child from the outset. Tell him that a new baby is on the way and he's going to have a new brother or sister. You might even ask him what his favourite names are. Make a list, put them up in the kitchen, and talk about them from time to time.

You should encourage your child to put his hand on your tummy as it gets bigger to feel the baby kicking. You could also tell him that your baby loves the sound of his voice and that he should talk to her through your tummy. If possible, he should sing her songs and nursery rhymes through your tummy. This, incidentally, isn't all hot air. Your developing baby does remember the voices of those around her and will bond with them after birth. So she will respond instantly on hearing her brother's or sister's voice once she's born, if she's heard it constantly during your pregnancy.

You could help your child to understand what's going on inside you by drawing together what's happening in your tummy month by month from pictures in this book (see pp.72–89) on large sheets of paper so that it's all very clear. Point out how the baby is developing then put the drawings round the wall at a height that your toddler can see and relate to. You can then make up stories about each stage of the new baby's development with remarks like, "Now your new baby's heart is beating, now your new baby can move his hands and legs and we can feel him kicking, now your new baby can suck her thumb, now your new baby is getting ready to be born, etc."

Try to encourage your toddler to take ownership of his new sister by using the word "your", as in "your baby", "your new sister". If you do, very soon he'll develop a sense of propriety, of ownership, and of a desire to take care of his new sister. He may think use of the words "our new baby" excludes him and makes him feel frozen out.

Your toddler will feel involved if you ask him to help with the preparations of his sister's nursery – helping to make up the cot, set out equipment, or even suggest that he try the baby bath first, with words like "Wouldn't you like to see what the baby bath feels like before your sister uses it?" All toddlers like to help and love to imitate your actions. So give your toddler small jobs to do and be very appreciative of all his efforts. You can show him all the new baby's tiny clothes and encourage him to feel special by saying how much bigger he is and how much he's grown since he needed them.

AFTER THE BIRTH

If you're going to be in hospital for several days try to arrange for your child to visit you and the baby as soon as possible after the delivery.

When your toddler visits, have eyes only for him. Ideally, the baby should be asleep in the bedside cot. Make a fuss of your toddler until he asks about the new baby. Only then show him his sister, but not for long, not with any fuss, and not paying too much attention to her. Make his visit short so that you can attend to your baby once he's gone.

Bringing the baby home   Try to help your toddler to feel secure and bond with the new baby.

• When you greet him, make sure someone else holds the baby so that you are free to cuddle him.

• For the first few minutes give him all your attention.

• Give your child a present from the new baby, something that he has really been looking forward to.

• In the first weeks set aside some time when the two of you can be together without any interruptions.

• Involve your child in the new baby's bathtimes, changing, and feeding times. Get him to fetch and carry and imitate your loving sounds with lots of ahhs and ooohs and words like "softly", "gently". Describe everything that your new baby is doing so that he can get to know her and relate to her.

• A newborn baby has a well-developed grasp reflex. Put one of your child's fingers into her hand – she'll grasp on to it very tightly and he'll interpret this as love from his newborn sister.

FATHER CARE

In many households, the father becomes the main helper when his partner arrives home with their new baby. Some men immediately involve themselves in caring for their partner and child, but others need to be prompted into action.

What you need from your partner more than anything else at this time is understanding, sympathy, and a readiness to let his routine relax and go along with you and the baby. This needs serious discussion before the baby is born. Otherwise your partner may find it hard to adapt and feel neglected, inadequate, and bereft of your affection and attention.

You may find it useful to divide the work between you. For instance, your partner could take over the cleaning, shopping, and laundry, leaving you free to concentrate on looking after yourself and the baby. Or you could simply share all the household and childcare work.

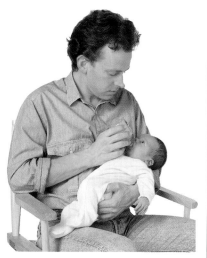

Help at mealtimes
If you are breastfeeding, express milk into a bottle (see p.327) so that your partner can also enjoy the pleasure of feeding the baby.

Arranging childcare

In the last weeks of pregnancy, it's a good idea for you and your partner to spend some time discussing and planning how you are going to run your domestic routine once you settle down at home with your new child. If your partner is able and willing to play a full part, you should be able to cope without too much difficulty; if not, you will need someone to help you, especially for the first few weeks.

The first few days of motherhood will be harder than you think. Labour and birth are physically and emotionally draining; you will feel you have very few reserves, and will be very fatigued. You will realize, once at home with your baby, that one job or activity succeeds another almost without respite, and in the middle of all this activity you are still learning about being a mother. Even if you have read every baby book going, you will find that your baby conforms to no typical schedule or plan, and that you have to work out your life around your baby's routine. Trying to impose a routine on your baby only causes you more work; you have to take your lead from him. As far as sleep is concerned, you have to get it when you can – new babies don't know night from day and require the same attention during the night as they do in the day.

During the first few weeks at home with your baby, try to get someone else to do the household chores, or simply cut back the amount you do to the bare minimum, until you get used to the schedule your baby follows naturally.

SOURCES OF HELP

Unless you want to become extremely tired, even depressed and weepy, you will need some help to tide you over at least the first few days, and preferably the first week or two. Don't be too proud to ask for or accept help – if you are reticent, you may soon come to regret it. Having help does not make you an inadequate mother. The best possible solution is some live-in help, so that your day can be split into shifts. That way you can at least make sure that you get sufficient rest and pay attention to your diet.

Family and friends Your mother and your mother-in-law are probably the people you trust most in the world when it comes to childcare. They have had children and are experienced at looking after babies, and they will give you lots of helpful support and advice. A good idea would be to get one of them, or another close relative who has the flexibility and time to come and live in your house around the time you go into labour. That way she can establish herself in your home with your family and partner, and be ready to receive you when you come home with the baby.

Such a helper is invaluable. You will feel confident that your household is ticking over quite normally. She should take off your shoulders all the administration and see to meals, laundry, shopping, and so on. This can relieve some of the responsibility from your partner, and so you can both devote more time to your baby. In addition, if your helper has had children of her own, she can be a fountain of information and advice.

Nannies   Nannies can either live with you or come on a daily basis. If you decide that you would like a nanny, try to arrange for her to be settled in with your family before the baby is born. This is a very good idea because you will get to know each other. Having a newborn baby in the house is quite a traumatic event, and it is important to have a helper who will fit in with your routines and lifestyle. You must also have confidence in her abilities and feel happy with her relationship with your baby.

You can find a nanny through personal recommendation, advertising, or through a really reliable nanny agency. I recommend you contact the Federation of Recruitment and Employment Services for the best one in your area.

But, no matter how you recruit your nanny, it is essential that you see her at least twice before you hire her, that you get two good references, and that you follow up these references with a telephone call to tease out any "between the lines" information. At the first meeting you could relax over tea or lunch or maybe go shopping together, and then follow this on another occasion with a formal interview. Both you and your partner should be involved in this process, because you will probably see different aspects of her character.

Draw up a contract of employment with a proper job description in which you cover all the tasks you expect her to undertake, and include the required approaches and attitudes. Your nanny should be prepared to bend her usual practices in order to fit in with yours. Remember that you are her employer and as such you are responsible for her welfare; she has the same employment rights as an employee in any other line of business.

Au pairs   These are young women (or occasionally young men) from abroad who help you with your baby in exchange for room, board, and a small wage. They are much cheaper than nannies but bear in mind that most have no childcare training and may speak little English. An au pair is supposed to live with you as part of the family; she is not an employee. It is not advisable (and not fair on your au pair) to leave her in sole care of a baby under one year for any length of time. In fact in the UK, au pairs are not supposed to work more than five hours a day, and their duties should only include babysitting and light housework, and you should give them time off to go to language classes if they wish.

MATERNITY NURSES

If you want short-term, live-in help, you can hire a maternity nurse. She will join your household just before or after the baby is born and will help you with all of the babycare.

As well as providing welcome help with the baby, maternity nurses are invaluable teachers. They will show you how to see to your baby's daily care: how to change nappies; how to breast- or bottlefeed him, how to know when he's had enough, and how to take the baby carefully off your breast to avoid soreness and cracked nipples, for example.

But it's up to you and your maternity nurse to work out what kind of regime you would like. You may decide, for instance, that you wish to have a night's sleep without interruption; the nurse will be on duty all the way through the night but you will take over at, say, 7 a.m. so that she can get some rest. Later in the day, she would be responsible for the baby's laundry, preparation of formula feeding, keeping the nursery clean, and looking after all the baby's needs and some of yours too.

As a general rule, a maternity nurse does not stay with you for more than four weeks, but you can arrange for her to stay for longer if your finances can stretch to it. Maternity nurses are expensive but will get you off to a good start if there is no one else to help.

The working mother

Vicky has decided to continue with a very demanding job while she has her second child. Accordingly, she has to fit the pieces of her life together like a jigsaw-puzzle – when to leave work, when to return, childcare, her family, and her health. She needs to make the well-being of herself and her baby the top priority in all her plans.

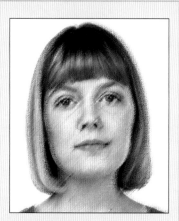

Name **Vicky Dyson**

Age **29 years**

Past medical history
Nothing abnormal

Obstetric history
One son aged six; everything normal

Vicky, a junior partner in a firm of accountants, is very keen to go on working while pregnant. She passed her accountancy exams while she was expecting her first child, so she knows she can cope. She also knows that she can combine work and mothering, having worked since shortly after the birth of her son. Her challenge now is to combine pregnancy with work, being a mother to a schoolboy, and maintaining a good relationship with her partner. The keys are time management and being sensitive to her own needs.

VICKY'S WORK SITUATION

Vicky's colleagues and senior partners are all men and she fears they will resent her taking a lot of time off either before or after the birth. I advised her to inform her senior partners immediately that she is pregnant and to make an appointment with them, for some time within the next three months, to discuss when she might leave work and when she might return (see p.64). I also advised her to make sure her diet gives her all the energy and nutrition she needs to keep working while her baby develops. She will also need extra rest and therefore should, if possible, take a nap in the afternoon – or at least rest with her feet up.

WHEN TO LEAVE

No two pregnancies are alike, so Vicky cannot know in advance how she will feel this time around. I advised her that she would be unwise to commit herself to staying at work beyond the 32nd week but perhaps she could arrange an informal option to do so if she feels well enough.

WHEN TO RETURN

This is a more complicated decision, as there are so many things to take into account.

Vicky's menstrual cycle may take only three months to get back to normal but her muscles and various organs need more time. The process takes a year altogether. Vicky has to make special feeding plans if she wants to go back to work before her baby is four months old. As she doesn't want to give her baby milk substitute, she will have to express her breast milk and freeze it (see **At the office**, opposite, and p.327). Vicky will need to allow time to build up an initial stock of milk, then a further six weeks for the baby to get used to the new arrangement.

I suggested that Vicky could choose a provisional date for her return to work, bearing in mind that she may feel quite different after the birth, and should consult her doctor as the date for her return approaches.

CHOOSING A CARER

When choosing a carer, she will need to check out all the available options well in advance – crèches, childminders, daytime nannies, au-pairs – until she finds a carer who's just right.

MAKING TIME

Once she is back at work, running her home, looking after her family, and mothering her new baby, Vicky will probably feel that time is very precious – and that she hasn't got enough of it.

She must have some time alone with her new baby every day, and her son, Jack, will need lots of reassurance at this stage. The best way to give him this is to let him have his own special time with her, so that he doesn't feel shut out. Vicky will also want to have time alone with her partner, Peter, so that their relationship doesn't suffer. She and Peter, with or without the children, will also want to spend time with their friends. Above all, Vicky will need some time to herself – even if it's only one free hour a week when nobody is making any demands upon her. Many mothers feel guilty about taking time to be alone or doing something for themselves but it's essential if a mother is to be relaxed and happy.

FINDING A ROUTINE

I suggested that Vicky would be likely to feel less overwhelmed if she has a routine to work to, and that the rest of her family would also feel happier if their days were structured. For example, her time with the baby could be when Vicky gets back from work. She could encourage Peter and Jack to bring her a cup of tea, make sure she is comfortable, then leave her alone with the baby while they go off and play together. Her special time with her son could be his bedtime, when she reads him a story and listens to him talk about his day. She and Peter could then have their evening meal together and chat, before the baby requires her late evening feed.

EXPRESSING HER MILK

I explained to Vicky that the main factor in maintaining a good supply of breast milk is the removal of milk from the breasts, either by feeding her baby or by expressing it regularly. Leaving milk in the breast discourages further milk production and supplies quickly dwindle. Vicky feels sure that she will have enough milk for her to be able to express some just after her feeds so that she can gradually create a stockpile of milk for future use.

AT THE OFFICE

I told Vicky she will probably find that her breasts will become full twice during the day, so she will have to make the time to express it during her working day.

Vicky told me that she intended to use a breast pump and, in spite of the fact that her firm is predominately male, there is a comfortable, clean ladies room where she can express her milk in private, as well as a refrigerator in her office where she can store it until she goes home in the evening, so she anticipates few problems. I reminded her that all containers must be sterilized and that breast milk can only be kept for up to 48 hours in the refrigerator (up to six months in the freezer).

As Vicky will be at work all day, the carer will be responsible for defrosting each day's supply of breast milk. This should usually be done in the refrigerator, although to defrost breast milk quickly, you can place the container under running lukewarm tap water. The baby's leftover milk must be thrown away and never kept or refrozen for later use.

VICKY'S BABY

As her mother is working, Vicky's baby will also have to adjust to a routine.

• She will have to accept the bottles of expressed milk, something she'll find easier if she's introduced to it before she is five weeks old.

• If she persistently refuses to accept milk from a bottle it's worth trying bottles with a different type of nipple.

• Six weeks before Vicky returns to work, the baby will start being weaned off the breast entirely for her daytime feeds. To start off, a single daytime feed will be replaced by a bottle until she is used to it.

• She will have to accept the person who looks after her all day while Vicky is at work.

• The baby will develop close bonds with her carer, who will become an important person in her life but this will in no way, however, affect her relationship with her parents.

• She must make the most of her time with her mother and the best time is when Vicky gets home from work; her breasts will be full of milk and the baby will be ready for a feed.

• She'll be quick to figure out that mummy is there all night and may become a wakeful baby, as two of my own sons did.

GETTING ENOUGH SLEEP

A good night's sleep is one of your top priorities in the late stages of pregnancy.

Aim to get eight hours of sleep a night, but you may suffer from irritating insomnia because, although your metabolism slows down at night, that of your baby does not. It keeps hammering away all through the night hours. If you cannot sleep, there are a number of ways to alleviate the problem:

• a warm (not hot) bath before going to bed is very relaxing and makes you sleepy and tranquil

• a hot milky bedtime drink helps you drop off; also, read a calming book, listen to music or the radio, or watch television

• deep breathing and relaxation exercises are excellent treatments for insomnia, so find a bedtime routine that you can rely on

• instead of worrying about your lack of sleep, get up in the middle of the night and do something – perhaps a job that you've been putting off for some time – or go into the nursery, look at things, touch them, rearrange them, and feel happy at the prospect of your forthcoming baby

• if you have worries that stop you sleeping, visualize each one as being written on a piece of paper. Then mentally screw it up and throw it away.

The late stages of pregnancy

Very little goes wrong in the last few weeks of pregnancy. From week 32 onwards, your doctor's main concern is the continued growth of the baby and your own health. Threats to your well-being could occur with an increase in blood pressure, which may herald pre-eclampsia (see p.224), or cessation of weight gain, suggesting that your baby isn't growing. Consequently, your doctor will want to see you more frequently, probably every three weeks from week 32 to week 36, and then fortnightly up to week 40.

One of the aspects of later pregnancy that you may be concerned about is your comfort. As your abdomen gets larger, sitting or lying in your usual positions becomes uncomfortable. If you lie flat on your back, the weight of your growing baby will press down on the major blood vessels and nerves that lie against the spine, causing numbness and tingling pain, and even dizziness and shortness of breath. Pay attention to your sleeping position in bed and make sure that you can be comfortable. Sometimes you will need cushions or soft pillows to support your body (see below).

TENSE AND RELAX TECHNIQUE

Good relaxation techniques combine the release of tension in the mind and body with deep, regular breathing, and it is helpful to practise these techniques so that towards the end of pregnancy they have become second nature.

Resting on your side
If you can't rest lying on your back, prop yourself up with plenty of cushions or pillows.

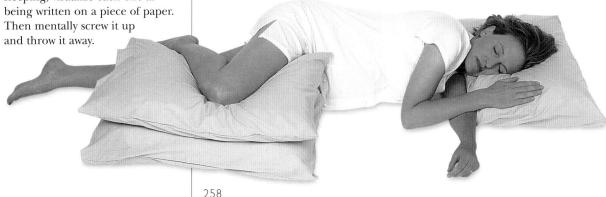

A good way to completely relax your whole body is to use the tense and relax technique. This is a pleasant aid to relaxation during pregnancy, and will also serve as a good preparation for labour, when it is a great help to be able to relax most of the muscles in your body, so that your uterus contracts without the rest of your body tensing.

The technique involves the tensing and relaxing of different parts of your body in sequence. Your partner can help by touching you where he can see you are tensing up: you respond to his touch by relaxing. It is best to practise this drill twice a day for 15–20 minutes if you can. Practise before meals or an hour or more after eating.

Find a comfortable position either lying on your back or propped up with cushions. Close your eyes and then try to clear your mind of any stressful thoughts, anxieties, or worries by breathing in and out slowly and regularly and concentrating all your attention on your breathing actions. Let pleasant, relaxing thoughts flow through your head, and if any worrying or nagging thought tries to recur, prevent it from doing so by saying "no" under your breath, then return to concentrating completely on your deep breathing. When your mind is totally relaxed and your breathing deep and regular, you can begin the tense and relax routine. Think about your right hand: tense it for a moment, palm upward, then relax it and tell it to feel heavy and warm. Work up through the right side of your body, tensing and relaxing your forearm, upper arm, and your shoulder. Then repeat the process on the upper left side of your body. Next, roll your knees outwards, and then in turn tense and relax your buttocks, thighs, calves, and your feet. Press your lower back gently into the floor or cushions, then release and relax.

Finally, relax the muscles of your head and neck. Relax the muscles of your face, eyes, and forehead, and smooth away any frowns.

Sitting in a chair
When you sit in a chair, sitting up straight will help strengthen your back muscles. If you need extra support, put a cushion at the small of your back.

YOUR BABY'S POSITION

As a baby reaches full maturity at about 37 weeks, he becomes heavier and tips head-down. Some babies, however, remain breech (see p.307) until term.

If a baby is in the breech position at term he may be delivered by Caesarean section (see p.308). If your baby is breech in the last weeks of pregnancy, though, you can be reassured that he will probably turn himself before labour actually begins:

• 30 percent of babies are breech at 30 weeks. Over half of these will turn spontaneously during the next two weeks

• 14 percent of babies are still breech at 32 weeks. There is a 60 percent chance that a baby that is bottom-down will turn of his own accord before labour starts

• Less than 5 percent of babies are still breech at 37 weeks. A quarter of these will turn on their own, although this is less likely if the legs are extended or there isn't much room in the uterus, for instance because it is a multiple pregnancy or the baby is large

• A few babies will kick themselves round once labour starts, as long as there is room

MONITORING THE OVERDUE BABY

Babies past their EDDs are monitored closely, and there are a number of different ways of keeping a check on your baby.

Fetal movement recording The most accurate sign that all is well with your baby is if you can detect regular fetal movements. Since mothers, and babies, are different, the amount of movement that is normal for each individual pregnancy varies. You are the best judge of whether your unborn baby is acting normally, and you can monitor his activity using a kick chart (see p.195).

Electronic fetal monitoring This may be used to check the baby's heartbeat by providing a continuous sound or paper recording (see p.275). If the heartbeat is satisfactory, it is usually judged unnecessary to perform other tests, or to induce labour.

Ultrasound You will probably be given an ultrasound scan to assess the volume of amniotic fluid. If this is becoming dangerously low, then you will be advised to have your pregnancy induced.

Are you overdue?

Only about five percent of all babies arrive on the actual date that they are expected. The expected date of delivery (EDD – see p.63) is only a statistical average, and studies have shown that as many as 40 percent of babies are born more than a week after the EDD. This 40 percent of babies that are "overdue" breaks down as follows: 25 percent of babies are born in the 42nd week of pregnancy, 12 percent in the 43rd week, and three percent of babies are born in the 44th week of pregnancy.

BEING OVERDUE

One of the main difficulties in deciding whether a baby is actually overdue or not is that the precise date of conception in any particular pregnancy is extremely difficult to pinpoint. Even if you have a regular menstrual cycle of 28 days (the standard on which the EDD chart is based), the date of ovulation is only known approximately (see p.63).

Apart from this uncertainty about the exact date of ovulation, every baby is different and therefore it is unrealistic to expect all babies to mature in precisely the same number of days. Moreover, since labour is initiated by your baby producing certain hormones as he reaches full maturity, it follows that the actual date of delivery can vary fairly widely – even in "textbook" pregnancies.

However, doctors do become concerned if a pregnancy continues much beyond the estimated date of delivery. This is because post-maturity and possible placental insufficiency pose some risks to the health of your unborn baby (see **Post-Maturity**, **Risks**, opposite). The longer the baby continues to grow inside the uterus, the larger he is likely to become, which, in turn, will increase the chances of a difficult labour, and the possibility that the placenta will not be able to continue to support the baby over an extended period (see **Your Baby's Placenta**, opposite).

Doctors also take into consideration whether you have a personal or maternal family history of longer than average gestations (43 or 44 weeks for example). If this is the case, your doctor will probably be more willing to allow you to go for more than two weeks overdue without inducing the labour – although you will be closely monitored in case any problems do develop and, in practice, most women are quite desperate to deliver by this stage of prregnancy.

Pelvic disproportion Labour may be delayed if your baby's head is too big to pass through your pelvis. This disproportion may prevent the baby's head from becoming engaged. If this is the case (see column, right) a Caesarean section may be required.

POST-MATURITY

An overdue baby is in danger of being post-mature. If a baby is post-mature this means that he will have lost fat from all over his body, particularly from his tummy. Consequently, his skin will look red and wrinkled as if it doesn't fit him, and it may have begun to peel. Very few babies are actually post-mature, however, because post-maturity depends not only on the baby's condition, but also on his placenta (see below), it is difficult to predict which babies will be at risk.

Risks These include a longer and more difficult labour, because the post-mature baby tends to be bigger than usual and the bones in his skull tend to be harder (which means that his descent through the birth canal is likely to be more traumatic for both him and for yourself) and there is also an increased risk of stillbirth (the risk of stillbirth doubles by the 43rd week and triples by the 44th week). A further risk is that a uterus that is slow to begin to start labour may also be relatively inefficient during the labour itself.

YOUR BABY'S PLACENTA

At term, the placenta – the organ that links the blood supplies of the mother and baby – looks rather like a piece of raw liver, is about the size of a dinner plate, and measures about 2.5 cm (1in) in thickness. The maternal side is divided into wedge shaped chunks called cotyledons.

The placenta has substantial functional reserves, readily adjusts to injury, repairs damages due to ischaemia (lack of oxygen) and does not undergo ageing. The widely held view that ageing occurs progressively during the course of a normal pregnancy is due to a misinterpretation of the appearance of different placental components over the duration of the pregnancy.

Unquestionably, however, there are changes in the character of the villi around the placenta as pregnancy advances, and by the 36th week of pregnancy there may be a deposition of calcium within the walls of the small blood vessels, and a protein deposit may appear on the surface of many of the villi. Both of these changes have the effect of limiting the flow of nutrients and waste across the placenta, but this is balanced by the proximity between fetal blood vessels and the villi, both factors enhancing the exchange of nutrients.

Risks If labour does not start at the right time (this varies from pregnancy to pregnancy, but is usually considered to be two weeks either side of the EDD), the placenta may then start to become relatively inefficient. However, this does happen slowly and at 42 weeks the placenta should still be capable of supplying your baby with sufficient nutrients. Problems occur when, occasionally, the placenta fails to nourish and support your baby adequately. This is known as placental insufficiency and would be a reason for inducing labour.

LATE ENGAGEMENT

When engagement is late in a first pregnancy, doctors worry in case disproportion is preventing your baby's head from engaging, as this could obstruct labour.

In order to check whether your baby's head will actually engage in, and pass through, your pelvis, your doctor will perform a simple test as follows:

Step 1

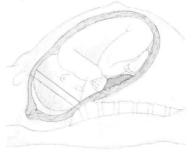

You will be asked to lie on your back. When you are in this position, your doctor will be able to feel your baby's head resting just at the pelvic brim.

Step 2

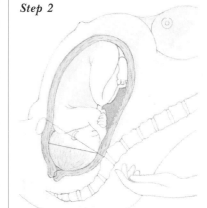

When you are propped up on your elbows, however, your baby's head slips easily into your pelvis, so showing there is no problem with pelvic disproportion.

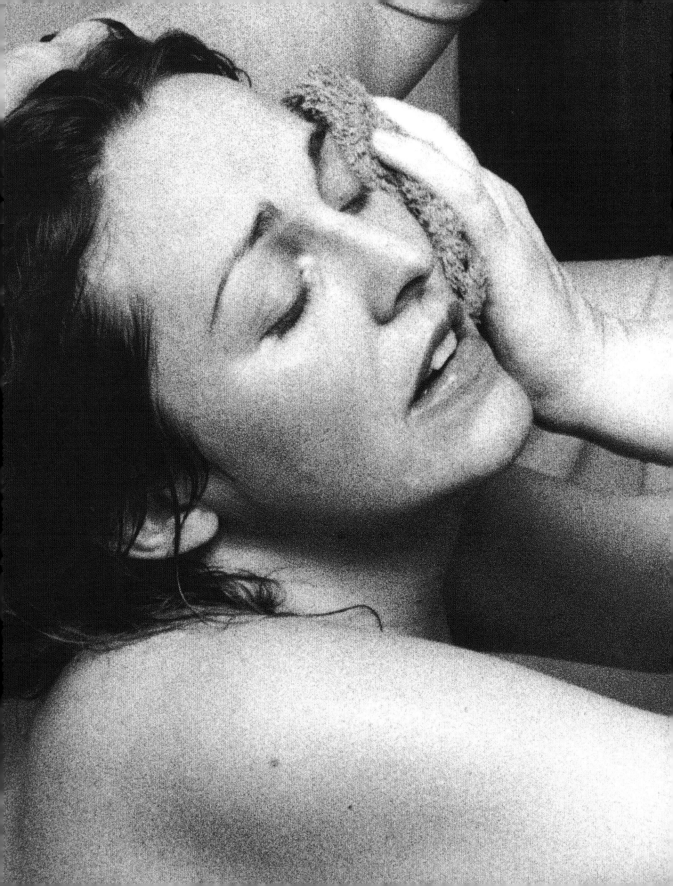

CHAPTER 13

Managing your
LABOUR

*Labour is the culmination
of your pregnancy. Very few
labours are pain-free, but there are
many methods and types of pain relief
available. The help and support of your
partner can be invaluable in making
your labour a smoother, more
comfortable experience.*

Preparing for a home birth

YOUR CHECKLIST

Although you can make most of your preparations well in advance, you will still have a few things that you need to take care of at the last minute.

When you go into labour (see p.270), you should:

- call your midwife

- make contact with your partner or birth assistant

- get in touch with whoever is going to care for your other children, if it is not your partner

- check that the room is ready

- check that your labour aids are conveniently to hand

- make yourself a hot, sweet drink.

When you opt for a home birth, your midwife will give you detailed advice on the preparations you need to make. Think about what you will need about four weeks in advance of your due date so that you do not have to rush around getting everything organized at the last minute, and you are at least partly prepared if your baby comes early.

ADVANCE PREPARATIONS

The room in which you intend to give birth should be arranged so that it is convenient and comfortable for you. Put the bed at right angles to the wall, with plenty of space on each side so that the midwife has easy access. A week or two before your due date she will deliver a home birth pack of medical equipment; don't try and open this as the contents will be sterile.

Protection Whether you wish to deliver your baby on to the floor or the bed, the bed itself and the floor area below and immediately around you will need to be protected during the birth. Have some old clean sheets, towels, and a large piece of plastic sheeting to hand so that it can be put down when the time comes.

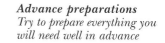

Advance preparations
Try to prepare everything you will need well in advance

Facilities for your midwife Ideally your midwife will need a small side table or a tea trolley next to the bed on which to put her instruments and other equipment, although a couple of tea trays will do, and a bright, adjustable reading lamp so that she can direct light on to your perineum. A torch (with spare batteries and bulb) would be useful to have at hand in case of a power cut.

You should also make sure that you stock up on food and drink in the few days before you are due. When you do this, remember that you will need food not only for yourself, your partner, and your other children (if you have any), but also for your midwife and for any visitors you may be expecting.

WHEN LABOUR STARTS

When your contractions are coming every 15 minutes, are about one minute long, and don't die away when you move around, telephone your midwife according to your arrangements. It is common for first labours to take a while to get going so, although your midwife will want to know that things have started happening, she is likely to advise you to try and relax and get some rest until you are in full labour because it is important to conserve your energy. All independent midwives are contactable by pagers or mobile phone, so it is easy to keep in touch.

Final preparations Make sure everything else that you and the midwife will need, for the birth and immediately afterwards, is prepared and ready to hand – including your comfort aids (see p.268), bowls for washing, a bedpan (or a clean bucket), clean towels, and large plastic bags for the soiled sheets, sanitary pads, and used dressings. Then put out a clean nightdress or large nightshirt for yourself, air your baby's clothes, and prepare her cot.

Your midwife Her equipment will include a sphygmomanometer to take blood pressure; Pinnard stethoscope or sonicaid (see column, p.178); Entonox (gas and air) cylinder; urine-testing sticks; local anaesthetic and syringes; scissors; suture material; mucus extractor; resuscitation equipment; intravenous equipment, in case of bleeding; Syntometrine. If you wish to have access to pain-relieving drugs she will give you a prescription in advance.

Unexpected hospitalization With the help of a skilled midwife or doctor, a home birth is completely safe for both you and your baby. But, as is also the case with hospital births, there can be complications, and if a serious problem arises you might have to go into hospital instead of giving birth at home. Should that happen, your midwife or doctor will accompany you.

Being unable to give birth at home, after all your preparation and anticipation, can be bitterly disappointing, but if you and your partner consider and discuss the possibility in advance it will be easier to cope with if it happens. It is better to tell yourself that you are going to start labour at home and see how it goes before deciding where your baby will actually be born.

WHEN NOT TO HAVE A HOME BIRTH

Normally, it is as safe to give birth at home as it is in a hospital, but in certain circumstances a hospital birth is your only option.

There are a number of factors that can make a hospital birth essential. Some, such as diabetes, will mean that you have to plan on a hospital delivery; other factors, such as pre-eclampsia, will mean that you have to abandon your plans for a home birth and go immediately to hospital.

The factors that rule out a home birth include:

• when you have had complications in previous pregnancies

• when your pelvis is too small for your baby's head to pass through it

• when your baby is presenting in the breech position

• when you have a medical problem that puts you, your baby, or both of you at risk, such as: high blood pressure; anaemia; diabetes; excess amniotic fluid; active herpes; placenta praevia; abruptio placentae; pre-eclampsia; eclampsia

• when you have a multiple pregnancy

• when your baby is premature

• when your pregnancy goes well beyond your EDD (see p.260).

Going to hospital

When your contractions begin, keep calm and do not rush: labour can last for as long as 12–14 hours for a first child and approximately seven hours for subsequent children.

When you go into labour you should:

• notify the hospital

• call an ambulance if you are not going to be driven to the hospital by your partner, birth assistant, or a friend

• contact your partner or birth assistant

• advise whoever is going to care for your other children, if it is not your partner

• check that your bag, your baby's bag, and your bag of labour aids are packed

• sit down and wait calmly for your transport to arrive

• make yourself a hot, sweet drink.

By getting everything ready and packing the things you will need to take with you to hospital, you won't have to worry about being caught unprepared.

WHAT TO TAKE

The items you will need with you in hospital fall into three categories: clothes and other personal effects for yourself; clothes and nappies for your baby; and your comfort aids for labour (see p.268). Contact your hospital to find out what you should bring with you, and what it will provide, such as nappies and clothing, for your baby.

For yourself You will need two or three maternity bras and front opening cotton nightdresses, a supply of breast pads, a dressing gown and slippers, underpants, and a supply of super-absorbent, stick-on sanitary towels (these may be supplied by the hospital). Pack an overnight bag with your hairbrush and shampoo, a couple of towels and facecloths, a small mirror, some make-up, face cream, hand cream, and tissues. If you have drawn up a birth plan (see p.122), remember to take it with you.

For your baby If the hospital does not provide nappies and baby clothing, you will need to do so. You will also need to take a nightdress, shawl, bonnet or hat, and a blanket in which to wrap your baby when you leave the hospital and go home.

Getting ready
Make sure that you have everything ready and packed well in advance

Is it time?

As you approach your due date, your body will begin to give you signals that it is preparing for the birth. You may experience the symptoms of pre-labour (see p.270) and, in some cases, labour. Although you don't have to rush to hospital when any of the following occur, you should be prepared for them happening and make your final preparations. The show normally comes first, and either the waters breaking or contractions will follow, although sometimes contractions precede the first two. A fuller explanation of each one will be found on page 270.

The show A plug of blood-tinged mucus, which has been sealing your cervix prior to birth, becomes dislodged during the early first stage of labour, if not before. It is usually easily recognizable.

The waters break Pressure due to contractions or the baby's head pressing on the membranes of the amniotic sac may cause it to rupture in advance of the start of labour. The amniotic fluid will then escape, either as a trickle or in a rush.

Regular contractions Whether or not you have been aware of any contractions previously, you start to experience them – in the form of severe cramp-like pains that come at regular intervals and last longer and longer. The interval between contractions gets shorter.

When to go

If, over an hour, you notice that your contractions are coming every 5–15 minutes, are about one minute long, and don't die away when you move around, or when you feel you cannot cope without pain relief, call your doctor or midwife according to prior arrangement. At this time, your first level of breathing (see column, p.282) will probably no longer be adequate, and you will be getting ready to use different types of breathing patterns. This is when pre-labour is easing into the first stage. There is still more than enough time to get to the hospital and it's early enough to complete all your last-minute checks without leaving you time to kill at the hospital.

There is absolutely no need to rush into hospital because the first stage usually lasts at least eight hours for the first baby. It is more comfortable at home anyway, particularly if you don't know whether your hospital is prepared to give you free rein to conduct your labour as you'd like. However, if you live a long way from the hospital or you are particularly worried about getting there in time, go as soon as you feel that you have to.

Transport You will probably travel to the hospital in an ambulance, by car, or by taxi. In any case, never try to drive yourself. If you call an ambulance or taxi, be sure to give your full address and, if necessary, a clear description of how to get to your house so that there is no unnecessary delay. If you plan to go by car, make sure that the car has had a recent service and keep an eye on the fuel gauge regularly from about week 38.

Your journey to hospital

If you are travelling to hospital by car rather than by ambulance, try to ensure that your journey will be both safe and comfortable.

In the weeks leading up to the birth, both you and whoever is going to drive you to the hospital should be thoroughly familiar with the route you are going to take. Find out how long the journey is likely to take at different times of the day, and work out alternative routes in case, on the day, you encounter exceptionally heavy traffic or other delays. Check to see if you need to take any money for the car park and make sure you have the right amount out ready. You should also check out the entrances to the hospital and find out how to get to the ward from them – especially during the night.

The car The bigger the car you travel in, the more comfortable you are likely to be. You will probably be more comfortable and safe in the back seat, and if it is large enough you can lie down on it rather than sit. If you have an estate car, you might find it more comfortable to kneel in the back, holding on to the seat back for support.

Sudden birth If your baby starts to arrive while you are still on your way to the hospital, try to remain calm. If you are close to the hospital, you have a good chance of getting there before the baby is actually born, but if you are farther away, it is best to stop the car at the nearest telephone, call for an ambulance, and then prepare yourself for an emergency delivery (see also p.304).

YOUR NOURISHMENT

Conserving your energy is important during the first stage, particularly in case you have a long and tiring labour.

Most hospitals advise against eating during labour in case there is an unexpected emergency that means you have to be anaesthetized. So take glucose sweets to suck, and high energy isotonic sports drinks to help you maintain energy levels.

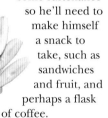

Your partner will also need some sustenance so he'll need to make himself a snack to take, such as sandwiches and fruit, and perhaps a flask of coffee.

Try to make sure there's enough for you to have later as you're likely to be ravenous after the birth and you'll want something to eat right away.

You will also need something to drink. A bottle or vacuum flask of diluted unsweetened fruit juice or cold water is ideal, although your partner might want some canned soft drinks.

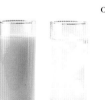

Comfort aids for labour

When organizing the things you will need for the birth, also get ready all the items that will make your labour a more comfortable experience. It's a good idea to prepare your comfort aids in advance so that you don't forget anything in the excitement when labour starts, and you won't be caught unprepared if your labour starts sooner than expected.

PROVISIONS FOR COMFORT

Your midwife or hospital attendants will give you advice about what comfort aids may be useful during labour. If you're having a home birth, keep all your aids together in the room where you intend to give birth. If you've opted for a hospital birth, pack them in a bag, and put it next to your case. Make sure your birth assistant knows where they are, and doesn't forget them in the excitement.

Distractions   Many women find the discomfort of labour can be alleviated with massage (see p.283). Counterpressure can be provided by your partner using his hands or a spinal roll, or even a tennis ball or rolling pin! A small amount of talcum powder or vegetable-based massage oil will stop your skin from being dragged or pinched. A hot water bottle or a hot pad placed in the small of your back can act as a compress to soothe backache.

In the early stages of labour, before it is really established, it is likely that you will find that for quite a long period of time nothing much seems to be happening. It will probably help to distract your attention and pass the time if you and your partner have to hand some books, magazines, playing cards, board games, and cassette tapes and a player.

PAIN-RELIEVING COMFORT AIDS

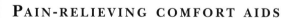

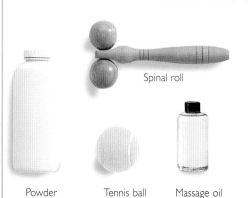

Spinal roll

Powder

Tennis ball

Massage oil

Hot water bottle

GENERAL COMFORT AIDS

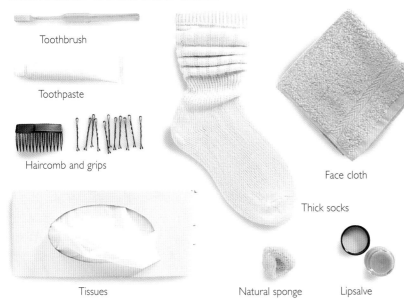

Toothbrush

Toothpaste

Haircomb and grips

Face cloth

Thick socks

Tissues

Natural sponge

Lipsalve

Keeping cool There will probably be times when you won't want anything to drink, but you really would like something wet and cool in your mouth. You may find it comforting to suck an ice cube or crushed ice, in which case you will need a portable icebox for storage if you are going into hospital. Alternatively, you may prefer moistening your lips and mouth by sucking on a small natural sponge that your birth partner has dipped in cold water.

Your face is likely to become very hot and sweaty, and you will probably find it refreshing to have it mopped with an absorbable face cloth. In addition, your birth assistant can create a slight breeze on your face by using a hand-held fan.

Keeping warm During the later stages of labour, and particularly immediately after the birth, some women begin to shake quite visibly with cold, so make sure that you have some leg warmers or thick socks in case this happens.

General comfort If your hair is long or falls in your face, a few hair grips, slides, combs, or a hairband will help to stop it from irritating you. Your lips are likely to become very dry because of breathing through your mouth, so include a lipsalve or chapstick that you can rub on to your lips to stop them from cracking.

If you feel nauseous and actually vomit, you will undoubtedly feel much better if you are able to clean your teeth, so don't forget to take your toothbrush and some toothpaste.

A box of tissues may come in handy, as may some scented wipes in single packs that can be opened when needed and used to cleanse the face, neck, and hands. For freshening up you may want to splash on some eau de Cologne.

YOUR CHECKLIST

Use the following checklist when you assemble your aids:

• food and drink

• spinal roll, or tennis ball

• massage oil or talcum powder

• hot water bottle

• magazines, board games, etc.

• ice, and storage if in hospital

• small natural sponge

• face cloth and hand-held fan

• leg warmers or thick socks

• haircombs, grips, or hairband

• lipsalve or chapstick

• toothbrush and toothpaste

• box of tissues or wet wipes

• eau de Cologne.

YOUR MOOD CHANGES

As you wait for indications that your baby is ready to be born, you may experience a number of differing emotions.

Contentment As your body changes in preparation for labour, you may respond to the ripening of your uterus in a sensual way. Particularly if it's your first pregnancy, you may feel a desire to enjoy these last days on your own indulging your whims, sharing moments of intimacy with your partner, or spending the time just day dreaming. Pamper yourself, and allow your feelings to flow naturally and easily.

Elation You may experience a sense of jubilation when your body alerts you to the moment that you have been anticipating with such excitement. Don't try to quench this feeling; share it with others as it may help to release any pangs of nervous tension.

Anxiety The signals of pre-labour may also evoke apprehension. You may worry about the pain you may suffer during labour and its effect on the baby, or whether you will be able to cope. You may feel nervous about your waters breaking in an embarrassing situation.

Impatience If your expected date of delivery comes and goes without any sign of impending delivery, don't be depressed. Remember the date is an approximation, and that most babies arrive either sooner or later than expected. This is particularly likely if you were born sooner or later than expected.

Pre-labour and labour

Medical definitions of labour divide it into three stages. In the first stage, the cervix opens fully to allow the baby to pass through; in the second stage the baby is born; in the third stage the placenta is delivered. All these stages are discussed in detail over the following pages. But, as well as these stages, most women experience pre-labour. Your experience of labour will be much more colourful and exciting than the above definition. Go into it believing very little can go wrong and very little will go wrong.

PRE-LABOUR

Before real labour begins, hormones secreted by your uterus and the baby prepare your body for birth in a number of ways. During the last few weeks, you will probably notice a few signs of your impending labour. However, just as each woman's experience of labour and birth is unique, so these pre-labour symptoms affect each woman in varying degrees of intensity. They provide useful signals that indicate to you that labour is imminent.

Engagement To position himself for the journey through the birth canal, your baby will move lower down so that his presenting part, usually the head, settles into your bony pelvis (see opposite). This is known as engagement and you will experience it as a feeling of lightening. If this is your first pregnancy, engagement will probably occur about two to three weeks before the onset of labour. If you've had previous babies, the baby's head may remain higher until just before labour starts, as your uterine muscles may have stretched and so will exert less pressure on your baby. You will know when engagement takes place because pressure on your diaphragm eases and breathing becomes easier. On the other hand, you will probably have to pass urine more frequently, as your baby will now be pressing down on your bladder.

Braxton Hicks' contractions Your uterus practises for the strong contractions needed in labour with weak, irregular contractions. Named after the doctor who first described them, the majority of women feel them during the last few months. If you place your hand on your abdomen, you may feel a hardening and tightening of your uterus, which lasts for approximately 25 seconds.

Unlike real labour contractions, these are usually painless, although a few women find them uncomfortable. If you feel any discomfort, sitting down quietly should help to ease them.

Runs of Braxton Hicks' contractions may become more frequent and intense as real labour approaches, helping to prepare the cervix for dilatation, and to increase the circulation of blood to the placenta. When you feel a run of Braxton Hicks', practise the relaxation techniques you intend to use during labour; the tightening and relaxing of your uterus will give you a good idea of how a contraction feels as it waxes, and then wanes.

Some mothers misinterpret Braxton Hicks' for real labour, arriving at hospital only to be told they can go home again (see **A false labour?** p.272).

"Nesting instinct" You may feel a surge of energy to make final preparations for the arrival of your baby. If you feel the urge to rush around cleaning or decorating the house, or cooking large meals, try to restrain yourself. You will need all this extra energy for coping with labour and delivery.

The show An obvious sign that labour is imminent is the appearance of the show – the plug of mucus that seals your cervix in pregnancy, providing protection against infection. Although the show often does not appear until labour is underway, the cervix may widen enough for the mucus plug to be dislodged up to twelve days before labour begins. This sticky substance may be slightly brown, pink, or blood-tinged from the capillaries that attached it to the cervix. The show signals dilatation of the cervix.

Premenstrual feelings Physical and emotional changes similar to those you experience premenstrually may occur. You may also feel crampy, with pressure in your rectum, and feel the need to empty your bowels and pass urine frequently.

YOUR BABY'S DESCENT

This is checked with an internal examination, and expressed as "stations", lines measured in centimetres from –5 to +5 in relation to the level of your ischial spines and your baby's head. When his head first enters your pelvis it is at station –5. When the top of his head is level with your ischial spines it is at station 0 (engaged). The other stations describe the head's position as it passes via the birth canal to the vaginal opening, station +5.

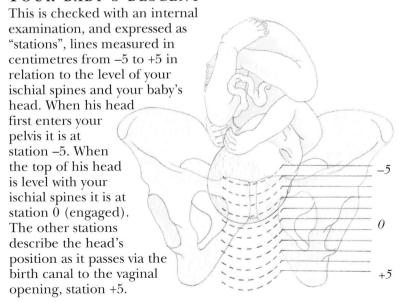

–5

0

+5

While no one actually knows for certain why labour starts, there is increasing evidence to show that the baby plays a major role.

Secreting hormones The onset of labour is triggered by the secretion of hormones – some pregnancy hormone levels drop, others rise. New hormones are secreted, one of which is produced by your baby.

Engagement Throughout your pregnancy, your baby will be floating in his amniotic sac above the pelvic brim. As his birth approaches, his head, or his bottom if he is in a breech presentation, will descend lower down into your pelvis and become engaged.

Kicking less You may notice that he is quieter than in previous months. From time to time you may feel a slight flurry of movement, although if his actions appear to have ceased completely, contact your doctor or midwife.

A FALSE LABOUR?

It's not always easy to distinguish false from real labour if it's your first pregnancy. As a general rule, if you're in doubt, you're not in real labour.

Although false labour is only a rehearsal, it is not a reason to be disappointed; false labour heralds real labour, and you won't have very much longer to wait.

There are some simple distinctions between the contractions of false and real labour.

Regularity False contractions never really settle down and become truly regular.

Frequency Contractions are sporadic. They may vary from 10 minutes to 20 minutes to 15 minutes, etc., with no steady pattern.

Effect of movement False contractions usually weaken or subside altogether if you get up and move around; real contractions increase.

Strength False contractions do not get progressively stronger. They may even weaken from time to time and disappear altogether.

Some women, especially if they are working, get overtired or overexcited, slip in and out of false labour for a few days before real labour begins.

Inform your doctor or midwife about the contractions. If they're not available, seek reassurance from your hospital. Go to hospital if you want to. If you stay at home keep on the move and stay upright to help labour progress.

The first stage

The months of preparing for your baby's birth have now reached their climax as you start to experience labour. In medical terms, the first stage begins when your contractions bring about dilatation and thinning of the cervix and ends when effacement (thinning) and dilatation (opening) are complete. At this point your midwife will confirm that you are fully dilated.

WHAT HAPPENS IN LABOUR

It is difficult to be sure about the onset of labour as it is different for each woman. However, certain classic signs – intense, uterine contractions, dilatation and thinning of the cervix, rupturing of the membranes – are taken to mean that labour is underway.

Contractions When true labour starts, the nature of contractions changes. They become more rhythmical, more painful, and occur at regular intervals. These contractions are not within your control and, once they have begun, will not stop until your baby is born.

You can time your contractions from the beginning of one contraction to the beginning of the next. In early labour, contractions are usually about 30–60 seconds long, at intervals of about 5–20 minutes. This can vary as some women may not notice their first contractions until they are closer together, say every five minutes. During the active phase, contractions usually last 60–90 seconds, at intervals of 2–4 minutes.

As the uterine muscles tighten, you may feel a sensation similar to menstrual cramps, spreading around your lower abdomen like a tight band. This is because the uterine muscle becomes short of oxygen as its blood vessels are compressed. The uterus is a huge muscle and needs a lot of energy during contractions.

Every woman feels contraction pains differently, but in early labour they may have the same character as dysmenorrhoea (menstrual cramps) or pain may be confined to mild backache. Some women experience persistent and severe backache (see p. 297). Very often a contraction feels like a wave of discomfort right across your abdomen that reaches a peak for a few seconds and then diminishes. At the same time, you can feel a hardening and tightening of the uterine muscle, which is held at the peak of its intensity for a few seconds before the muscle begins to relax.

Women assume that contractions will get steadily longer, more frequent, and stronger. This is not so; don't be disturbed if your contractions seem to vary. It is as normal for a strong contraction to be followed by a weaker one that doesn't last quite as long, as it is for contractions to follow one another relentlessly.

The cervix dilates and thins The cervix is usually a thick-walled canal about two centimetres long (three quarters of an inch), and firmly closed. In the last few weeks, pregnancy hormones may soften your cervix, but the intense contractions of first-stage labour are needed to dilate and thin it. Dilatation is measured in centimetres from 0–10 (up to four inches). Your cervix will only dilate about four centimetres (one and a half inches) during the *latent phase*, then progress to eight centimetres (three inches) in the *active phase* (see below). The pain increases as it becomes fully dilated during transition. Eventually, the whole cervix opens up and is made one with the body of the uterus, thus creating a continuous channel through which your baby can emerge.

The waters break The membranes of the amniotic sac may rupture painlessly at any time during labour, although this usually occurs towards the end of the first stage. Fluid may leak or gush out; the flow depends on the size and site of the break and whether or not the baby's head is plugging the hole.

Usually, if the membranes rupture spontaneously near term, labour occurs within a short time, although occasionally it is delayed – if the baby's presenting part is not engaged, or if the baby is presenting abnormally. Delay also occurs in normal cases. When this happens, you will be advised to have labour induced.

HOW LONG DOES LABOUR LAST?

Every woman's experience of labour varies greatly, and the time span of each can't be predicted. An average labour lasts about 12–14 hours for first-time mothers, and about seven hours for subsequent labours. If your labour lasts longer than 12 hours the first time, or nine hours in subsequent labours, your doctor will look for the cause of slow progress, and may intervene.

The first stage of labour can be further divided into three separate phases. The *latent phase* is the longest, lasting about eight hours for first babies, and you will feel contractions occurring with increasing frequency and length, but they won't be too distressing. Try to conserve your energy during this time as your body will be warming up for the more demanding phases to follow. The next, *active phase*, will be shorter, lasting about three to five hours, but this is when your contractions become more painful, and you may seek pain relief (see p.280). The final, *transitional phase*, is the shortest and most intense of all, usually lasting just under an hour, and comes just before the delivery.

Transition This is the most intense phase of the first stage. Your contractions will now be lasting about 60–90 seconds, with intervals of only 30–90 seconds. As the contractions become more forceful, you may find it difficult to relax. This is the time you may feel the most discomfort. You may also feel a very strong urge to push, but should not do so unless told you are fully dilated. The intense pain may make you feel extremely irritable, to the point of being ill-tempered with your birth partner. This is natural, and you must not feel that you are failing if you think you haven't the energy to go on any more; you will find hidden resources of energy to help you cope. Try to bear in mind that this phase means your baby's birth is now just minutes away.

YOUR CERVIX DILATES

During the first stage of labour the cervix, which is normally tough, must be stretched thin and needs to open wide before your baby's head is able to pass through.

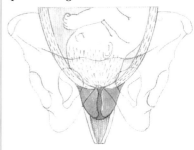

Latent phase
Your cervix remains about 2cm (¾ in) long until contractions start thinning it out (effacing).

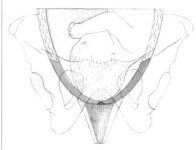

Active phase
When the cervical canal is fully effaced, further contractions will widen (dilate) your cervix.

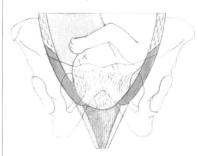

Transitional phase
At full dilatation the last part of your cervix at the front has opened to 10cm (4in).

When you arrive at the hospital, the midwife will prepare you for the birth. There are certain routine examinations that you will undergo.

• While consulting your notes the midwife will ask you questions about your labour's progress – whether your waters have broken and how frequently your contractions are coming.

• You will then be examined; the midwife will palpate your abdomen to feel the baby's position; she will listen to the fetal heartbeat, take your blood pressure, pulse, and temperature and give you an internal examination to see how far your cervix has dilated.

• You will be asked to give a urine sample to test for the presence of protein and sugar.

• You'll be asked when you last moved your bowels. You won't be given an enema or a suppository unless you request it.

• You then have a shower or bath and settle in to your delivery room. If you have any questions or you want to make your feelings known to the staff, now is the time to remind them of some of your preferences.

Hospital procedures

Each hospital has its own set of routine procedures for labour. You will probably have a good idea what regulations your hospital staff follow if you have visited the hospital beforehand, met the staff who will be looking after you, looked at the labour and delivery rooms, and had some idea of what the ward routine is like. Hospitals can be intimidating but are much less so when you get to know them.

Admission to hospital Once you've arrived in hospital you may be put in a wheelchair to transport you from the hospital entrance to the labour ward. If your labour is well advanced, you'll welcome a wheelchair, but if not, you will be able to walk comfortably and you should make sure you are allowed to do so.

You should have outlined in your birth plan (see p.122) how you wish your labour to proceed, and once you've met your midwife or doctor, this is the time to make sure they have a copy that you can look over with them. They will also make some checks and ask you various questions about your labour (see column, left, and p.116).

If you aren't happy with any procedure, if equipment, lights, and needles frighten you, or if you are upset by a staff member, act at the time. Don't wait so that your fears and anxieties fester and grow. Your birth assistant can voice your feelings if you aren't feeling strong enough to be assertive.

Examinations Your baby's heart will be regularly monitored by a sonicaid, or an electronic fetal monitor (see right). You will probably have an internal examination every two to four hours during the first stage to check the dilatation of your cervix but there's no hard and fast rule.

Each time you have an internal examination, ask how you are progressing. It is very comforting to know how far your cervix has dilated between examinations. If you're asked a question while you are having a contraction, concentrate on your relaxation techniques and answer the question when the contraction is over.

Pain relief After the admission procedures, the anaesthetist will visit you if you have opted for some form of medical pain relief (see p.280). If you are having epidural anaesthesia, the procedure will be set up now. This usually takes 10–20 minutes. The anaesthetist may then leave you with your birth assistant and midwife, but will return later to check whether the anaesthetic needs topping up. If you have decided not to have medical pain relief, you will be left with your birth assistant and a midwife who will stay with you throughout your labour.

ELECTRONIC FETAL MONITORING

This high-tech replacement for the ear trumpet is used to track the baby's heartbeat. All mothers are given 20 minutes' electronic fetal monitoring (EFM) for legal reasons, but there's no need for continuous monitoring for a normal labour, and it will be done externally, without the need for a fetal scalp monitor. In all high risk pregnancies, EFM will be used throughout for your own and especially your baby's safety. You will have EFM if you are being induced or your labour is being accelerated for any reason, or if you have opted for epidural anaesthesia. Its main function is that it gives warning of fetal distress.

What it is There are two kinds of electronic monitors, external and internal. An external monitor will be used for routine short periods of monitoring and it is sometimes used in pregnancy when it is felt necessary to monitor the baby's heartbeat over a period of time. Belts are strapped round your abdomen with sensors that record the baby's heartbeat and the uterine contractions, which are then printed out on a graph. The internal monitor is slightly more accurate. You'll have belts strapped around your body and a tiny electrode will be clipped on to your baby's scalp once your cervix is 2–3cm (2–2½in) dilated. There is also a video display unit (VDU) that records the contractions and heartbeats as visible waves, punctuated by flashing lights.

The latest type of EFM, known as telemetry, uses radio waves and allows you to walk around as the baby's monitor is attached to a transmitter strapped to your thigh. The older equipment confines you to a bed or chair.

How it works During a contraction, blood flow to the placenta is reduced for a few seconds, and your baby's heart rate dips. The heart rate returns to baseline when the contraction passes. If the return to baseline is delayed, your baby may be distressed and action can be taken early to protect his well-being.

How it helps doctors EFM provides medical staff with a second-by-second report on the condition of your baby. It will warn the doctors if your baby is in distress so they can intervene before anything untoward has happened. If your doctors decide that you and your baby would be better off with EFM, try to see it as something that gives reassurance that your baby is doing fine.

Disadvantages EFM increases the amount of electronic equipment in the delivery room, making the atmosphere very clinical, and the staff may concentrate more on the machine than on you. As staff are aware of any tiny changes that may occur, they are more likely to intervene rather than letting labour take its natural course.

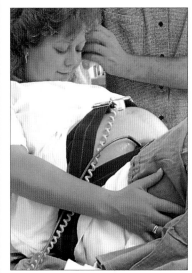

Monitoring in labour
Contractions are recorded by an external monitor strapped to your abdomen. An internal monitor is attached to your baby.

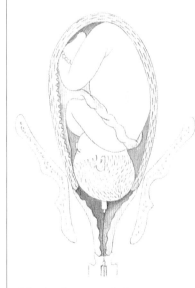

Monitoring your baby
The electrode is attached to his presenting part, usually his head, by piercing the skin and provides an electrical contact that picks up his heartbeat. Some babies' heads will be bruised or have a rash where the electrode was attached to them. However, many mothers find EFM reassuring as they can watch their baby's heartbeat throughout labour.

Partner's role in labour

The more comfortable and relaxed a mother feels during labour, the better her ability to cope with pain. She can find this security with loving support from a birth assistant. A partner is the natural choice, as he will probably be closely involved throughout pregnancy, and eager to share the experience of his child's birth. Most hospitals welcome fathers, friends, or relatives to support the mother.

UNDERSTANDING YOUR ROLE

Like many partners, you may be nervous. You may worry about feeling squeamish, or being inadequate at offering sufficient support. You can help to combat this by preparing yourself. It's important you know as much as possible so you can effectively help the mother meet the physical and emotional demands of labour. At antenatal classes there will be demonstrations to describe labour's onset and the effect of contractions, and you will be taught techniques to help her relax.

If it's going to be a hospital birth, visit the hospital's labour and delivery rooms and introduce yourself to her hospital attendants so you won't feel like an outsider when the time comes. If the birth is to be at home, make sure you know the route to hospital in case of an emergency, and find out what will be expected of you; trust will create a calmer atmosphere.

HOW TO HELP DURING LABOUR

You may have a very active role throughout the labour and birth, but sometimes your presence is all the mother needs. Make sure you are familiar with her birth plan and the alternative version (see p.122). You need to be aware of her wishes in order to provide her with the best care and attention during labour.

Use your intuition You need to judge the situation, observing the mother's moods and fitting in. She may want to stay quiet, going through contractions alone without being touched. Alternatively, she may need much verbal or physical encouragement, or to be distracted.

Supporting your partner
If your partner leans back against you, you can support her weight and cuddle her at the same time.

Provide emotional support   Remain as intimate as possible using loving words, and keep your movements slow, quiet, and steady. Be positive: offer praise, never criticism. If she wants to hear your voice, constantly tell her how well she is doing (how far dilated), how she can relax herself, what others such as the midwife are doing to help her, and what will soon happen. Also, help her to see how much she has achieved already – it's easy for her to be overwhelmed by how far she thinks she has to go. Massage and stroke her slowly, but if she just wants to hold your hand, you can offer encouragement by using facial expressions, and lots of eye contact. Sometimes just the expression of love in her partner's eyes can help a woman bear the pain of contractions.

Combat fatigue   Before labour, advise her to rest as much as possible, particularly if she seems to spend a lot of energy cleaning during the nesting period. If she has a long, tiring labour, try to help her relax between contractions to conserve her energy for the second stage. If she's not feeling nauseous, provide her with as much nourishment as she wants (see also p.268).

Help her cope with pain   It's hard to see someone you care about in pain, but try not to reveal your anxiety as she will become discouraged. On the other hand, don't discredit her suffering. Acknowledge it positively, telling her each contraction is bringing your baby's birth nearer, and offer different suggestions for relief. Don't let her feel embarrassed about expressing her discomfort – encourage her to be as uninhibited as possible. A woman in labour should never be ashamed of needing pain relief.

If she feels particularly anxious during a contraction, try to calm her fears by discussing how she felt before the next one starts. Try not to be upset if she becomes critical or aggressive as this often happens when the pain is very intense.

Assist with breathing   You will probably have practised the mother's preferred method in antenatal classes, but allow her to follow her own rhythm. If she seems to lose control, stay close by and slowly guide her through the pattern until she has enough reassurance to carry on alone. Be prepared to adapt – very few people follow exactly what they practised at antenatal classes.

Offer comfort   You can be a great help in relieving her discomfort. Suggest different positions (see p.278) and support her with cushions or blankets, or let her lean against you while you cuddle, and rock together. Look out for signs of tension in her neck, shoulders, or forehead, and gently stroke these areas. Massage will offer some relief, and if she's using visualization techniques, gently talk her through them. She will probably find having her face and hands wiped very soothing, and offer her ice cubes to suck. If she feels cold, help her put on socks, or leg warmers. As labour progresses she may want to talk less, but you can communicate by touching or caressing, or by using eye contact.

HOW YOUR PARTNER CAN HELP

A birth partner can do a lot to help during labour, not only providing you with comfort and reassurance, but also dealing with staff on your behalf. Bear in mind that although the hospital uniforms and equipment may appear daunting, the medical team is there to support both of you.

Your birth partner can:

• answer questions for you (if allowed to by the staff), which saves you having your concentration disturbed

• support you in the positions you choose for pain relief and/or to give birth

• stroke and massage you if you find it comforting

• change the atmosphere (dim the lights, change the music) for you

• ask people to leave if too many build up in your personal space during a home birth, and request that any students present at a hospital delivery are removed if they are inhibiting you

• be the one you can really rely on to interact with the staff on your behalf and to stand by your decisions regarding pain relief – whether to accept it or not, and if so, when and how much. If you do decide to ask for relief, he should encourage you to have a breathing space of about 15 minutes before it is administered, as things can change very quickly and you may find you don't need it after all.

First stage positions

There are many different positions that you can adopt to ease your discomfort. Some women prefer to stand up and move around during labour, as this helps to strengthen contractions, which then accelerates labour. As the contractions proceed, you may instinctively choose a sitting or kneeling position, but if not, try using cushions, chairs, or your partner for support.

Massage your partner's back as she rests against you. You may also find rocking together helps

Standing
Lean forward and rest against your birth attendant, or a wall. The weight of your baby will be taken off your spine and the contractions will be more efficient. Rotate your hips. Your birth attendant will be able to help you breathe correctly.

Let your shoulders drop. You can rest against a cushion during contractions

Make sure your back is straight

Sitting
If you find it more comfortable to sit down, try leaning forward with your legs wide apart. You can sit facing the chair back, resting on a pillow or cushion. Alternatively, to keep your body supported, you may prefer to lean against your birth attendant, who can rub your back.

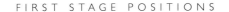

Kneeling

As the contractions strengthen you may find it less tiring to go down on to your hands and knees. This helps to alleviate backache. Keep your legs wide apart, and rock your pelvis. Make sure your back is straight and don't allow it to arch. Between contractions, lean forward on to your folded arms or sit back on your heels.

Rock your pelvis backwards and forwards during contractions to relieve backache

During transition

If your cervix is not fully dilated towards the end of the first stage, just before giving birth, use gravity to slow down the baby while the cervix continues to dilate. Lean on to a pile of cushions with your legs wide apart, or kneel with your head down and your bottom raised.

Kneeling on the floor with your bottom raised and your head on the floor may relieve backache

Take the pressure off your lower back by leaning forward with your head on a pillow

Lying down

There may be times during labour when you find it comfortable to lie down. If so, try lying on your side, and place cushions under your head and upper thigh. Keep your legs wide apart.

Relax your shoulders, and concentrate on your breathing with your eyes closed

279

HOW DRUGS AFFECT YOU

Apart from offering pain relief, drugs can affect your experience of childbirth in other ways. Make sure you opt for the type that will help to enhance, rather than detract from, the pleasure of your baby's birth.

Drowsiness This is a common side effect of gas and oxygen, tranquillizers, and narcotics. Some women enjoy the sensation of drifting, but sometimes the sleepiness can make mothers feel they lack control. After using narcotics, a few women have become so lightheaded they were unaware of what was happening around them, and gave birth without realizing it had happened.

Dizziness Pethidine and other narcotics can sometimes induce a feeling of confusion, or disorientation, and some mothers have even had hallucinations.

Nausea The sensation of nausea is usually quite slight with gas and oxygen, but is quite common after using pethidine and other narcotics, and a few mothers may suffer attacks of vomiting.

Your state of mind can have a major effect on the intensity of pain experienced during labour. So if the use of drugs will make you less anxious, there is no point in depriving yourself, as excessive tension may affect the uterus, slow down labour, and adversely affect your baby (see column, opposite).

Pain relief

For many women, particularly first-time mothers, anticipation of their baby's birth may be overshadowed by worry about pain during labour. Labour invariably involves pain, but you can build up your confidence by preparing for the intensity of contractions, by understanding your own limits of pain tolerance, and by learning about different methods of pain relief. If possible, try to view the pain as a positive element of labour – each contraction brings the birth of your baby nearer.

COPING WITH PAIN

The kind of pain you'll experience during contractions can vary. Very often, it feels like a thick band being squeezed around your abdomen as the uterine muscles harden and tighten for a few seconds before relaxing. Some women describe it as being like severe menstrual cramp, others experience backache, but there may be a combination of sensations as the contraction reaches its peak, culminating in a wave of discomfort, which then subsides.

Individual response You may prefer not to use drugs during labour as they can dim your awareness of what is happening and deprive you of the sensation of giving birth. However, it is difficult to know your pain threshold, particularly if this is your first baby. Some women are surprised by the overpowering intensity of their contractions, others may worsen pain through fear and anxiety. Analgesia in childbirth can offer complete relief of pain as in epidural anaesthesia or reduction of pain to bearable levels as with gas and air and narcotics. Many people opt for no drugs in the early part of the first stage, then have a low dose of gas and air towards transition. Don't be self-critical if you opt for pain relief with drugs, it isn't a sign of cowardice. Remember your labour isn't a test, and the use of drugs may even be essential for you to deliver your baby.

If you haven't made up your mind about the use of painkillers, you may try to do without drugs for as long as possible. If so, a useful tip is to wait 15 minutes after you feel you want pain relief before having it. During that time your labour may progress well, and it gives you and your birth assistant time to discuss whether or not you can get by with encouragement, or whether you really do feel the pain is increasing to the point where relief is necessary.

If you wish to have full participation in your baby's birth without dimming your consciousness of the physical and emotional sensations, there are alternatives to drugs for pain relief. Also, your body can provide its own brand of painkiller and relaxant, endorphins. The more natural your labour, the more quickly your own endorphins will be produced and your pain threshold increased.

A clear choice   Find out as much as possible about the types of pain relief that will be available. Have a discussion with your doctor, midwife, and hospital attendants, and then outline your choices in your birth plan (see p.122) with an alternative version available in case any complications arise.

Many doctors and midwives seek to make labour and delivery as pain-free as possible with the aid of drugs. Unless you state your preferences very clearly, you may find certain analgesics are used automatically whether you want them or not. Don't hesitate to question their use, or to request a smaller dosage.

PAIN-RELIEVING DRUGS

Some types of pain relief will only be available in large or teaching hospitals, others are widely available in all hospitals. Your midwife will also be able to offer certain types for a home delivery.

Regional anaesthetics   These remove sensation from part of your body by blocking the transmission of pain from nerve fibres. Caudal anaesthesia is administered by an injection into your spinal area around the sacrum, and numbs your vagina and perineum. This may be used for short-term relief if the birth involves a vacuum extraction, or forceps delivery.

To administer a pudendal block, anaesthesia is injected straight into your vagina near the pelvic region, blocking the pudendal nerve. This numbs the lower part of your vagina, and may be used if you have an episiotomy, although it is used infrequently.

The most widely used form of this type of anaesthesia is the epidural block (see below). This prevents pain spreading from your uterus by acting as a "nerve block" in your spine. A well-managed epidural removes all sensation from your waist to your knees, but you remain alert. It may be particularly recommended

HOW DRUGS AFFECT YOUR BABY

Most drugs will cross the placenta to affect your baby once they are in your bloodstream. There will be a higher concentration in your baby's blood than in your own.

Drowsiness Pethidine can make your baby drowsy after the birth which may affect his ability to suckle and to respond to you after he is born.

Breathing difficulties Narcotics can depress your baby's respiration. If you take pethidine late in your labour it will remain longer in your baby's bloodstream. Drugs used in epidural anaesthesia cannot enter your baby's blood. A baby born after epidural anaesthesia therefore stands a very good chance of being alert and of breathing well.

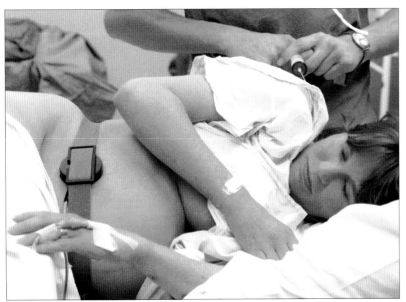

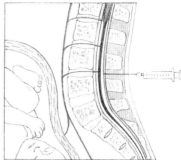

Epidural anaesthetic
Once you have had an injection of local anaesthetic in your back, (to numb it), the anaesthetist will insert a fine, hollow needle into the epidural space – the region around the spinal cord inside the spinal column (see above).

WAYS YOU CAN BREATHE

Relaxing your body and focusing on your breathing will help to alleviate your anxiety and let you ride out your contractions. Practise breathing patterns beforehand with your birth assistant so he or she can guide you during labour, if necessary.

Slow breathing During the early stages, calmly and deliberately breathe out through your mouth as the contraction begins. Then slowly breathe in through your nose. Sustain the same steady pattern throughout the contraction, which may last about 45–60 seconds.

Light breathing As your contractions become more intense and frequent, you may find it easier to breathe above them. Take light, short breaths that seem to involve only the upper part of your body, and not your abdomen where the contraction takes place.

You will probably find that you will use different breathing techniques at different stages of your labour.

---

if you have a difficult labour, pre-eclampsia, or severe asthma, or if you have a forceps delivery. Most mothers who have a Caesarean have an epidural instead of a general anaesthetic, which means they are able to stay awake during the birth. First of all, a local anaesthetic will be given in your back to numb the area for the injection. A fine, hollow needle is then inserted into the epidural space (see previous page) and a thin tube known as a catheter is threaded down inside the hollow needle. The needle is removed, leaving the catheter in position. The catheter is then taped firmly in place. Anaesthetic is syringed down the catheter, which is then sealed, although it can be topped up if necessary. You need to let the attendants know in advance that you wish to have an epidural as it has to be given by a skilled anaesthetist, and it usually takes 10–20 minutes to be set up. The anaesthetic will take effect within a few minutes.

Inhalation analgesics This is a gas that you administer yourself using a face mask, and includes Entonox (gas and oxygen). You inhale deeply as the contraction starts, and carry on until the contraction peaks or you have had enough. You then put the mask aside and breathe normally. Gas works by numbing the pain centre in the brain, and can make you feel as though you're floating. You may be able to practise this in an antenatal class.

Narcotics Now considered rather old-fashioned, the most commonly used is pethidine, which is derived from morphine, and is given by injection in the thigh or buttock in varying dosages during the first stage. It dulls the sensation of pain by acting on the nerve cells in the brain and spine. If you choose to take a narcotic, it is probably wise to ask for a small dose (50–75 mg) to see how you are affected. Narcotics take about 20 minutes to work.

RELIEF WITHOUT DRUGS

It's important that you have mastered your chosen pain-relief method, and familiarized your birth assistant with the technique, before you go into labour. If special equipment is required, make sure it is available at home or in hospital. One method on its own may not be enough – you may need a combination for more complete relief.

Positions Walking around, leaning against your partner or the wall, and rocking your pelvis will probably feel much more comfortable than lying on your back. There are some positions that you will probably find more comfortable than others, as these will relieve the pressure on your back (see p.278).

Massage This is a wonderful way to get reassurance from your partner and relieve discomfort, whether you're lying, standing, or squatting. It can help particularly if you have backache in labour, as around 90 percent of women do (see column, right), or if you suffer from a backache labour (see p.296).

Water Lying in warm water can be very relaxing and soothing. Immersion in water renders you virtually weightless and this brings relief between contractions. For these reasons birthing pools are increasingly being used by mothers under supervision (see p.107). Many hospitals are installing special birthing pools or there may be the facility to hire a pool. It is worth checking early in pregnancy so that you know it is going to be available for you to use when you go into labour.

Visualizing Creating images in your mind can be a very effective way of calming fear and reducing pain. As your contraction begins, imagine something that you find particularly soothing, for example warm, bright sunshine. Contractions in the first stage are opening the cervix and you may find the image of the bud of your favourite flower opening very slowly, petal by petal, helpful. Many women find thoughts of waves very comforting, matching the flow of the waves with their own contractions.

Sounds You can help to diffuse the pain and anxiety of labour by vocalizing in the way you feel most helpful. Sighing, moaning, groaning, grunting are all ways of releasing tension, and you shouldn't be inhibited, or worry about disturbing others.

Many women find that listening to music is very effective. Your birth assistant can play different pieces on a cassette recorder, according to how you are feeling. A light, uplifting piece of music may help you rise above your contraction. When your contractions intensify, more dramatic pieces of music, building up to a crescendo, may help you to cope with them.

Hypnosis This isn't something that you should try on a whim as you need to be able to respond to hypnosis very easily. Women who go into a deep trance have been able to have a forceps delivery, stitches, or Caesarean without feeling pain. A period of practice sessions is advisable, and both you and your hypnotist should be completely familiar with what you will have to do during labour and delivery.

Acupuncture You should only opt for this method if you have already found that it can relieve pain in other situations. In addition, your acupuncturist must be familiar with labour and delivery. This may not stop you feeling any pain at all, but it will certainly reduce it, and also helps to stop nausea.

TENS (Trans-cutaneous Electrical Nerve Stimulation.) Pain impulses conducted by nerves are blocked by an electric current, which also stimulates the production of endorphins. A battery-powered stimulator is connected by wires to electrodes that are placed on either side of the spine. You are then able to use a handset that regulates the amount of stimulation, enabling you to control the amount of pain-relief that you receive. Ask your midwife or obstetric physiotherapist if this method is available.

RELIEVING BACKACHE

Many women suffer from backache during labour, sometimes because of the baby's head pressing against the sacrum. Your birth assistant can help to relieve the discomfort by gently massaging your lower back during labour.

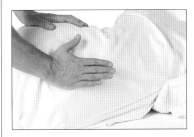

Rubbing the sacrum
Using the heel of your hand rub all around the mother's sacrum and lower back.

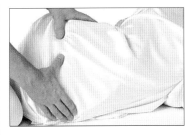

Circular pressure
Press your thumbs over the sacrum and move them gently in a circle. Rest your hands on the mother's hips for support.

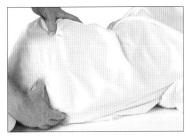

Deep pressure
Press your thumbs into the middle of each buttock. Make sure she is focusing on her breathing to help her relax.

BREATHING IN THE SECOND STAGE

You will be taught breathing exercises in antenatal classes. The importance of good breathing techniques during the second stage of labour can't be overestimated. It gives you the sensation of being in control of your own body and this is very empowering.

As you begin the second stage, you may want to accelerate your breathing. This is the most shallow form of breathing you should use in labour. Instead of using your chest and throat, focus on breathing only through your mouth. Breathe lightly in and out through your lips, starting slowly and gradually quickening. Be careful not to breathe out too deeply or you will start to hyperventilate. If you begin to feel at all dizzy, place your hands lightly over your nose and mouth while you are breathing.

Into the second stage
Full dilatation occurs at the end of the first stage of labour. The first indication that this has happened is a tremendous urge to push. Always ask an attendant to check your cervix – don't hang on and fight the urge even if it isn't long since you were checked because the final few centimetres of dilatation can be reached in seconds. Once full dilatation is confirmed you are able to push with force. Your mood will change and you will feel re-energized and positive as you work hard towards the birth of your baby, which is now only a short time away.

The second stage: delivery

Delivery is the main event: it's what you've prepared for over the last nine months. Your expectations are realistic – a manageable labour, not necessarily painless but happy and relaxed with your chosen birth assistant, staff whom you know, and with equipment and familiar surroundings. The most important factor in your being happy and relaxed is that everyone around you is a familiar friend.

CONTRACTIONS AND PUSHING

The second stage is the expulsive stage when you push your baby out. It lasts from the full dilatation of your cervix until the baby is born and, for a first baby, it generally doesn't take longer than two hours (the average is about one hour) and it may be as little as 15–20 minutes for subsequent babies. Contractions are at this time 60–90 seconds long and occur at two- to four-minute intervals.

You will almost certainly feel the urge to push down, known as bearing down, which is caused by your baby's head pressing down on your pelvic floor and rectum, and which is quite involuntary. Your pushing should be smooth and continuous; all the muscular effort should be smooth and slow so that the vaginal and perineal tissues and muscles are given enough time to stretch so they will be able to accommodate your baby's head.

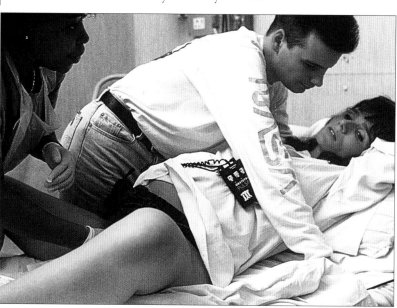

Upright is the most efficient position to be in when you're pushing, whether you sit on a birthing stool, stand with your arms around your partner's neck, or squat. This means that the downward muscular force of your body and the downward force of gravity are working in unison to expel your baby.

Be sure that you are not delivered lying on your back, even if you're supported by pillows, because in this position you're pushing your baby out uphill against the force of gravity. This is much harder work, and accordingly delivery is slower.

During pushing, the pelvic floor and the anal area should be fully relaxed, so make a conscious effort to let go of this part of your body. You may lose a little stool or urinate, but don't be embarrassed; it is very common and your attendants have seen it all before. When you've finished a push, make two slow, deep breaths, but don't relax too quickly at the end of a contraction. The baby will continue to maintain its forward progress if you relax slowly. If your second stage is considered to be prolonged, the delivery of your baby could be assisted by forceps (see p.306).

NORMAL DELIVERY

The first sign that the baby is coming is the bulging of your anus and perineum. With each contraction, more and more of the baby's head appears at your vaginal opening, until it doesn't slip back at all between contractions. This is known as crowning.

You will probably feel a stinging or burning sensation as the baby stretches the outlet of your vagina. As soon as you feel it, try to stop bearing down, pant, and allow the contractions of your uterus to push the baby out on its own. This may be difficult as you may still be feeling like pushing, but if you continue to push you increase the risk that you will tear or need an episiotomy. As you stop pushing, lean back and try to go limp. Make a conscious effort to relax the muscles of the perineal floor. The stinging or burning sensation only lasts for a short time and is followed by a numb feeling as the baby's head stretches your vaginal tissues so thin that the nerves are blocked, having a naturally anaesthetic effect. If the medical staff feel you are going to tear badly, this is the moment they may do an episiotomy (see p.110).

When her head has been delivered, your baby will be face down, but almost immediately she will twist her head so that she is facing your left or right thigh. The midwife or other attendant will then wipe your baby's eyes, nose, and mouth, and clear any fluid from her nose and upper air passages. The midwife will also check that the umbilical cord is not round the baby's neck – if it is, she will gently lift it over the head, make a loop through which the baby can be delivered or, if it is very tight, she may clamp and cut it.

After delivery of the head, your uterine contractions will stop for a minute or so. When they restart, the first contraction will usually deliver one shoulder and the next will deliver the other. Once both shoulders are delivered, the rest of your baby will slide out quickly and easily. Your attendants will hold her firmly as she will be slippery with blood, amniotic fluid, and *vernix caseosa*.

WHAT YOUR BABY DOES

Her body goes through several twists and turns as she descends through the birth canal, all of which are aimed towards achieving a smooth, safe birth.

Your baby has a pliable body but a fairly firm, oval head. Both these parts have to adapt themselves to a curved lower birth canal made up of the lower part of the uterus inside the pelvis, dilated cervix, and stretched vagina. There are various adjustments that your baby makes as labour progresses.

• She will bring her chin down on to her chest as she descends through the pelvis.

• She will rotate her head.

• She will extend her head backwards so that the back of her head touches her back as she emerges from the birth canal and vagina.

• She will make a little sideways wriggle so that her head turns to one side or the other; the shoulder of that side can then be delivered through the vagina.

• She will make another little wriggle to swing her head all the way round so that the other shoulder is delivered. (If you imagine this in quick succession, it's like a shrug of one shoulder after the other: during delivery this is so fast that you hardly perceive it).

• Her trunk, buttocks, and legs follow her head out through the birth canal.

Giving birth

Your baby's journey down the birth canal lasts about an hour on average. You will probably feel swept along by an unbelievably strong, fundamental urge to bear down and push your baby out of the uterus, although if you have had an epidural anaesthetic the urge to bear down may be somewhat reduced.

The urge to push out your baby is usually an overwhelming and irresistible feeling

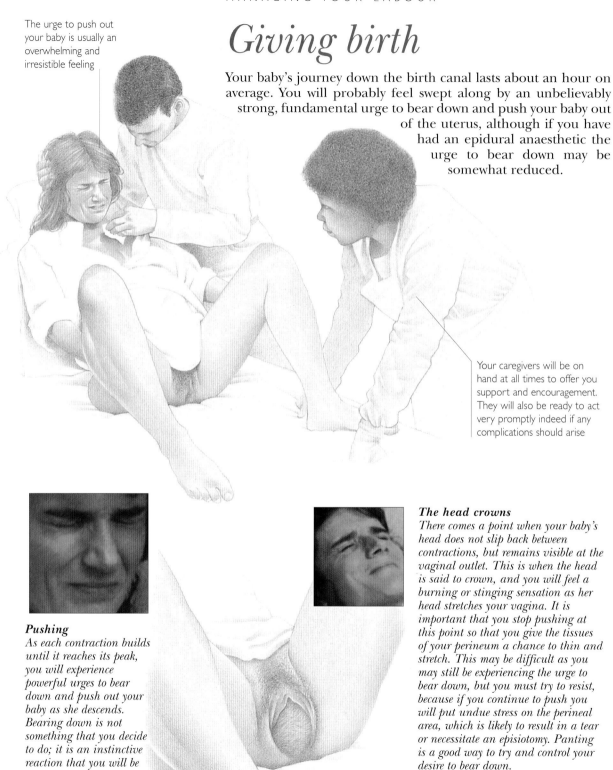

Your caregivers will be on hand at all times to offer you support and encouragement. They will also be ready to act very promptly indeed if any complications should arise

Pushing
As each contraction builds until it reaches its peak, you will experience powerful urges to bear down and push out your baby as she descends. Bearing down is not something that you decide to do; it is an instinctive reaction that you will be powerless to resist.

The head crowns
There comes a point when your baby's head does not slip back between contractions, but remains visible at the vaginal outlet. This is when the head is said to crown, and you will feel a burning or stinging sensation as her head stretches your vagina. It is important that you stop pushing at this point so that you give the tissues of your perineum a chance to thin and stretch. This may be difficult as you may still be experiencing the urge to bear down, but you must try to resist, because if you continue to push you will put undue stress on the perineal area, which is likely to result in a tear or necessitate an episiotomy. Panting is a good way to try and control your desire to bear down.

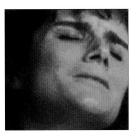

The head emerges

As her head is born, she will immediately turn her head sideways. Your contractions will probably pause for a few moments at this point, and your caregivers will feel around your baby's neck to make sure that the cord is not present. If it is, they will either lift it up over her head or make a loop through which she can be born. Her shoulders will be delivered in the next contraction.

Once her head is born, she turns it immediately so that she is facing towards the inside of one of your thighs

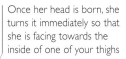

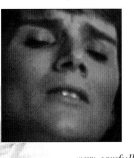

With a couple of almost imperceptible shrugs, her shoulders are born and she slithers out into the hands that are waiting to catch her

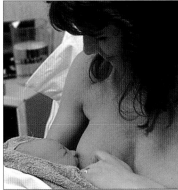

The baby is born

As soon as her shoulders are free, the rest of her body will be born immediately. As she slithers out of your vagina she will usually be followed by a great gush of amniotic fluid. Your caregivers will hold her very carefully as she will be slippery. She may be breathing and crying already.

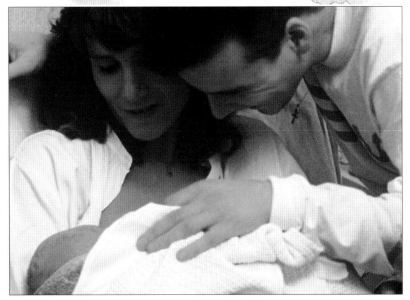

The first cuddle

Your caregivers will usually wrap or cover her in a blanket to keep her warm and then give her to you to hold in the first few minutes after her birth. She may start to suckle spontaneously.

RECORDING THE BIRTH

Photographs of the baby's birth can provide great joy for all involved and other family and friends. However, it's important to bear a few things in mind.

• Remember to seek special permission from the doctor and midwife before labour begins.

• If you intend to take more than a few photographs, or if you want to videotape the event, it would be better for a friend or relative to do this. The mother will need you to be sensitive to her every need, not rushing around clicking the camera or focusing on the best image. You may alienate yourself from her, not to mention the doctor and midwife, if you are constantly behind a piece of equipment.

• The room's atmosphere will have a great effect on the mother's labour. The lighting should be dim enough for her to feel relaxed, so use high-speed film (400 ISO) instead of brightening the room. Many hospitals will not allow direct flash to be used as it is irritating for the mother, distracting for the midwife, and may damage the baby's eyes.

Partner's role at birth

By this second stage of labour, your role in providing loving support for the mother will be well-established. You have now passed through the most painful phase and have reached the climactic stage of delivery.

SECOND STAGE JOBS

Many of the jobs you performed during the first stage – making her comfortable, supporting different positions, providing refreshment, giving moral support – may also be needed at this stage. However, this is when you will also have to encourage her to push. All this will make the mother's job very much easier and help her feel emotionally secure and relaxed.

If there is a medical emergency and staff have to move quickly, it may be advisable to be prepared to leave the delivery room, although you're unlikely to be asked to leave. However, you cannot guarantee that you will not be in the way, so be sensitive to the situation.

Helping with the delivery position Your partner, having been through the first stage of labour, will probably know by now which position she finds the most comfortable. You can offer valuable support to help her through the pushing stage, but don't hesitate

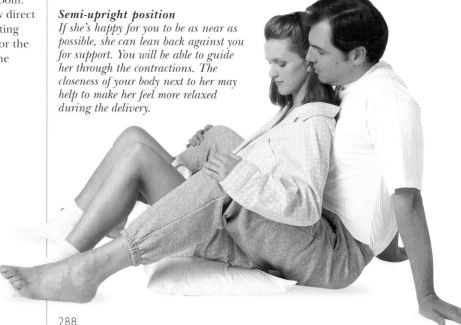

Semi-upright position
If she's happy for you to be as near as possible, she can lean back against you for support. You will be able to guide her through the contractions. The closeness of your body next to her may help to make her feel more relaxed during the delivery.

to ask the midwife for advice if you're not certain what to do. If she doesn't want to be held, you can offer suggestions for other positions that she may find comfortable, and place pillows or cushions underneath and behind her for support. Try to practise different ways of sitting or squatting before labour so that you are both familiar with them; if you are feeling uncomfortable this may make your partner nervous.

If your partner is happy sitting in bed or on the floor, suggest that she try the knee-chest position, which many women find comfortable in the second stage. She should drop her chin on to her chest while holding on to her knees. Between contractions, suggest that she relaxes against the pillow to conserve her energy.

Helping her with breathing and pushing To help her through these last few contractions tap out a rhythm for the different kinds of breathing, using words like: breathe, breathe, pant, pant, blow. As she's pushing, gently remind her to relax her pelvic floor.

At the peak of contractions, suggest that she takes two or three deep breaths and pushes as hard as she can. She should push in a strong and steady way, and you can remind her that each push brings the birth of your baby nearer.

Encouraging her to relax Between contractions make sure she relaxes as she needs to conserve strength for pushing her baby through the birth canal. Massage her back (see p.283) if she has backache or needs comforting and reassuring. If she is hot and bothered, mop her brow or spray her face with a water spray.

Standing by Once the baby's head has crowned, you may have a more passive role and become an observer. The midwife will guide your partner through this pushing stage. Don't be disappointed if the mother doesn't communicate with you during the birth and seems to rely more on the midwife. She will be fully preoccupied and involved, and may not notice you for some time.

Showing her the baby When the baby's head is emerging, hold a mirror nearby so that she can see his head crowning and then his whole body slithering out. Encourage her to reach down and touch his head as he is born.

Loving reception With the assistance of the midwife, you may be able to catch your baby as his body emerges. After you have greeted him for the first time, place him on your partner's stomach. You can then cuddle them both to help to keep them warm and to let them know that you're there.

Be prepared for your own and the mother's reactions – relief, tears, awed silence, exhausted collapse, whoops of joy. You may even feel squeamish at the sight of his bloodied, greasy, tiny body. Whatever your reaction, it's all perfectly understandable, and it marks a new phase in your family's history.

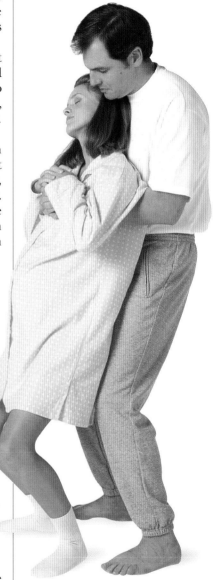

Supported squat
If your partner wants to deliver standing up, you can help support her by taking her weight on your arms. When she is supported in this position, her pelvis will be completely open and she will be able to take full advantage of gravity. Her legs should be wide apart.

WHAT THE PLACENTA LOOKS LIKE

The majority of first-time mothers are very interested in seeing their baby's placenta.

The placenta measures about 8–10in (20–25cm) in diameter and weighs about 1lb (0.5kg). It is disc-shaped, and its surfaces are very different in appearance.

The fetal side was contiguous with the wall of your uterus and covered by membranes. It is flat and smooth and is bluish gray in color, with blood vessels radiating out from the umbilical cord. The maternal side was embedded in the wall of your uterus and is made up of wedges (cotyledons) so that the surface area is increased for gaseous exchange. This side is dark red and looks like several pieces of raw liver joined together.

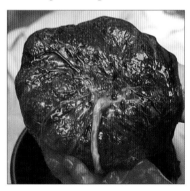

The fetal side
The side of the placenta that was facing your baby is flat and smooth. Note the umbilical cord emerging from its center and the prominent blood vessels.

The third stage

Once your baby has been born, your uterus rests for about 15 minutes. It will then start to contract again in order to expel the placenta. This is the third stage of labor and is comparatively painless – you probably will hardly notice it.

THE THIRD STAGE

During the third stage of labor the placenta becomes detached from the uterine wall and is delivered by expulsion down the birth canal. The large blood vessels, which are about the thickness of a pencil and which run to and from the placenta, are simply torn across. However, bleeding is rare because the muscle fibers of the uterus are arranged in a crisscross fashion, which means that when the uterus contracts, the muscles tighten around the blood vessels and prevent them from bleeding. This is why it is absolutely essential that the uterus contract into a hard ball once the placenta has been expelled. The uterus can be kept tightly contracted by massaging it intermittently for an hour or so after the third stage is complete. Normally the third stage lasts about 10 to 20 minutes, but with active management it can be much shorter.

THE PLACENTA IS DELIVERED

Traditionally, no attempt is made to deliver the placenta until there are clear signs that it is separating from the uterine wall and moving downward into the vagina. The signs that your attendants will look out for are the resumption of contractions a few minutes after the birth of your baby, which indicates that the placenta is about to separate, and a desire to bear down on your part, which indicates that the placenta has separated from the uterine wall and is pressing down on your pelvic floor.

When these signs have appeared, delivery of the placenta is encouraged by pulling gently on the cord and at the same time pressing above the rim of the pelvis to control descent. The placenta is expelled from the vagina, followed by the membranes. Rarely, a retroplacental blood clot will also be expelled.

Delivery There are two different ways in which the placenta may pass through the vulva. The first is when the center of the placenta comes out first, pulling the membranes behind it. In the second way, the placenta presents by an edge and slips out of the vulva sideways. Most women want to see the placenta – this is very understandable, as it is an amazing organ that has been the life-support system for your baby for nine months (see column, left).

After delivery Once the placenta is delivered, medical staff carefully examine it to make sure that it's complete and that none of it has been left behind. If any of the placenta has been retained by the uterus, it can be a cause of hemorrhage later on, so it should be removed as soon as the diagnosis is made. In cases of doubt, an ultrasound scan will probably show whether the uterus is completely empty. The membranes should form a complete bag except for the hole through which the fetus has passed. The cut end of the cord will be examined to check that the umbilical blood vessels are normal.

After the placenta is delivered, the whole of the vulval outlet will be carefully examined for tears; anything other than a minute one must be stitched immediately.

ACTIVE MANAGEMENT OF THE THIRD STAGE

Using a hormonal drug known as ergonovine maleate, many hospitals and obstetricians now actively manage the third stage of delivery. When given at the time of birth or imediately afterward, this drug can reduce the number of cases of excessive bleeding, which is the loss of more than a pint of blood (500ml).

Ergonovine causes prolonged contraction of the uterus without a period of relaxation, and while the uterus is contracted there is not likely to be any bleeding.

Syntocinon The placenta separates very quickly from the uterine wall once the uterus starts to contract, thereby shortening the third stage of labor. Nowadays most attendants use a combination of ergonovine and oxytocin because ergonovine on its own takes effect rather slowly and can cause nausea. Using it with Syntocinon, a synthetic oxytocin, which acts quickly to stimulate uterine contractions, gives a better result. The drugs are given by intramuscular injection just when the head is crowning or with delivery of the first shoulder.

Oxytocin is a hormone naturally produced by your body in response to seeing and touching your baby and to putting her to your breast. It does the same job as ergonovine, but it is less reliable.

HOW YOU WILL FEEL

Shivering and shaking can be quite profound after delivery of the placenta. After delivery of my second child I was shivering so much and my teeth were chattering so much that I couldn't speak or breathe properly. My own explanation for this reaction is that for nine months I had a little furnace inside me, producing quite a lot of heat, and my body had adjusted to take account of that heat production by turning my own thermostat down slightly. When my baby left my body, I was deprived of that heat and my body temperature probably dropped a few degrees. The only way the body can raise its temperature is to generate heat through muscular work. That's exactly what shivering does; by rapid contraction and relaxation of muscles, body heat is produced. The shivering usually passes in about half an hour, during which time the body temperature is brought back up to normal and your own thermostat reset.

POSTPARTUM HEMORRHAGE

This is rare, largely because the uterus has a self-protecting device to stop it from bleeding.

Once the uterus is completely empty, it contracts down to about the size of a tennis ball. The contraction of the uterine muscles nips the uterine arteries so that they cannot bleed. Under normal circumstances, therefore, little bleeding occurs after the delivery. What bleeding there is appears as the lochia – the usual postpartum vaginal discharge, which is red for 2–3 days, then turns brown, and disappears within 2–6 weeks.

A uterus in which remnants of the placenta are retained will bleed; this bleeding is called postpartum hemorrhage. If a small fragment of placenta is left in the uterus, it is usually diagnosed by examining the placenta and finding that a portion is missing. The mother is given a general anesthetic, and the placenta is gently scraped away (curettaged) from inside the uterus.

If bleeding occurs more than 24 hours after delivery, the lochia may become bright red again. This can occur as a result of being too energetic. Consult your doctor, who will probably advise you to rest for several days. Recurrent or heavy bleeding or passing blood clots can indicate infection or retention of a small piece of placenta. Contact your doctor immediately.

THE APGAR SCORE

When your baby is born, she is checked to see whether she is fit and healthy. Within a minute of her birth, 5 simple tests are carried out. These are scored on the Apgar scale (named after Dr. Virginia Apgar, who devised it). The Apgar score includes the following checks:

Pulse/heart rate This measures the strength and regularity of the heartbeat. 100 beats per minute scores 2; below 100 scores 1; no pulse scores 0.

Breathing This reveals the maturity and health of the baby's lungs. Regular breathing scores 2, irregular 1, none 0.

Movements An indication of the baby's muscle-tone. Active movements score 2; some movements 1; limp scores 0.

Skin colour This shows how well the lungs are working to oxygenate the blood. Pink skin scores 2, bluish extremities 1, totally blue skin scores 0.

Reflexes Crying and grimacing can reveal that the baby responds to stimuli. Crying scores 2, whimpering 1, silence 0.

Most babies score between 7 and 10. A second test is done about 5 minutes later.

Your brand new baby
As you hold her you will experience the glow of motherhood – a mixture of love, pride, awe, and wonder, mixed with the all-encompassing tiredness that comes with a hard job well done.

Baby's first hours

Once your baby is delivered, all of the attention will be given to her, not to you, and rightly so. She may cry first when delivered and will be crying lustily a few seconds after birth. She will probably be a bluish-white colour at first and may be covered with vernix caseosa. She will have streaks of blood on her head and body and, depending on your delivery, her head may look slightly pointed after her journey down the birth canal.

HER FIRST MOMENTS

If her breathing is normal, there's absolutely no reason why you should not hold her immediately. If there's a danger of her being cold, you can be covered with a towel or blanket. Your gentle stroking movements and the sound of your heartbeat and voice will reassure your baby. Her eyes will almost certainly fasten on your face and she may scrabble as if trying to swim towards you.

Cutting the cord The first procedure is the clamping of the cord. Some practitioners believe that the baby benefits from the return of placental blood through the umbilical cord, and that the cord should not be clamped until it stops pulsating. However, others believe that this could cause the baby to develop anaemia. At the appropriate time, two clamps are applied to the cord, one a short

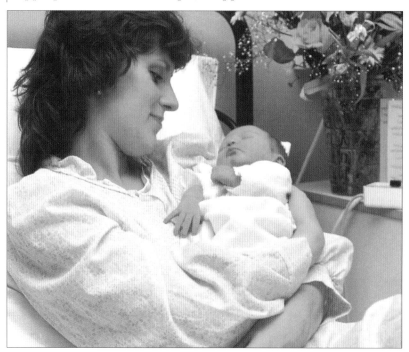

distance from the navel, the other about an inch away. These clamps prevent the cord from bleeding; the one closest to the baby being the most important. The cord is then cut between the clamps. It may have been clamped and cut during delivery if it was looped tightly around the baby's neck. This is quite common.

Her general condition The midwife will check your baby's general condition. She will remove any remaining fluid in the baby's mouth, nose, or air passages by sucking it out with disposable plastic tubing. If the baby doesn't start to breathe immediately, the midwife will take her and give her oxygen.

WELCOMING YOUR BABY

Once the well-being of you and your baby is established, by all means ask the nursing and medical staff to leave if you wish to be left alone in the warmth of your house or hospital birthing room with your partner and your baby. However, you may have to wait until after you have been stitched; your midwife or doctor will be able to make a much neater repair if you are stitched as soon as possible after the birth before the tissues swell. Once this is done, you can relax after your hard work and mutually enjoy this amazing new experience. It's a good idea to put your baby to the breast immediately because it stimulates the delivery of the placenta, even if your baby isn't hungry at first.

These initial few moments should be spent in concentrating on your baby, getting to know her, learning to recognize her face, cooing at her so that she can hear the sound of your voice. You should hold her about 20–25 centimetres (8–10 inches) away from your face because at this distance she can make out your face quite clearly. Smile and talk gently in a sing-song voice, because newborn babies are attuned to high vocal pitches.

Within half an hour of birth your partner should be given his baby to hold for the first time. Men have the potential to bond as deeply and as quickly with their newborn children as women do.

After this initial bonding process, you will be washed down and asked to pass urine to make sure that everything is in working order. You can then change and the midwives will give your baby a more thorough check over.

CHECKING HER THOROUGHLY

Shortly after birth (in addition to the Apgar score, see column, left), the doctor or midwife will carry out specific checks on your baby. The doctor will check that her facial features and body proportions are normal. She will be turned over to check that the back is normal and there are no indications of spina bifida. Her anus is checked, as are her fingers and toes. The number of blood vessels in the umbilical cord is recorded; there are usually two arteries and one vein. She will then be weighed, and her head circumference and possibly her body length measured. This preliminary examination takes only a few seconds in the hands of an experienced doctor or midwife.

YOUR BABY'S IDENTIFICATION

Before your baby leaves the delivery room, she will have some form of identification fastened to her, so that all the staff will know that she is yours.

Plastic bracelets will usually be sealed around both your baby's wrist and her ankle. The identifying bracelets must remain on your baby at all times while she is in hospital. These bracelets are usually marked with:

• your surname (she will be referred to by the staff as "baby Brown" for example)

• her date of birth

• an identification number (an identification number is used by most hospitals for both you and your baby)

In addition to the above:

• her footprints may be taken

• her cot may be marked with her name and number.

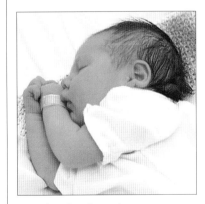

Keeping her bracelets
Like many mothers, you may want to keep your baby's identity bracelets as souvenirs. As your baby grows day by day, it will soon seem astonishing that her wrists and ankles could ever have been quite so tiny.

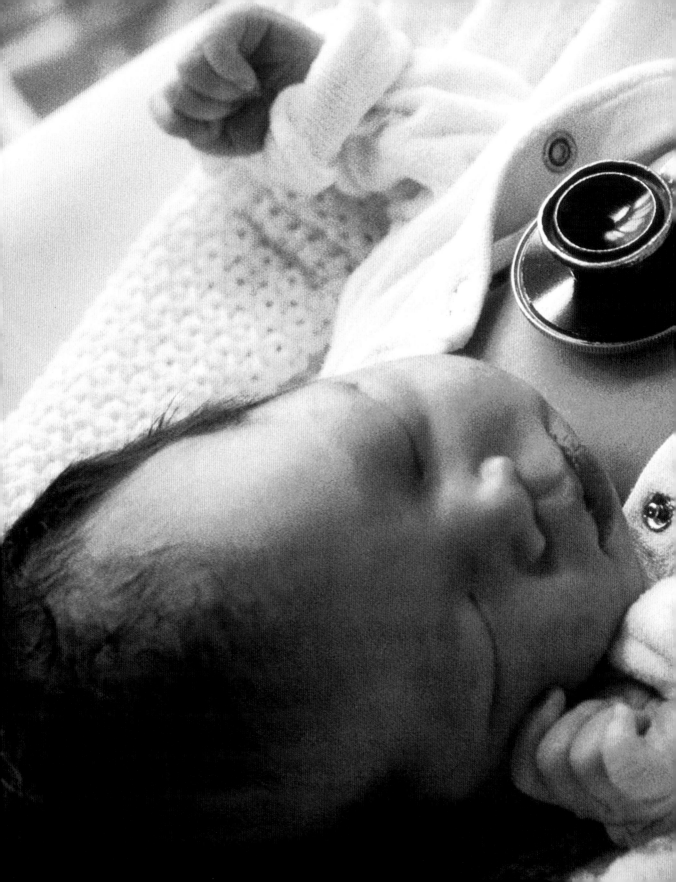

CHAPTER 14

Special
DELIVERIES

As a rule most babies are delivered without a hitch
and are fit and healthy. Nonetheless labors vary
enormously. No two labors are alike, even for the same
woman. From time to time some require a
special approach and a few will require intervention.
They turn out just as well for mother and baby.

Special labours

Most labours are quite straightforward, but occasionally a complication arises that calls for a special approach. With vigilant antenatal care, potential difficulties should be anticipated and easily avoided. Now and then the first stage is underway before a problem becomes apparent.

BACKACHE LABOUR

Occasionally, the discomfort of uterine contractions will be experienced primarily as low back pain. This is usually due to stretching of the cervix as it dilates. It may also occur if your baby lies in the posterior position with the back of his head up against your spine (one in ten babies lie in this position; it is not abnormal). In this position, your baby's neck may not be properly flexed and a larger proportion of the head than normal presents, which may prolong labour. Most of the time, your baby will rotate the 180 degrees into the anterior position and labour will proceed smoothly. If, as occasionally happens, the baby fails to rotate to the anterior position, this is no cause for alarm, although your doctor may deliver him using forceps or, more rarely, vacuum extraction. This kind of labour may start slowly and be protracted, so it can be very tiring. There are various ways in which you and your birth assistant can relieve your backache.

Counterpressure This is the most effective way of relieving backache (see p.283). However, if being touched by someone else is irritating, for example during transition, you may prefer to use your own knuckles by placing a hand underneath each buttock.

Change in position When you are lying flat on your back, your baby is pressing down hardest on your spine and its nerves. Try to stay upright and walk around as much as possible. You can also relieve the pressure of your baby on your spine by sitting tailor-fashion (see p.150), leaning forward, or by rocking your pelvis. If you feel more comfortable lying down, lie on the side that your baby is turning towards (your midwife will be able to advise you which side that is).

Application of heat You may find it helpful if, during or between contractions, your birth assistant places a heating pad or hot water bottle against the lower part of your back. A hot shower, if directed particularly on to your back, may also provide some relief.

PROLONGED LABOUR

Labour is said to be prolonged when strong uterine contractions fail to bring about the expected delivery. This may be due to the inability of the cervix to dilate, or failure of the baby to descend through the birth canal. Doctors keep a very careful eye on the

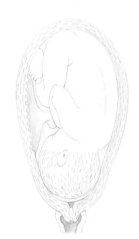

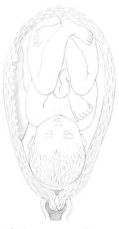

Your baby's presentation
The way your baby is presenting can affect your labour and birth. The usual presentation is when your baby's spine faces outwards (top), but if your baby's head is facing outwards (bottom), labour might possibly be delayed. Most babies, however, rotate to the correct position before passing down the birth canal.

length of each stage of labour. When labour appears to be progressing more slowly than normal, your obstetrician may suspect obstruction and take an early decision to intervene – with a forceps delivery if it's suitable, or a Caesarean section.

No woman is allowed to go on with a difficult birth for much over the accepted times (see p.273) as this may lead to maternal exhaustion and fetal distress.

Obstruction can be more quickly detected in a mother who has had several children. However, your doctor or midwife will be monitoring your general condition throughout labour, and they will be alerted to possible obstruction if your condition appears to deteriorate and you look tired and anxious.

With a very long labour, when you are foregoing food and rest, you might become too tired or distressed to push adequately. Your doctor and midwife will not allow this to happen.

Failure to dilate When contractions are weak and infrequent with the cervix dilating slowly, the uterus may be failing to coordinate muscular activity. One way in which your doctor and midwife will be able to see exactly how your labour is progressing is by plotting a partogram (see below). If the failure of the uterus to contract efficiently is the only reason for the lack of progress, your doctor may begin special procedures to speed up effacement and dilatation. The membranes may be artificially ruptured and then Syntocinon may be administered intravenously with a drip or with a pump. The dosage will be carefully increased until strong contractions are occurring regularly about every three minutes.

CAUSES OF FETAL OBSTRUCTION

Certain fetal conditions may exist that cause you to have an obstructed labour. Fortunately, problems can usually be detected beforehand so everybody is well-prepared.

• Your baby is too large.

• Your baby is lying in a transverse or oblique position.

• Your baby is in a breech, face, or brow presentation.

• Your baby is lying in the posterior position.

• Your twin babies are entwined.

• Your baby has a congenital abnormality such as hydrocephalus.

YOUR LABOUR'S PROGRESS

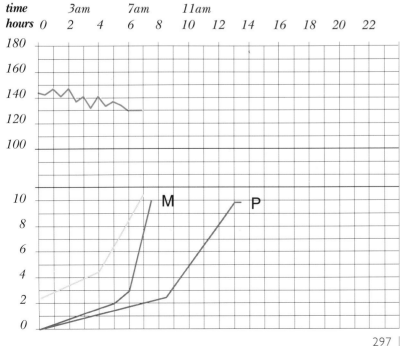

Plotting your partogram
The partogram records the baby's heart rate and the mother's cervical dilatation. The other lines on the graph depict the expected dilatation of a multiparous (more than one pregnancy) woman (M) and a primiparous (first pregnancy) woman (P), which are compared with the mother's actual progress. This chart represents a multiparous mother who got off to a slow start, although labour eventually became normal.

———— fetal heart rate
beats/minute

—————— mother's dilatation

———— expected dilatation

MATERNAL CAUSES OF OBSTRUCTION

If your labor is failing to progress normally, there may be reasons why your pelvis or uterus is obstructing the descent of your baby.

• Deformity or disproportion of the bony pelvis.

• Pelvic tumors such as fibroids or an ovarian cyst.

• Abnormalities of the uterus, cervix, or vagina.

• A contraction ring of the uterus, which is when the uterus pulls in excessively, creating a band of tight muscle. This can stop contractions from passing all the way down and may result in constriction of the uterus or cervix. Fortunately, it is very rare unless the uterus has been overstimulated by oxytocin or prostaglandin, such as during induction (see p.300). A Cesarean section is almost always required.

doctor will pay close attention throughout to ensure that there are no unexpected increases in the strength or frequency of your contractions.

Failure to descend I have already mentioned breech and posterior presentation as causes of obstruction. One other reason for an obstructed labor is disproportion. Disproportion is a result of the size of your baby's head and the size of your pelvis failing to match up. If your pelvis is too small relative to your baby's head, disproportion results. It is easy to understand how your baby might fail to descend in such circumstances (see also p.176).

If you're a first-time mother and your baby is still high and nonengaged during the last few weeks of your pregnancy (see column, p.261), your doctor may suspect disproportion. This will also be taken into account if the baby's head remains high during labor despite strong contractions.

If the disproportion is very slight, your doctor may let you try to have a trial of labor (bear in mind that it is your uterus on trial, not you), provided there are no other irregularities and the baby's head is felt to be descending. Once the baby's head has entered the pelvic cavity, a vaginal delivery usually occurs. If the disproportion is major, doctors will perform a Cesarean section.

Rest assured that most of the abnormalities that cause obstruction and a prolonged labor (see column, left, and p.297) will be picked up during your pregnancy, so early treatment is possible and a plan of action can be made by the doctors and midwives before labor begins.

PREMATURE LABOR

A premature labor is one that occurs at less than 37 weeks of gestation. In about 40 percent of cases the cause is a mystery. It is, however, known to occur in the following instances: premature rupture of the membranes; multiple pregnancy; preeclampsia; cervical incompetence; and uterine abnormalities. Overwork, stress, and some maternal diseases, such as anemia or malnutrition, may also have an effect.

Knowing whether you've actually gone into premature labor is almost as difficult for your doctors as it is for you (see column, right). The diagnosis is not easy, and criteria differ at different centers – showing that often it's quite arbitrary. As a general rule, a premature labor begins without any warning; the first sign may be rupture of the membranes, the beginning of uterine contractions, or some vaginal bleeding. There is no stopping labor if your membranes have ruptured and labor has begun, but you or your doctor can take certain precautions while the membranes are intact or before labor really gets going.

What you can do If your membranes have ruptured (see p.273) but labor hasn't started, you should go straight to the hospital. The risk of ascending infection is great, and both you and your preterm baby will be vulnerable. The doctors will monitor you closely for signs of infection, such as a fever, and will give you antibiotics if necessary. Labor is unlikely to be suppressed once the membranes have ruptured spontaneously; if contractions do not begin on their own within a day or so, oxytocin usually will be given in order to encourage them to start.

What the hospital will do If labor starts between 24 and 34 weeks, the aim is to delay your labor to allow time to mature the baby's lungs with steroid medications and bed rest. A preterm baby (see also pp.344 & 345) has an increased risk of developing respiratory distress syndrome, and the shorter the gestation period, the greater the risk. Bed rest can also improve uterine blood supply so that your baby will get enough oxygen and be as well nourished as possible.

Additionally, being in the hospital allows your doctor to check for evidence of infection in cases of premature rupture of the membranes and to monitor your baby's condition. It also ensures that your premature baby can be looked after in intensive care immediately after delivery. If your local hospital does not have a neonatal intensive care unit that can handle very premature babies, you may even be moved to another hospital farther away. This is unfortunate in that it may make it harder for your partner, friends, and family to visit you, but you can be assured that the unit will be able to give your tiny baby the best possible start in life (see p.344).

Drug treatments Because all of the drugs used cause some side effects, they are suitable only for certain cases of premature labor. The main criteria for drug treatment are that you be healthy, have no heart disease, diabetes, high blood pressure, or an abnormally placed placenta, and, of course, that your baby is alive, with no evidence of a congenital defect.

If you are very anxious, you may be given a mild sedative, but morphine and certain other drugs should not be administered during labor unless your pain is extremely severe. These drugs may make your uterine muscles more irritable rather than calming them down; they may also have a detrimental effect on your baby.

Managing labor Once the membranes have ruptured, labor will proceed as normal (see p.270). As a general rule, premature labor tends to be shorter and easier than full-term labor, mainly because the baby's head is smaller and softer. However, an episiotomy is usually given to protect the baby's head from pressure changes within the birth canal. For the same reason, almost all premature babies are delivered with the assistance of forceps. You will probably be offered an epidural anesthetic instead of analgesic drugs because the latter can depress the fetal respiratory system. Doctors will take special care to avoid hypoxia (lack of oxygen to the tissues) throughout labor and delivery. Cesarean delivery in premature labor is used in some situations, particularly if fetal distress occurs.

ARE YOU IN PREMATURE LABOR?

Here are some useful pointers for diagnosing whether or not you're in premature labor.

• You are less than 37 weeks into your pregnancy.

• You've observed uterine contractions for at least an hour.

• Contractions occur every 5–10 minutes.

• The contractions last for 30 seconds and persist over the period of an hour.

• A vaginal examination by your doctor or midwife shows that your cervix is more than 1in (2.5cm) dilated and therefore more than three-quarters effaced.

According to these criteria, two-thirds of all patients who are thought to be in premature labor will actually be found not to be in real labor, and no treatment will be required. This will be quickly confirmed if you go straight to the hospital so that staff can observe uterine activity very carefully.

Induction of labour

Towards the end of pregnancy
obstetricians are always on the
look out for signs of placental
insufficiency as the baby
outgrows its food supply.

The issue of when induction
of labour is necessary if you're
overdue is controversial, so it is
worth having a discussion about
this at one of your antenatal
checks. Of course induction is not
always necessary. A mother who
reaches her estimated date of
delivery, given that she and the
baby are perfectly normal, should
be allowed to go into spontaneous
labour. I would very much
advocate, however, that you
cooperate with the frequent
monitoring of your condition and
that of the baby once the EDD has
been passed and, if there is any
sign of fetal distress, agree to have
medical intervention.

REASONS FOR
INDUCTION

**Anything that makes the uterine
environment unhealthy is a
reason for induction. Your
labour may be induced if:**

• you have hypertension,
pre-eclampsia, heart disease,
diabetes, or antepartum bleeding

• there are signs of placental
insufficiency (so that the baby is
in danger of not getting enough
nutrients and oxygen from the
placenta)

• your membranes have ruptured
(see p.273) but labour hasn't
started within 24–48 hours

• your pregnancy is prolonged
beyond 42 weeks.

**Induction starts off labour artificially with rupture of the
membranes and oxytocin or prostaglandins being given to
stimulate uterine contractions. The same techniques are used
to accelerate labour if the contractions are weak and progress
slow. If your induction is not done for the medical reasons
below (see box) or as an emergency, you will have an elective
induction. An appointment will be made for you to be
admitted to hospital at a certain time. Your partner will be
able to be with you at all times. If you're in any doubt about
why your doctor is suggesting induction of labour, ask for a
detailed explanation – this should cover all of the alternatives.
The ultimate decision rests, of course, with yourself.**

THE HISTORY OF INDUCTION

Forty years ago when drugs first became available, the induction
of labour was often used for hospital or social convenience. It was
sometimes planned to suit working hours or a woman might ask
to be induced so that the birth could fall on her birthday. Such
reasons are no longer accepted as valid.

When induction first became fashionable, there was not today's
technological back-up, such as ultrasound and amniocentesis, for
doctors to establish fetal maturity, and babies might be born too
early with respiratory problems. The rate of Caesarean section
also rose. Nowadays, fewer than one in five labours are induced.

However, only five percent of babies actually come on the due
date and it can be hard for some doctors and quite a lot of
mothers, to remain philosophical when that magic date passes.
There may be concern that the placenta is becoming inadequate
and that the baby is outgrowing its environment.

If you feel anxious when you learn that your labour is to be
induced, I'd like to reassure you that induction is a great asset
provided it is done strictly for medical reasons. You shouldn't
worry unduly, as it's being done either for your well-being or the
baby's. Don't be angry with yourself if your birth does not turn
out the way that you had planned or imagined it to be.

HOW IT IS DONE

Most obstetric units will normally use a combination of three
different methods to induce labour.

Prostaglandin pessaries One of the more modern methods of
induction is by use of prostaglandin pessaries, which affect the
pregnant uterus, causing it to go into labour. Pessaries are inserted
into the vagina during the evening and you may be lucky enough
to be in labour by morning. This is a very satisfactory method of
induction as you can move freely around the labour room.

Artificial rupture of the membranes (ARM) Also known as amniotomy, this method of induction, often accompanied by an oxytocin drip (see below), involves the use of an instrument not unlike a crochet hook. It is inserted through the cervix into the uterus to make a small opening in the membrane so that the waters escape. For most women this is a painless procedure because the amniotic membranes are entirely insensitive. So long as the uterus is contracting at the time it is performed, labour usually reaches full intensity quickly after ARM because the baby's head is no longer cushioned and presses down hard against the cervix, encouraging the uterus to contract and the cervix to dilate. If left alone, the waters don't usually break until late in the first stage.

Amniotomy is not just a method of induction. It will be performed if an elecrode needs to be attached to the baby's scalp to monitor its heartbeat (see p.275). It will also be performed if the baby's heart rate goes down because of distress. In this case, traces of meconium, the baby's first bowel movement, may be seen in the amniotic fluid.

Oxytocin-induced labour The natural hormone from the posterior pituitary gland in the brain, oxytocin, will stimulate labour and the synthetic form is used for inducing labour.

Although it used sometimes to be administered in tablet form, oxytocin is now only given through a drip because it is easier to regulate. Ask for it to be inserted in the left arm if you are right-handed, and check that you can have a long tube connecting you to the drip. You will then have more room to move around, even if this is just on the bed; some drip stands are on wheels so that you can still move around the room and change position if you wish, which will help you control the more intense labour pains. The oxytocin drip can be turned down if you go into strong labour quickly and the cervix becomes half dilated. The needle won't be removed from your arm until after the baby is born because the uterine contractions help to expel the placenta.

Contractions brought on by an oxytocin drip are often stronger, longer, and more painful than normal contractions, with shorter periods of relaxation between them, and an increased need for painkilling drugs. As the blood supply to the uterus is temporarily shut off during each strong contraction, it's thought that this may be detrimental to the fetus. Today, obstetricians believe that only a small percentage of deliveries actually need an oxytocin-induced labour.

EXPECTATIONS OF INDUCED LABOUR

If properly handled, induced labour need not be more painful or difficult than natural labour and, using oxytocin, your doctor or midwife should be able to get you to the stage where you will have a normal labour. You can still do all your breathing exercises and push the baby out at your own pace if you prefer to have a completely natural childbirth. If the induced labour does become too painful, which it may, you can always request an epidural anaesthetic or some other form of pain relief (see p.280).

AMNIOTOMY AND YOUR BABY

The membranes usually rupture naturally towards the end of the first stage of labour.

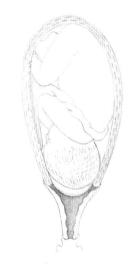

Intact membranes
The bag of waters provides a cushion for the baby's head as it presses against the cervix.

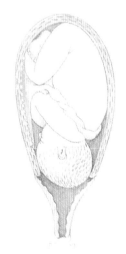

Ruptured membranes
Contractions increase in intensity pressing the baby's head against the cervix helping it to open.

Breech baby

Joanna was a firm believer in home delivery, but when her baby was diagnosed as being breech, I advised her to have the baby in the hospital. While most breech labors proceed smoothly, she would want to have her obstetrician, as well as an anesthesiologist and pediatrician, present at the delivery in case there were complications.

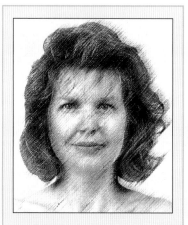

Name **Joanna Rolfe**

Age **33 years**

Past medical history
Nothing abnormal

Obstetric history **Two children, ages seven and four, both normal pregnancies, normal deliveries in the cephalic (head-down) position**

Joanna is American, married to an Englishman, David. When her baby was found to be breech, Joanna was glad she had decided to have her baby in the UK; British and European obstetricians do not automatically advise Cesarean delivery of breech babies, whereas American obstetricians do. There is evidence that most mothers have breech babies by vaginal delivery without very much difficulty; statistically, however, babies born by Cesarean section do have a slightly better survival rate.

EXPECTATIONS OF THE BIRTH

Most babies are in the breech position until around the 32nd week of pregnancy, when they usually turn upside down of their own accord, but Joanna's baby was still breech at 36 weeks. Some doctors and midwives try to turn the baby externally, by manipulation of the mother's abdomen, but Joanna's caregivers did not attempt this.

I advised her of recent findings that show a very slightly lower mortality rate with Cesarean section (see p.308), but Joanna was eager to have a vaginal delivery and her obstetrician was willing to comply with her wishes. Even so, I advised her to expect special measures. Since her baby's bottom would be smaller, softer, and more squashable than the head, Joanna's vaginal and pelvic tissues might not be stretched enough to allow the head, the largest part of her baby, through the birth canal. Forceps would probably be necessary to protect the head in the narrowed birth canal, and an episiotomy would make this easier. I also told her the obstetrician would be very concerned about the position of the cord, as this may appear before the baby and become compressed. External fetal monitoring would be carried out at the beginning of labor, and this would be continued via a fetal scalp monitor (see p.275) as soon as the membranes ruptured.

I also warned her that the first stage of labor could be rather prolonged because the buttocks aren't as efficient as the head at dilating the cervix. However, Joanna made excellent progress.

A GOOD START

Joanna's labor started with simple backache, which went on for four hours until her contractions began. On arriving in the hospital she was examined by a midwife, who found the baby's buttocks pressed against the cervix with five centimeters (2in) of dilation. Shortly afterward, Joanna's backache became very severe, but she was able to get some relief by kneeling on all fours. However, when the contractions became more painful than she felt able to cope with, Joanna requested an epidural anesthetic.

Because a baby's bottom is smaller than its head, the second stage of labor may be shorter in a breech delivery, and Joanna's doctors expected an imminent birth once she entered the transition stage. For the birth, Joanna propped herself up in a sitting position. Just prior to delivery, the obstetrician rapidly gave Joanna a local anesthetic in the perineum (rather than topping off her epidural, which was wearing off) and then performed a large episiotomy in order to assist the birth of the baby's head. After he had examined her again, the obstetrician told Joanna that a foot was presenting ahead of the buttocks and he could feel the projection of the heel.

THE BABY APPEARS

With the next contraction, both feet and legs presented, and the doctor gradually eased them out. The buttocks started to appear soon after: first the uppermost buttock and then the one lying behind. Joanna's obstetrician advised her not to push, but to allow the power of the uterine contractions to ease the baby's buttocks out very gently. He was particularly good in reassuring her that they had plenty of time available and she was going to be able to deliver the baby quite easily. And, with the next uterine contraction, the baby was born to the level of the shoulders.

To help deliver the shoulders, the obstetrician rotated the baby's body gently through 180 degrees, keeping her back upward. An arm appeared underneath Joanna's pubic arch and was easily delivered, as was the second arm after rotation back through 180 degrees in the opposite direction.

A PROBLEM OCCURS

Delivering the head was not so easy. It was rather slow, too slow for the obstetrician, especially when he saw that the baby's heart

rate was slowing, a sign of mild fetal distress. The baby's chest was free and she was making attempts to take her first breath.

Joanna's obstetrician reached his hand into her vagina and over the baby's face. Putting a finger on either side of her nose, he attempted to flex her head and

Forceps delivery
Forceps are slipped into the vagina, one tong on either side of the baby's head. This guards the head as it is carefully drawn through the pelvis and delivered. Once the nose and mouth are free, they are usually suctioned to clear them of mucus, since a breech baby often attempts to breathe while the head is still in the birth canal.

bring her out over the perineum. This manouver proved unsuccessful, and forceps were applied. An assistant held the baby's feet while the doctor applied the forceps around the sides of her head. The baby's head was delivered within seconds, and she cried immediately.

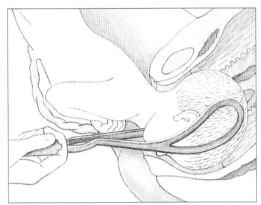

JOANNA'S BABY

There are three main breech presentations. Joanna's baby, Grace, was diagnosed as being complete – her buttocks were presenting and her feet were low in Joanna's pelvis.

In flexed or complete breech, the thighs are flexed against the body and the knees are bent. This was

the position that Joanna's baby was in. In frank breech, the thighs are flexed but the legs are extended upward. The baby's arms are often wrapped around the legs. In footling breech, the thighs are poorly flexed and the feet are above the cervix – they drop down after the rupture of the membranes.

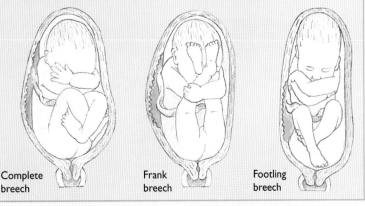

Complete breech   Frank breech   Footling breech

ON YOUR WAY TO THE HOSPITAL

If the urge to bear down comes as you are driving to the hospital, use your breathing techniques to avoid pushing; try to stay calm.

Assess the situation with your partner. If the urge is too strong for you to control, your partner should pull the car over and stop. If possible, cover the back seat and car floor with a thick layer of newspapers or towels. You can then lie down and deliver the baby on the back seat into his hands.

Follow the procedure for the birth in the main text. Once the baby is born, it is essential that he is kept warm, so wrap him in a blanket or towel (or in your partner's shirt, jumper, or coat, if no other covering is available) and hold him close against your skin. If the placenta arrives before you reach hospital, wrap it up with the baby as this provides him with much needed extra warmth. Do not cut the umbilical cord.

Sudden birth

Sometimes labour progresses so quickly that the birth happens away from medical assistance, whether at home or on the way to hospital. If this happens, the following information will help you and your partner deliver your baby safely. This is not intended to be used as a guide for an out-of-hospital birth without a professional attendant being present, as this can be very risky indeed. However, it is reassuring that the majority of emergency births that happen at home rarely suffer any complications.

WHAT YOU SHOULD DO

As you get the urge to push, try to pant or blow for as long as you can in order to delay your baby's birth. However, the contractions alone are usually enough to expel the baby when he is coming this fast, so this will not delay things for long, although it may be long enough for your midwife or the ambulance to arrive. Never try to hold your legs together to delay delivery, or allow anyone else to do so, as it may result in your baby having brain damage. If you cannot comfortably delay your baby's birth, don't try to interfere. Deliver the head slowly. There is a greater chance that your vagina and perineum will tear if you push along with the force of your uterus, so pant lightly with each contraction.

Prolapsed cord If a loop of the umbilical cord washes out when the membranes rupture and your partner can see a piece of grey-blue shiny cord bulging out of your vagina, this means that you have a prolapsed cord and you must get help as soon as possible as your baby's oxygen supply is in danger of being cut off. Don't panic; you have time. Get on to the floor on your knees, with your chest to your knees, your head on the floor, and your buttocks in the air. This will help to take the pressure of the baby's head off your cervix. If the cord is still protruding, your partner should cover it with a wet, warm, very clean towel while he rings the hospital or goes for help. Do not touch or put any pressure on the cord and stay in the knee-chest position even on the way to hospital, because it reduces pressure on the cord. A prolapsed cord always necessitates a Caesarean delivery, unless the cervix is fully dilated, in which case forceps or ventouse will be used.

WHAT THE BIRTH ASSISTANT SHOULD DO

If it looks as if your baby will be born at home without medical assistance, you should telephone the hospital or your midwife if you haven't done so already. If you haven't got a telephone, on no account should you leave the mother alone. However anxious and overwhelmed you feel, you must stay calm and reassure your partner – she needs to feel confident and relaxed. Bear in mind that the vast majority of sudden births are entirely uncomplicated. Encourage your partner to take up any positions in which she feels comfortable (see p.278) and to eat and drink if she feels like it. Speak quietly and keep other people at bay. Between contractions turn up the heating in the room if at all possible. Wash your hands thoroughly in soap and water, and then fetch as many clean bath towels as you have and place them conveniently to hand. Fold one and put it on the floor so that you have something soft on which the baby can be laid.

Then fill several bowls with hand-warm water, and collect as many clean hand towels, face flannels, and tea-towels as you have, to be immersed in the water and used as wipes for the baby and mother during and after delivery.

The birth Your partner will know when the baby is coming because she'll feel a stinging or burning sensation as the baby stretches her vagina. Look to see if you can see the top of the baby's head in the vaginal outlet (known as crowning – see p.285). Remind your partner to pant or blow, so that her vagina and perineum have time to thin and stretch, which might help to avoid tearing.

The baby's head will probably be born in one contraction and the rest of his body in the contraction afterwards. When the head is born, wipe each of the baby's eyes from inside to outside with separate pieces of moist linen, and then feel round his neck to see if the cord is present. If it is, crook your little finger underneath it and pull it very gently over his head, or lift it so that his body can be born through the loop.

Do not interfere with the cord because it may go into a spasm and deprive your baby of oxygen. If the membranes are still present over the baby's face, gently tear them off with your fingernail so that your baby can breathe. Be careful to hold him firmly as he is born, as he will be slippery with blood, mucus, and *vernix caseosa*. Never pull on his head, his body, or his cord.

Once he is born, he will probably give a couple of gasps, a cry, and then start to cry properly. If he doesn't cry at once, place him across your partner's thigh or abdomen, with his head lower than his feet, and then gently rub his back. This helps any mucus to drain away and usually causes a change in blood pressure, which brings about his first breath. Talking to him lovingly also helps.

After the birth Once he is breathing, pass him to your partner so she can put him to her breast, and keep him warm against her skin. If he is interested in feeding, the nipple stimulation will release oxytocin, which will encourage your partner's uterus to contract and expel the placenta.

Keep your partner and the baby warm with blankets or towels, especially the baby's head, as most heat is lost from here. Bear in mind that the normal colour of a baby at birth is a bluish-white. He will gradually become pink in the first minutes as oxygen enters his body; his hands and feet will take somewhat longer. Do not try to wash off the vernix, and never cut the umbilical cord.

THE DELIVERY OF THE PLACENTA

If the placenta is born before an attendant arrives:

• never pull on the cord

• do not cut the cord

• after the placenta is born, massage the mother's uterus firmly, with a deep circular motion, gently pushing downwards 5–7cm (2–3in) below the navel and rubbing. This is important to make sure the uterus contracts and stays hard after the birth so that there is no haemorrhage

• it's normal for a couple of cups of blood to be delivered when the placenta comes out

• getting the baby to nurse immediately will help contract the uterus and minimize blood loss

• if your baby won't suck, get the mother to gently massage her nipples as a substitute way of releasing oxytocin into her system.

FORCEPS ASSISTED DELIVERY

Forceps look like large sugar tongs and are designed so that they will fit snugly over the sides of the baby's head, covering the ears. They're rather like a cage that protects the head from any pressure within the birth canal.

The decision to use forceps is a medical judgement on the part of your attendants. Forceps are only applied when the first stage is complete, the cervix is fully dilated, and the head is in the birth canal.

Why it is done Forceps are applied when the baby's head has descended into the mother's pelvis but fails to descend further; when the baby presents in a posterior position; in a breech delivery (see main text); when the uterus fails to maintain contractions; and when the mother lacks the strength to push. Occasionally, forceps may be used for a quick delivery early in the second stage if the baby shows signs of lacking oxygen, even if the birth is not imminent. Nowadays, most premature babies are delivered by forceps to protect their delicate skull bones from being compressed in the birth canal.

How it is done If you're going to have a forceps delivery, your legs will be put up in stirrups. A local anaesthetic will be injected into your perineum, and an episiotomy (see p.110) performed. Then the forceps will be inserted into your vagina one at a time. A few gentle pulls on the forceps, 30–40 seconds at a time, will bring your baby's head down on to your perineum. You should feel no pain. Once his head has been delivered, the forceps are removed and the rest of his body will be delivered as normal.

Complications at delivery

The usual course of delivery is set out on the previous pages. Certain factors, however, may complicate a delivery and special procedures may be required. Sometimes a delivery is special because the complicating factor may not have been anticipated and forceps or a vacuum extractor will have to be used. On the other hand, multiple and breech births are special but are usually diagnosed well in advance.

ASSISTED DELIVERY

Occasionally, labour and delivery do not proceed as smoothly as expected, so your obstetrician will require assistance to complete a vaginal delivery. Forceps (see column, left) can be used to protect the baby's head or, along with vacuum extraction, may be used to accelerate the baby's progress through the birth canal.

Vacuum extraction The vacuum extractor, or ventouse, is a gentler alternative to forceps, and is widely used throughout Europe. It consists of a metal plate or cone-shaped cup of synthetic material. This plate or cup is placed over the baby's scalp and, using an attached pump, a vacuum is created that makes the plate or cup adhere. This instrument then becomes a "handle" with which the obstetrician can both rotate the head and apply traction. Although it leaves a conspicuous bruise on the baby's head, it has many advantages (see column, right).

MULTIPLE DELIVERIES

The delivery of twins is always approached as if there were two single babies; if one has a vaginal delivery it does not follow that the other will. You will probably be advised to have the babies in hospital in case they are not presenting properly. However, the commonest way for twins to present at birth is for both to be head down. The second one usually arrives eight to ten minutes after the first. Your obstetrician may suggest an epidural anaesthetic (see p.281) as twin labours can be prolonged, or the second baby may have to be turned. This is done by rupturing the second baby's membrane and manually moving him.

Twin deliveries have become much safer in the last few years because the exact position of the second baby and its condition can be confirmed by ultrasound and fetal monitors. If there should be three or more babies, it is more likely that you will have a Caesarean section, although some doctors will deliver triplets vaginally if they have great experience in this procedure.

BREECH BIRTH

If your baby is in a breech position, and your obstetrician decides that he can be delivered safely without a Caesarean section, he will usually be born buttocks first. The breech birth should not be thought of as an abnormal birth – it is better to think of it as a variation of normal, because four out of every hundred babies are born in the breech position.

In a breech birth, the buttocks are usually delivered first, then the legs. Before the head is delivered, you will almost certainly have to have an episiotomy because the head is the widest part and your baby's rump will not have stretched your birth canal sufficiently for his head to pass through it unpressurized (see **Case Study**, p.302).

Once the baby's body is born, his weight pulls the head down to the vagina. His body is then lifted upwards and slightly backwards by the midwife, and one push is usually enough to deliver him. Forceps may be used to protect the baby's head. It is now fairly common practice for you to be given an epidural if you are having a breech birth. This is to prevent pushing against an incompletely dilated cervix, but also means that if you need a Caesarean section it can be done quickly and simply without further anaesthesia.

VACUUM EXTRACTOR

Because the device takes up less room in the vagina, and is easier to apply, it offers several advantages over forceps.

• It can be applied to the lowest part of the baby's head.

• The shape of the baby's head is unaffected. (Although it does result in an unsightly bruise, which will fade within a week or two of the birth).

• An episiotomy is not always necessary.

DELIVERING A BREECH BABY VAGINALLY

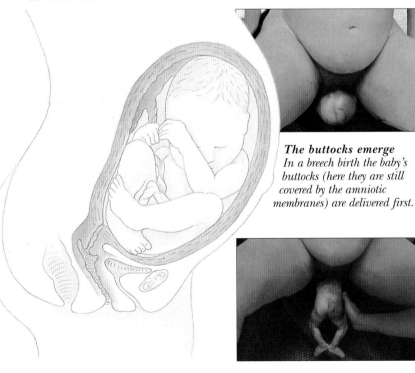

The buttocks emerge
In a breech birth the baby's buttocks (here they are still covered by the amniotic membranes) are delivered first.

Breech position
Before the labour begins, the baby's breech (buttocks) has not engaged within his mother's pelvis and her cervix is uneffaced.

Legs and body
Once the baby's buttocks are clear of the birth opening, the membranes rupture and the baby's legs and body are delivered.

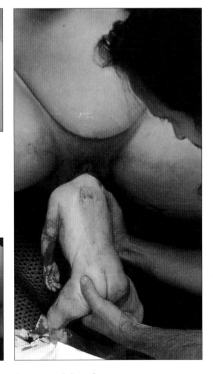

Arms and head
In the final stages of a breech delivery, the baby's arms emerge and then his body will be gently supported as the head is guided out.

A Caesarean operation usually takes 45–60 minutes, but the baby is delivered within the first 5–10 minutes; the rest of the time is spent stitching you up.

Preparation Before the operation begins, your pubic hair is shaved, you are given an epidural anaesthetic or spinal block, and an intravenous drip is set up to supply you with fluids during the operation. Then a catheter (a thin, flexible tube) is inserted up your urethra and into your bladder to drain it of urine. A small screen is placed in front of your face so you don't have to watch the operation. Your abdomen is swabbed to prevent any infection. If time is a factor, for instance, in the case of serious fetal distress, you may be given a general anaesthetic, even if you already had an epidural in place.

The operation The obstetrician makes a short, horizontal incision along the "bikini line" at the base of your abdomen, then makes a similar incision in the lower segment of your uterus. The amniotic fluid is drained off by suction, and the baby is gently lifted out. Then the cord is cut, the placenta is removed, and your uterus and abdomen are stitched.

Caesarean section

When a normal vaginal delivery is considered dangerous or even impossible, your baby will be delivered by Caesarean section – small horizontal incisions are made in your abdomen and uterus, and your baby is delivered through them. (The old-fashioned vertical cut is not used nowadays because of the risk of it retearing during a subsequent labour.) The percentage of babies delivered by Caesarean section has increased rapidly and is currently around 25 percent in the United Kingdom, of which two-thirds are emergency and one-third elective. This is partly because doctors are worried about being sued if a difficult birth causes complications that could have been avoided by Caesarean section, and partly because the operation is now so safe that it can be less risky than some other forms of delivery.

Very often, when a Caesarean section is necessary, the need for it will be apparent before labour begins, which means that you, your partner, and the obstetrician have time to discuss and plan for it. This type of planned Caesarean, known as elective, is in contrast to an emergency Caesarean, where its necessity may only become evident once labour is under way.

ELECTIVE CAESAREAN SECTION

The most common reasons for electing to have a Caesarean include the baby's head being too large to pass through your pelvis, the baby being in a breech position (see p.307) or lying across your pelvis; placenta praevia (see p.222); and certain medical conditions such as diabetes or active herpes type II infection. It may also be necessary if you have previously had a Caesarean. This was once thought essential, because it was feared that the scar of the previous Caesarean section would open up during labour. But experience has shown that this does not happen with the horizontal or "bikini" cut, and so hospitals often allow a vaginal delivery to begin and, if there are no problems, to proceed as normal – a "trial of labour".

Elective Caesareans are often carried out under an epidural anaesthetic (see p.281). This has several advantages over a general anaesthetic: it is safer for your baby; you have no post-operative nausea or vomiting; and because you are conscious, you can hold your baby as soon as he is born. In addition, it is usually possible for your partner to be with you during the operation, just as he could be if you were having a vaginal delivery.

When you have had a Caesarean, you may feel disappointed or even cheated that you did not have a vaginal delivery. Such feelings are perfectly natural, and the best thing you can do is talk about them with your partner. It will probably help if he can describe the birth to you in detail – this will help you to visualize and accept it.

It also helps, of course, to prepare yourself in advance for this type of birth. With your partner present, find out from the obstetrician what the operation entails, the procedures that will be used, and whether your partner is allowed to be present. Ask if you can see a video so you will know what is going to happen to you. If at all possible, talk to other women who have had Caesarean sections. They will provide useful information and valuable reassurance.

EMERGENCY CAESAREAN SECTION

This is often needed when something goes wrong during labour, such as a prolapsed umbilical cord, placental haemorrhage, fetal distress or serious failure to progress in labour. Emergency Caesarean sections may be carried out under epidural and the hospital may not allow your partner to be present at the operation.

AFTER A CAESAREAN SECTION

As is the case with any major surgery, it takes time to recover from a Caesarean, but even so you will be encouraged to get up and walk around a few hours afterwards to stimulate your circulation. You will be given painkillers if you need them, and the dressings will be removed after three or four days. Your internal stitches will be made with absorbable sutures, which will dissolve away naturally, and your external stitches will be removed within about a week.

CAESAREAN UNDER EPIDURAL ANAESTHETIC

THE EFFECTS ON YOUR BABY

Not having to pass through the birth canal is both a benefit and a drawback for the baby born by Caesarean section.

Unlike a baby born by vaginal delivery, who initially has a rather squashed appearance after being squeezed through the birth canal, a Caesarean baby has smooth features and a rounded head. But often the Caesarean baby needs more time to adjust to the outside world because of his sudden entry into it, and because he has missed the journey through the birth canal that helps to clear amniotic fluid from a baby's lungs and stimulates his circulation.

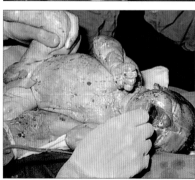

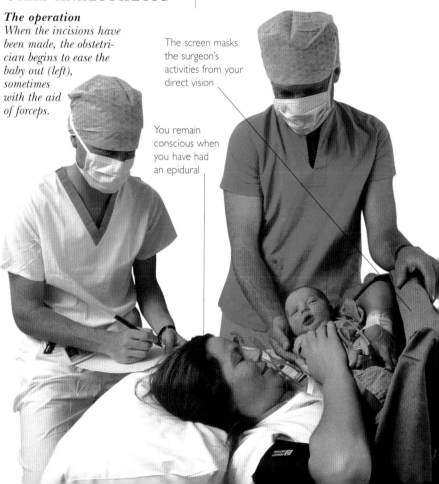

The operation
When the incisions have been made, the obstetrician begins to ease the baby out (left), sometimes with the aid of forceps.

The screen masks the surgeon's activities from your direct vision

You remain conscious when you have had an epidural

The delivery
Within 5–10 minutes of the incisions, the baby is delivered (above right) and the umbilical cord clamped and cut. As the placenta is delivered and the incisions stitched up, you can hold your baby.

An emergency Caesarean

About 25 percent of babies in the UK are born by Caesarean section. A Caesarean is either planned, known as an "elective" Caesarean, or one may need to be carried out as an emergency because it's essential to deliver the baby quickly. Fran was glad she'd taken the trouble to find out about Caesarean sections in advance.

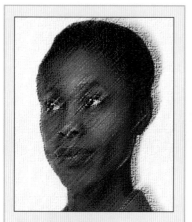

Name **Frances Ward**

Age **27 years**

Past medical history
Nothing abnormal

Obstetric history **One child aged three, pregnancy and delivery normal**

Fran's second pregnancy was uneventful. She and the baby were both doing well. Three days before her expected date of delivery, she went into labour which proceeded normally until the end of the first stage, when Fran was suddenly told she would have to have a Caesarean section.

WELL-INFORMED PARENTS

Fran had been surprised when I told her how frequently Caesarean sections are performed. Her antenatal classes did not cover the subject in any depth so she and her husband, Jonathan, decided to find out as much as possible about it for themselves. They like to be well-informed about anything they plan to do, whether it's visiting a foreign country or having a baby. They questioned clinic staff, read books, and watched videos on all types of birth, including Caesarean deliveries.

AN UNEXPECTED EMERGENCY

Fran's waters broke halfway through the first stage of labour, when her cervix was only four centimetres dilated. Following the rule that every mother must have an internal examination as soon as her membranes have ruptured, the midwife examined Fran at once. She discovered a prolapsed cord – a loop of the umbilical cord coming through the cervix into the vagina in advance of the baby. This is an extremely dangerous situation because as the baby's head presses down on the undilated cervix, the prolapsed section of the cord

is squeezed tighter and tighter, cutting off the baby's blood and oxygen supply.

The midwife touched the cord and could feel that it was pulsating. This was reassuring as it meant that the baby was still receiving an adequate blood supply. However, within the next couple of minutes the sonicaid picked up that the baby's heartbeat was starting to dip and was showing signs of considerable fetal distress. Fran's obstetrician told her it was essential for the baby that it be delivered by emergency Caesarean section.

AVOIDING DISASTER

While the operating theatre was prepared, Fran was asked to lie with her legs up in stirrups so that the baby would slip backwards, up into the pelvis, relieving the pressure on the cord. Meanwhile, the midwife inserted three fingers into Fran's vagina in order to keep the baby's head pushed up away from the cervix.

Fortunately Fran had elected to have an epidural anaesthetic early in labour, so she didn't need to have a general anaesthetic or intragastric suction to prevent inhalation of vomit. There was the added bonus that she would be alert during the whole procedure.

THE OPERATION

Fran had chosen her particular hospital because it encouraged fathers to participate in their baby's births. She was pleased that Jonathan was able to watch the operation, because it meant that, even if she couldn't see the baby being born, at least Jonathan would see their child's entrance into the world.

The surgeon made a standard transverse incision (see column, p.308) through which Fran's baby was gently lifted out. As soon as the baby's head was delivered, the anaesthetist gave Fran an injection of Syntometrine. This stimulates uterine contractions, making it easier for the placenta to separate from the uterine wall and follow the baby out through the incision.

While Fran was being sewn up, the baby was handed to Jonathan so that he could hold her before taking her for her mother to see for the first time. Although Fran was disappointed about not having a normal vaginal delivery, Fran and Jonathan had still shared the experience of Eleanor's birth and Fran had been able to hold and bond with Eleanor in the first few minutes after her birth.

After the operation, Fran returned to the postnatal ward with Eleanor where she could concentrate on feeding her and getting to know her better.

RECOVERING FROM THE CAESAREAN

Fran found getting back to normal was almost the hardest part. I suggested she could join a self-help group for post-Caesarean mothers, where she would get useful advice on how to handle the postnatal period. Fran also worried that her next baby would have to be delivered by Caesarean, too. I reassured her that most mothers have normal deliveries following Caesareans, although there may be clear-cut reasons for having another one.

Rest and healing

Fran had undergone abdominal surgery, so she needed plenty of rest and time for her scar to heal. When her stitches were removed, five days after the operation, she was told that the scar would heal in three weeks and would fade after six months. Fran was surprised to find herself losing blood from her vagina, just as she did after her first child, which was a vaginal delivery, but I reassured her that this is quite normal.

Breastfeeding

I told Fran that if she was going to breastfeed sitting up, it was important for her to sit up straight. Her abdominal wall was tender so she used pillows to prop up Eleanor level with her breasts. She also found it comfortable to breastfeed lying on her side, resting on one elbow, with Eleanor on a pillow next to her.

Moving about

Fran found standing up quite difficult because her stomach hurt, but I advised her to try and stand up perfectly straight as soon as she got out of bed, and to place her hands over her wound, supporting it, whenever she wanted to laugh or cough. I told her that the more she managed to move around, the speedier her recovery would be. After her stitches were removed, she was allowed home but was advised to rest and to be very careful when lifting anything, including picking up her other child for cuddles or carrying any shopping. She also had to refrain from strenuous exercise and driving for at least six weeks.

FRAN'S BABY

Her birth was very different from that of a baby who is pushed down the birth canal.

- Once the incision was made, the surgeon slipped a hand under her head and applied forceps

- Her head was gently pulled out with the forceps

- Her shoulders were manoeuvred carefully through the incision

- Her body was gently pulled out – she was now delivered

- She was held with her head downwards while her mouth and pharynx were cleansed of fluid with a soft catheter attached to suction apparatus

- She took her first breath

- Her cord was clamped and cut

- She was checked to make sure that all her systems were functioning properly (see Apgar Score, p.292)

- As soon as she was breathing normally, she was handed to her father for a cuddle

**The death of a baby will be as
painful for the father as it is for
you. However, he may express his
grief very differently, and this can
lead to tension in the relationship.**

If a father grieves in a different
way to his partner, it does not
mean his grief is any less intense.
Some men feel they should hide
their grief and throw themselves
into work in order to find some
relief from the pain they are
feeling. Fortunately, all of us are
learning that it is more healthy
to express feelings than to
suppress them, and men should
be encouraged to let their true
feelings show, especially to their
partners.

Support groups for bereaved
parents can put fathers in contact
with other men who have lost their
babies. By being with such other
men, a father may learn to express
his grief, anger, and all the other
possible emotions he may feel, in
whatever way is appropriate. What
is essential is that he is able to
express his grief in his own way.

If a baby dies

**The death of any child is always a tragic event, but the death
of a baby before, during, or very soon after birth can be
especially distressing. Today, the number of babies who are
stillborn after 24 weeks or who die within the first few weeks
of life has fallen to about one percent in the Western world,
largely owing to improved obstetric and paediatric care.**

WHY BABIES DIE

Perinatal deaths can be divided into three main groups: stillbirths
– babies who die before labour begins; intrapartum deaths –
babies who die during labour; and neonatal deaths – babies who
die within four weeks of their births.

Stillbirth Approximately 45 percent of perinatal deaths are
stillbirths, and in about a third of these cases the precise cause is
not known. Of the rest, the most important causes are severe fetal
defects (see also p.196) and a placenta that is not entirely healthy.
It could be that the placenta failed to develop adequately, became
diseased in some way, or became unable to continue to support the
baby (see p.260). Whatever the cause, the placenta was unable to
provide adequate nutrition for the baby. It might even have begun
to separate from the wall of the uterus before labour started. Other
less common causes of stillbirth include Rhesus incompatibility
(see p.202), and maternal diabetes that is not carefully controlled.

The first thing that happens when a baby dies in the uterus is
the almost complete disappearance from your blood of
pregnancy hormones, oestrogen and progesterone. As a result,
many of the signs and sensations of being pregnant fade quite
quickly. One of the first indications may be lack of fetal
movement, and the uterus may diminish in size due to absorption
of the amniotic fluid. This could result in very rapid weight loss,
which is why loss of weight or a lack of weight gain is taken very
seriously indeed throughout your pregnancy. If your doctors or
midwives suspect that your baby has died, an ultrasound scan will
be done in order to detect your baby's heartbeat.

Labour usually starts within two to three days of a baby's death,
although many women want to have their babies removed as soon
as they find out that they have died. If you find yourself in this
unhappy situation your wishes should be respected; usually
induction of labour will be offered.

When you go into labour, there will be no physical difference
between this labour and a normal one. You will require a great
deal of sympathy and support, and will be offered as much pain
relief as you want. Everybody involved will recognize that your
attitude to this labour will be severely affected by the fact that you
are not giving birth to a live baby.

Intrapartum death This is exceptionally rare but the death of a baby during labour is usually due to a lack of oxygen as happens in arrested labour. Another possible cause is injury to the baby during labour and delivery, although this is far less common than it was in the past, thanks to high levels of modern obstetric care.

Neonatal death Death of the newborn is often due to breathing difficulties, especially in babies born preterm (see pp.344 & 348), who are post-mature, or who are suffering from severe fetal defects. Fatal neonatal infections, once a significant cause of the deaths of newborn babies, are now very rare because of improved hygiene standards and modern antibiotics.

COPING WITH A DEATH

It is very important for both partners to come to terms with their grief, to be open about the death of their baby, to accept it, and to go through the grieving process.

It is common for bereaved parents to feel isolated, angry with themselves, each other, the staff, or the unfairness of life, and often guilty about something they did or didn't do. These emotions are absolutely normal. However, accepting that everyone involved did everything possible and that nobody is to blame, while acknowledging how you feel, will help to speed the healing process.

Having a photograph of the baby can also help, and holding him after he is born is often a consolation. It is also a good idea to give the baby a name, to bury the baby formally, and to be present at the burial. Another important form of solace is to get in touch with other parents who have had stillbirths (see **Addresses**, p.370). Details of support groups are usually available from your hospital. Don't be afraid to ask for help from a counsellor if you need it.

Emotional effects The emotional and physical effects on the mother are due not only to the shock and grief of losing her baby but also to the sudden withdrawal of pregnancy hormones. This can affect her mood, bringing on tearfulness, depression, insomnia, appetite loss, and withdrawal. The comfort and generosity of her partner, family, and friends will be vital.

It is also important that both partners try to be open with each other and share their grief so that they can offer each other support and comfort. In addition, the hospital should be able to provide a counselling service for both parents.

GETTING PREGNANT AGAIN

Grief over the death of a baby should have subsided before another pregnancy is contemplated. This usually takes at least six months and sometimes a year or more. Many women, however, find the key to normality and a return to happiness is through conceiving again. Once partners have decided to try for another baby, they may find that worry about losing this baby will be hard to shake off. However, the risk of a recurrence is very slight. Where a predisposing cause is determined, subsequent pregnancies are carefully managed.

LOSING A TWIN

The death of a twin or triplet is just as tragic to the parents as the death of a singleton, and carries additional problems.

The loss of a twin or triplet results in a complex emotional situation of the parents having to mourn the death of the lost baby, while celebrating the life of the surviving twin or triplet(s). Faced with this impossible combination of emotions, many parents postpone their mourning, although some find they cannot attend to the needs of their living baby or babies properly because of the intensity of grief for the dead baby.

The loss of a twin or triplet may also cast a shadow over the life of the surviving twin or triplet(s), and birthdays may be particularly difficult for the first few years.

It must be stressed that a mother who's had a multiple pregnancy continues to think of herself as the mother of twins or triplets, regardless of whether any have died.

Parents who have lost a twin or a triplet may be told that they are "lucky" because they've still got their other child(ren) – no other parent is expected to find comfort from the death of a child in the survival of its siblings.

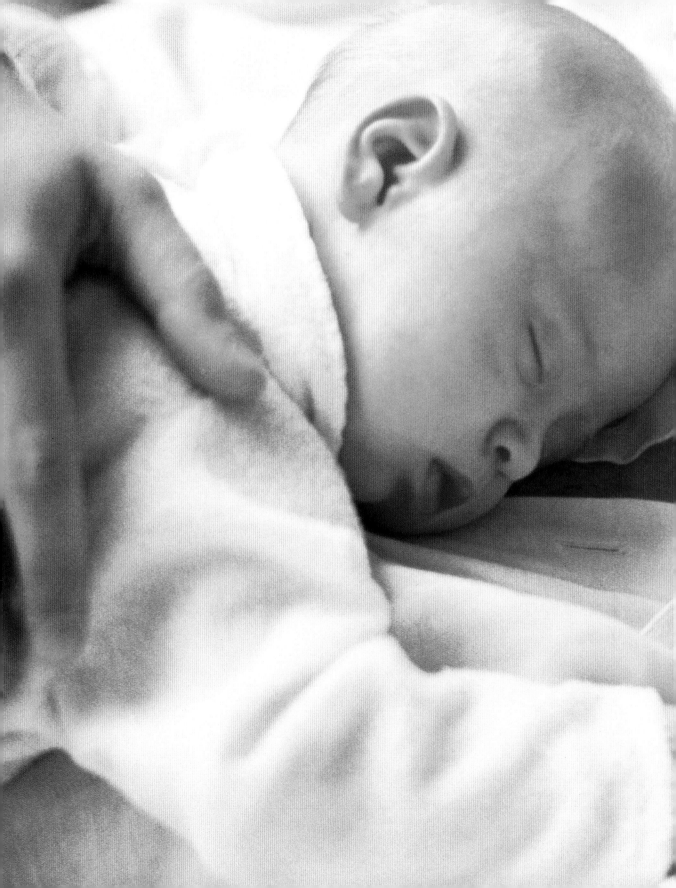

CHAPTER 15

Getting to know your
NEWBORN
BABY

Nurturing a relationship with your baby begins the second she is born. As you both learn how to care for her and meet her needs, your relationship will deepen and grow, and what she can do will amaze you.

YOUR FIRST REACTION

Your newborn baby's appearance may startle you at first glance. With his wrinkly skin you may think he looks more like an old man than a baby.

A few parents are worried about their feelings when their baby actually arrives: he doesn't seem to be quite what they'd expected.

Unless you've had a Caesarean, his head may be slightly squashed with some bruising; his eyelids may be puffy, because of the pressure of passing through the birth canal.

He may seem quite messy as he will be coated in a greasy substance (see right), possibly mixed with some of your blood, and have patches of body hair. His limbs may also have a slightly bluish tint, and his genitals will seem huge.

Don't be disappointed if his initial appearance doesn't immediately or automatically inspire feelings of love and tenderness. These will develop as you get to know each other.

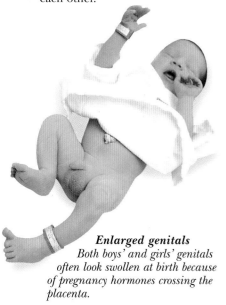

Enlarged genitals
Both boys' and girls' genitals often look swollen at birth because of pregnancy hormones crossing the placenta.

Your new baby

Hold your baby soon after birth so that you can establish strong emotional bonding. Your baby will start to learn about you, and how much you love him, by hearing your voice, smelling and feeling your skin, and being cuddled and suckled.

A newborn baby's tiny, vulnerable body and complete dependence on you will arouse many new emotions. Your initial responses and behaviour are probably the most important interactions that will ever occur between you and your child.

Research has shown that parents who are given unrestricted contact with their babies immediately after delivery later tend to be more sympathetic to their children's needs than are parents whose babies are taken away at birth. A lack of initial contact can make some mothers feel alienated from their new babies, and so less attentive.

WHAT YOUR BABY LOOKS LIKE

There are huge variations in what is considered normal for the weight and length of a newborn baby. Average weights are between 2.5–4.5 kilograms (5lb 8oz to 9lb 12oz), and average lengths vary from 48–51 centimetres (19–20 inches).

Head This is still large in comparison with the rest of his body – it is one-quarter of your baby's length. The younger a baby is, the larger his head is in proportion to his body. The average circumference of a newborn baby's head is about 35cm (14in). Measuring head circumference is regarded as a vital part of examining a baby because the growth of the head reflects the development of the brain.

The head usually has a pointed shape because it has been moulded as it came through the birth canal. Moulding is caused by the skull bones overriding each other. Sometimes this pressure also causes swelling on one or both sides of the baby's head. This swelling leaves the brain unaffected and it subsides within a few weeks.

There may be slight bruising if your baby was delivered by forceps. You will feel a soft spot on the top, called a fontanelle, where the skull bones have not yet joined together and won't until your baby is 18 months.

Skin Some babies are born completely covered in a greasy, white substance called *vernix caseosa*, others only on their face and hands. Vernix eases the baby's delivery and offers protection against minor skin infections. In some hospitals it is cleaned off immediately, whereas in others it is left to be naturally rubbed off the skin, which happens within two or three days.

Your baby's circulation takes some time to stabilize. This may cause the top half of his body to look paler than the bottom half. There is nothing to worry about.

You may notice downy hair on your baby's body, which is known as lanugo hair; it covered your baby's body while he was in your uterus (see p.80). Some babies only have it on the head, while on others it covers the shoulders. Both are quite normal and the lanugo hair usually rubs off within a couple of weeks. More permanent hair will appear later. Some babies are born with a full head of hair; others are completeley bald. However, the hair on your baby's head when he's born may not be the colour he eventually ends up with.

Newborn characteristics

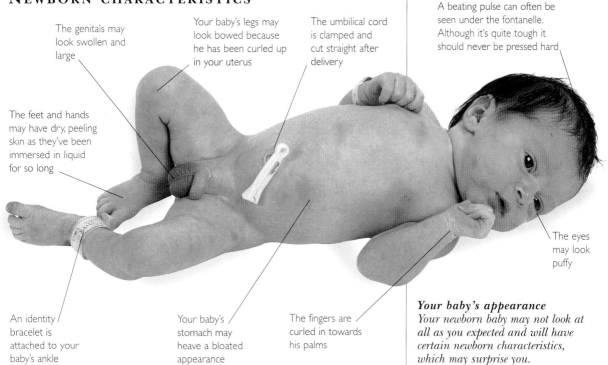

The genitals may look swollen and large

Your baby's legs may look bowed because he has been curled up in your uterus

The umbilical cord is clamped and cut straight after delivery

A beating pulse can often be seen under the fontanelle. Although it's quite tough it should never be pressed hard

The feet and hands may have dry, peeling skin as they've been immersed in liquid for so long

The eyes may look puffy

An identity bracelet is attached to your baby's ankle

Your baby's stomach may heave a bloated appearance

The fingers are curled in towards his palms

Your baby's appearance
Your newborn baby may not look at all as you expected and will have certain newborn characteristics, which may surprise you.

Hands and feet   These are always slightly more bluish than the rest of his body because of his primitive circulation. There may be dry patches with peeling skin, which will disappear in a few days. His fingernails may be long and sharp; you can gently nibble off the tips if he's getting scratched, but don't cut them.

Eyes   Your newborn baby may not be able to open his eyes straight away due to puffiness caused by pressure on his head during the birth. This pressure may also have broken some tiny blood vessels in his eyes, causing harmless small, red, triangular marks in the whites that need no treatment and will disappear within a couple of weeks. He may have a condition called "sticky

YOUR BABY'S BIRTHMARKS

A group of small blood vessels under the surface of the skin may appear as a small blemish on your baby's body, but won't usually need any treatment.

Stork bites These are mild pink patches; they are very common and usually appear on the nose, eyelids, and neck under the hair-line. They take about a year to disappear.

Strawberry birthmarks These first appear as tiny red dots and may increase in size up to the end of the first year. They almost always disappear by 5 years of age.

Mongolian spots These are blue and are found on the lower backs of babies with dark skin tones (nearly all black and Asian babies, and some Mediterranean babies, have them). The spots look like bruises, but they are harmless and fade away naturally.

Port wine stains These are large, flat red or purple marks on the baby's skin. They are often found on the face and neck. These marks are permanent, so if you are worried consult your doctor.

eye" – a yellow discharge around the eyelids. This condition is quite common, and although it is not serious it should always be treated by a doctor.

Your baby may squint or look cross-eyed because although he can see clearly to a distance of 20cm (8in) or so, he cannot focus both eyes at the same time beyond that. These conditions should gradually clear up as his eye muscles grow stronger (usually within a month); you should consult a doctor if he still squints at three months. If he is reluctant to open his eyes at first you should never try to force them open. Try holding his head above your head so that he opens them naturally. All babies are born with blue eyes, and their adult eye colour may not develop until about six months.

Umbilicus The umbilical cord is clamped with forceps and then cut with scissors. A short length of cord remains, which will dry up and become almost black within two to four hours after the birth. The cord doesn't separate from the navel until about ten days after the birth. Some babies have umbilical hernias (small swellings near the navel) but these usually clear up within a year. If the hernia persists or enlarges consult your doctor.

Breasts In both boy and girl babies, the breasts may be slightly enlarged and leak a little milk, owing to pregnancy hormones. This is quite normal, and will subside in a couple of days.

YOUR BABY'S CARE

Whether you leave hospital after 12 hours or a few days, your baby will have been thoroughly examined by a paediatrician to make sure that everything is going well and that there are no problems. Your doctor or midwife will also want to check that your baby is feeding well and that her stools are normal. She will be given a blood test, usually by means of a tiny heel prick, to check for phenylketonuria (PKU), a rare metabolic disease, and for thyroid gland underactivity.

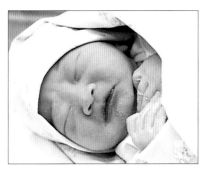

Puffy eyelids
Your baby's eyelids may be quite puffy because of the constriction of the birth canal, but this swelling will subside in a couple of days.

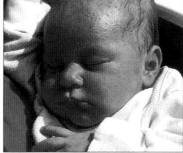

Spotty skin
Small white spots, called milia, are caused by blocked sebaceous glands that lubricate the skin. They will soon disappear.

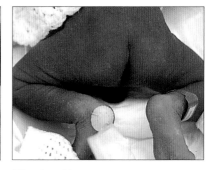

Blotchy skin tone
His circulation hasn't yet stabilized. You may see red and white blotches on his body, and his legs may be a different colour.

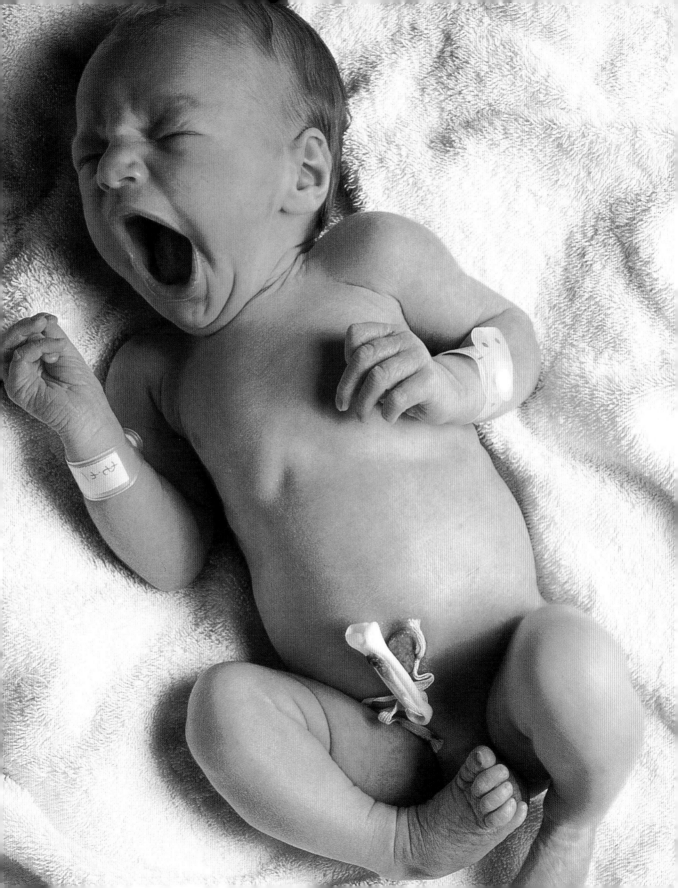

Make time to play with your baby as much as you can; this is vital to her development.

Try to recognize her needs She will have many expressions that you will soon find easy to interpret. When she's content she will appear tranquil and quiet, and she'll look rather red and flustered when she's feeling miserable or uncomfortable.

Playing together Don't be self-conscious; when cuddling her, pull silly faces and use funny, high-pitched tones telling her how much you love her. She will respond by nodding, moving her mouth, maybe sticking out her tongue, and jerking her body.

What your baby can do

Your newborn baby has her own distinctive personality and may surprise you with her behaviour. Spend as much time as you can studying her, and you will discover, and grow to understand, her unique expressions and responses.

POSTURE AND SENSES

Your baby's head is too heavy for her back and neck muscles to support, so all her postures when not lying down are governed by her gradual ability to control her head. If your baby is placed on her back, she will probably turn her head to one side, extend the arm on that side, and flex the opposite arm in towards her chest. By the time she is a week old, she will raise her head in small jerks when supported on your shoulder, and at six weeks she will probably be able to hold up her head for more than a minute.

At birth, her senses of sound, smell, and taste are fairly acute. She will soon recognize you by smell, and within two weeks by sight. At first, her mouth is her main instrument for touching. When you hold your baby close to you for the first time, she will focus on your face, and look into your eyes. Babies like looking at faces more than anything else. Hearing high-pitched human voices gives her great pleasure, and she will prefer yours, and your partner's deeper one, to all others. She'll also respond to sounds with a change in her breathing, and be startled by loud noises.

REFLEX ACTIONS

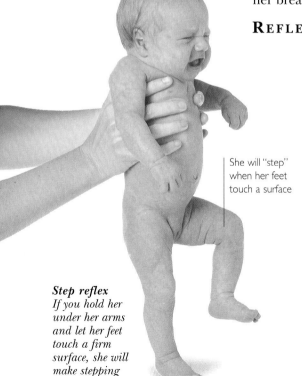

She will "step" when her feet touch a surface

Step reflex
If you hold her under her arms and let her feet touch a firm surface, she will make stepping movements.

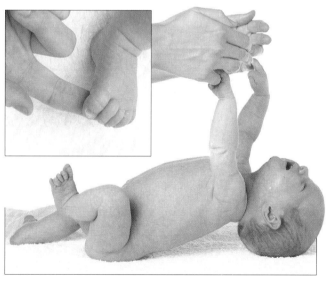

Grasp reflex
Your baby's fingers will tightly grasp anything that is placed in her palm. The grasp is so strong that her whole body *weight can be supported if she grabs your fingers with both of her hands. The soles of her feet will also curl over if they are touched or tickled.*

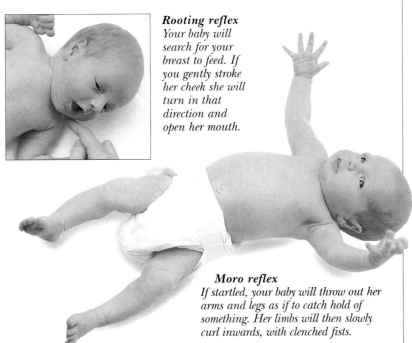

Rooting reflex
Your baby will search for your breast to feed. If you gently stroke her cheek she will turn in that direction and open her mouth.

Moro reflex
If startled, your baby will throw out her arms and legs as if to catch hold of something. Her limbs will then slowly curl inwards, with clenched fists.

All babies use certain reflexive movements to protect themselves. They usually last until about three months after which time your baby will lose them. Your baby will close her eyes reflexively if you touch her eyelids. All babies have a sucking reflex when pressure is put on the palate in the baby's mouth. The sucking is more like chomping, is very strong, and lasts for some time. The swallowing reflex is inherent in all babies at birth as they will have used it when swallowing fluids in the uterus. This enables them to swallow colostrum or milk the instant they are born. If she swallows too much liquid, her gagging reflex will immediately occur in order to clear her breathing passages.

WHY YOUR BABY CRIES

Crying is her only way of signalling to you. You'll soon learn to recognize all the different kinds of cries, and how to respond to them.

• Your baby's first cry may sound more like a whimper, or splutter, before escalating to a full blown cry. Before bellowing forth, she will take a deep breath, her body will tense, her face will grimace and become bright red, and she will open her mouth wide and literally scream. Distressing as this is, it shows that she is perfectly healthy.

• She will cry when she's hungry, and usually won't stop until she's put to your nipple or given a bottle. Some babies will cry sooner than others when hungry.

• Tiredness, uncomfortable clothing, being too hot or too cold, or being undressed are all reasons why she may cry.

• One of the main causes for distress is loneliness. Babies thrive on physical contact; if they feel abandoned they will cry until picked up and cuddled.

SOUNDS YOUR BABY WILL MAKE

BREATHING

Your baby's breathing will seem very light in comparison to your own. At times it may be fast and noisy or irregular. She may snuffle trying to draw air through her small nasal passages. Don't be alarmed if at first you cannot detect her breathing; it will get stronger every day.

SNEEZES

Your baby's sensitivity to bright lights makes her sneeze because light stimulates the nerves to her nose as well as her eyes. A sneeze will clear out her nasal passages, preventing dust getting into her lungs. Sneezing is quite common – it doesn't mean she has a cold.

HICCUPS

Your baby will often hiccup and this is perfectly normal. Hiccups are often caused by sudden, irregular contractions of the diaphragm, and are a sign that the muscles involved in breathing are getting stronger, and are also trying to work in harmony.

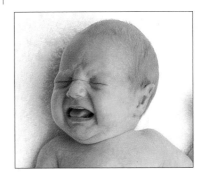

A cry for attention
Sudden movements, very bright lights, loud noises, or feeling too hot or too cold may all make your baby start to cry.

GOING HOME

Make sure the hospital is informed of how long you intend to stay. The routine for checking out will vary from hospital to hospital. Some women leave quite soon after the birth, others are in for over a week. The normal stay is usually between one and three days. Before you are discharged:

• a midwife or doctor will examine you and this will include checking to see that your uterus is returning to its pre-pregnant size, that your stitches (if any) are healing, and that your breasts are okay. The flow of lochia will be checked for colour and amount, and to see if you have passed any clots. Clotting accompanied by persistent bleeding may indicate that some placental tissue has been retained

• if you have had a Caesarean, your incision will be checked and non-absorbable sutures removed

• you will be asked about your contraception plans, and given a prescription for the pill if necessary

• if you weren't immune to rubella (German measles) during your pregnancy, you will be immunized

• a nurse or a midwife will show you how to clean your baby's umbilical cord

• you will be given a date for your postnatal check-up, and advised to take your baby to the clinic for a 6-week check-up

• when you leave, dress your baby warmly as she will not be efficient at regulating her temperature. You will need some loose clothing, as your breasts will enlarge when your milk comes in and your stomach will not return to its pre-pregnancy flatness until some months after the birth.

Your stay in hospital

Your hospital care routine will vary, depending on whether you had a vaginal or Caesarean delivery (see p.306), which hospital you are in, how long you stay for, and the condition of both you and your newborn baby.

YOUR CARE

Immediately after delivery, your temperature will be taken, and your pulse rate and blood pressure recorded. They will continue to be recorded every four hours for the first day or so, then twice daily during the rest of your stay in hospital, or your first week to ten days at home. There may be slight shifts in your pulse rate but these are normal, so there is no need for you to worry.

Medical staff will also check that any stitches or tears are healing properly and that there is no infection. They may also advise you about applying ice packs to the area to prevent swelling and ease pain, and may prescribe painkillers during the first few days for afterpains.

The amount and appearance of lochia will be regularly monitored by staff. They will want to make sure that there are no abnormal blood clots or excessive bleeding. The condition of your uterus and cervix will be checked to ensure that they are starting to return to their pre-pregnant condition. Your doctor will also examine your legs for signs of thrombosis and check your general emotional state.

Regaining mobility New mothers should move about as much as possible soon after delivery. Early mobility will help you regain your strength more quickly and facilitates bowel and bladder function (see also p.354).

Unless you're very tired and simply want to sleep you can get up to go to the toilet, shower, or walk about any time after the birth. It is wise to ask for assistance initially, as you could feel a little faint or weak. Blood tests are often routinely taken on about the fourth or fifth day after delivery to ensure that your haemoglobin is returning to normal.

Caesarean births About 20 percent of women have Caesarean births in Britain and, if you have had a general anaesthetic, you will probably feel sick and wobbly. The incision will be painful and the stitches will be covered by a soft dressing. You will probably have an intravenous drip in your arm and will be given analgesics to help you sleep. If your baby is in good condition there is no reason why she can't be with you all the time.

If your stitches are not self-absorbing, they will be removed about five days after delivery. This will cause you only mild discomfort. After a Caesarean, you will usually stay in hospital for about five days if everything is normal (see also pp.306 & 308).

HOSPITAL PROCEDURES

Hospital routines can be a little annoying especially if you're woken for meals or routine checks by the midwives when you'd rather be asleep. However, where breastfeeding is concerned, think about your own and your baby's needs above all else. Make sure that you give yourself sufficient time to feed your baby and ask for help if you're finding it difficult. Start slowly with only short periods of two to three minutes on each breast so that the nipples have a chance to harden up, which will prevent soreness and cracking. Your baby may not seem very interested initially – he may be tired too, but after the first day, try to put him to the breast whenever he seems to want it.

Maintaining good nutrition and replenishing your reserves for breastfeeding is important. Hospital food can sometimes be bland and unappetizing, as well as being rather nutritionally inadequate, and on top of this the helpings can be pretty meagre. It's a good idea to have special packages brought in by your visitors, or ask a friend to visit you around mealtime and bring in the food of your choice.

Visitors Welcome though they undoubtedly will be, bear in mind that visitors will tire you out more than you will imagine, so try to limit each visit to a maximum of half an hour. You should try to get everyone except your partner and your other children to stick to visiting times. Generally speaking, partners are allowed unlimited access; however, this policy does vary from hospital to hospital.

Social contact There is quite a lot to enjoy while you are in hospital. You will have the company of other mothers and can share your experiences, observations, and worries with them. A pleasant social life often develops between mothers with new babies. In sharing your learning experiences and working out plans together, you may find that you form friendships that will last well after your confinement ends.

Feeling unhappy If you find that ward life doesn't suit you and you are unhappy in hospital, you could ask for an early discharge. Many busy maternity units are happy for mothers and babies to go home just six hours after the birth if all is well, and your stay is unlikely to be more than 48 hours long. However, even this can seem a long time if you're feeling homesick and anxious. You could try confiding in one of the midwives on the hospital staff or in another more experienced mother, and remember that you, your baby, and your partner will all be home together as a family very soon.

REGISTERING YOUR BABY'S BIRTH

By law, every birth must be notified to the Registrar within six weeks in England, Wales, and Northern Ireland, and within three weeks in Scotland.

The hospital will be able to give you the address of their nearest local registry office (which may not be near where you live). The Registrar will ask the name and place of birth, and the father's occupation. If partners are unmarried, both need to be present in order for both parents' names to appear on the baby's birth certificate.

In Scotland and Northern Ireland, the mother's maiden name will also be needed, and in Scotland, the date and place of the marriage as well, if applicable.

A short form birth certificate, stating the child's name and sex, and the date and place of birth, will be issued free. A full certificate can be obtained later for a small fee. You will need the birth certificate for claiming benefits for your baby.

Do register your baby as soon as you can because child benefit is only paid from the date of registration, not the date of birth.

The Registrar will also give you a form with your baby's National Health Service number on it. You need this form to register your baby with your doctor. Fill it in and take it to your GP's surgery.

BENEFITS FOR YOU

From the moment your baby is born you can develop a special feeling of intimacy by holding him close to your bare skin.

Skin-to-skin contact enables you to become intimate with your baby. You will enjoy "skin bathing" with your baby – the feel of his soft, warm skin against yours, and the wonderful smell of newborn baby.

When you are feeding, whether by breast or bottle, don't let a barrier of clothing always come between you. You will both benefit from him being held close against your bare skin (see column, right) – not least because he will begin to recognize your smell (an important step in the bonding process, especially if you are not breastfeeding).

Holding and handling

A newborn baby can appear very fragile and, at first, many parents are quite scared to pick up and handle their baby because of the feeling that he is so breakable. However, your baby is actually very resilient and, as long as you support him firmly, there's no need to be afraid.

FIRM SUPPORT

Even if he's crying to be picked up, don't use jerky or quick movements when lifting him – do it as slowly, as gently, and as quietly as you can. Most babies like to be handled in a firm way; it makes them feel more secure. He won't be able to support his head for several weeks so you will have to support it so that it doesn't loll. Always hold your baby close, keeping your arms close to your body, and bending over the place you are lifting from or putting down. You will gain confidence very quickly.

To put him down, just reverse the process of picking him up, always making sure to support his neck. When you lay your baby down, it's safest to put him on his back, or his side, if propped.

PICKING UP YOUR BABY

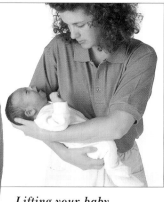

Lifting your baby
Slide one hand underneath his neck and head, and slide the other behind his lower back (left). Lift him gently so that his head doesn't fall back. Remember to support his head in the crook of your arm (above) so that it does not loll around.

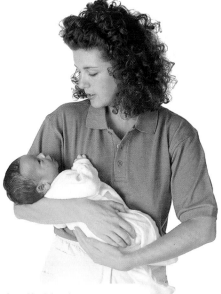

Cradle him in your arms
Your baby will feel secure cradled in the crook of your elbow, his head and limbs well supported.

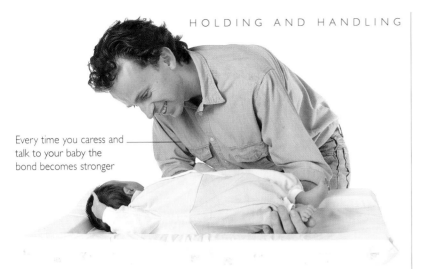

Every time you caress and talk to your baby the bond becomes stronger

BENEFITS FOR YOUR BABY

Recent research has shown that the more physical contact babies have, the healthier and happier they become.

You can appeal to your baby's sense of rhythm by rocking and swaying him. Skin-to-skin contact stimulates his senses of touch and smell, and even helps him to grow. Human skin sends and receives warmth that has a positive effect on other human skins. Snuggling together will evoke a feeling of sensuous contentment.

Loving support A mother often feels prime responsibility for her newborn baby, but most partners are keen to be fully involved as early as possible. Both your baby and his father will develop a better understanding of each other through cuddling, handling, and carrying, and the more tactile their relationship, the more loving it will be.

All through the day, especially when changing him, you can discover ways to gently explore and caress his body. The best way to cuddle together is by lying naked in bed. In this way he can smell your skin, feel its touch and warmth, and hear your heart beating clearly.

Your baby will be comforted by the familiar beat of your heart

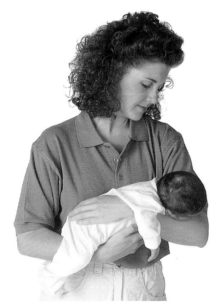

Hold him face down
Your baby may like being held face down in your arms, his cheek resting on your forearm.

Hold him against your shoulder
Held upright like this, your baby feels secure. Take his weight with a hand under his bottom, and support his head with the other hand.

PRODUCING MILK

The changes to your breasts during pregnancy prepare them for the production of milk, which begins a few days after you have given birth.

Each female breast contains 15–20 groups of milk-secreting glands, connected to the nipple by the milk ducts. During pregnancy, the placenta and ovaries secrete high levels of the hormones oestrogen and progesterone, which stimulate the glands to produce colostrum. Colostrum provides your baby with water, protein, sugar, vitamins, minerals, and antibodies to protect him against infection. The production of colostrum ceases, and that of milk begins, about 3–5 days after the baby is born.

Stimulating milk
Your baby's sucking stimulates nerve endings in the areolae, which send messages to the brain to produce prolactin and oxytocin.

Pituitary gland

Hypothalamus

Beginning to breastfeed

Pregnant women who are planning to breastfeed for the first time often worry that they will not produce enough milk, or that their milk will not be sufficiently nourishing. These understandable fears are usually groundless. Bear in mind that every woman is equipped to feed her baby. No breast is too small and, in most cases, supply will automatically meet demand.

FEEDING ON DEMAND

A baby can digest a full feed of breast milk in about an hour and a half to two hours (half the time it takes for a bottlefed baby to digest a full feed of infant formula). Breastfeeding on demand thus means frequent feeding, but this will not deplete your milk resources – research has shown that mothers who breastfeed their babies on demand produce more milk than those who feed their babies at regular but less frequent intervals.

One study compared babies breastfed on demand with those fed only every three or four hours. The babies fed on demand got an average of nearly ten feeds a day, compared to an average for the others of just over seven. However, the more frequent feeding didn't mean that a daily amount of milk was being divided into more but smaller feeds – the opposite, in fact.

Better fed The fed-on-demand babies got an average of just over 73 millilitres per feed (725 millilitres per day), while those fed at fixed intervals got only 68.8 millilitres per feed (502 millilitres per day). As a result, after two weeks the fed-on-demand babies had gained more weight than the others, an average of 561 grams compared to 347 grams.

MAINTAINING YOUR MILK SUPPLY

Milk production is quite a complex affair and many factors can affect it, including your emotions, health, and diet.

Producing milk The change from colostrum to breast milk is initially triggered by hormonal changes after the birth, but the continuation of milk production depends on the sucking action of the baby. When he sucks, this stimulates nerve endings in the areolae, and these nerve signals go to a part of the brain called the hypothalamus. When the hypothalamus receives these signals, it in turn sends out signals to the pituitary gland instructing it to release a hormone, prolactin, that stimulates milk production.

Consequently, this response to the baby's sucking is known as the prolactin reflex. The pituitary gland also releases oxytocin, a hormone that causes the muscle fibres around the milk glands to contract, squeezing the milk from the glands into the milk ducts. This is called the milk ejection or "let down" reflex and, when your breasts are full, it can be triggered not only by sucking but also by your baby's hunger cries or even simply his proximity to you.

A good milk supply The most important factor in maintaining your milk supply is frequent feeding, so that the prolactin reflex and the milk ejection reflex are initiated frequently and engorgement (swelling of the milk-producing glands by milk) is prevented.

If the glands do swell, they are unable to make milk efficiently. At the same time, you will tend to avoid feeding because it is painful, and for these reasons the reflex that promotes the release of prolactin diminishes and so milk production slows down. You can relieve the engorgement by expressing milk (see column, right), and prevent recurrence by regular and frequent feeding.

As well as regular feeding, at each feed wait until your baby empties the first breast before switching him to the other. This will ensure that he gets not only the thirst-quenching, low-fat foremilk that is delivered from the breast first, but also the highly nourishing, fat-rich hindmilk that follows.

It is important to eat a nutritious diet at this time, as your body will be under even more nutritional stress than during pregnancy. You don't need any special foods for breastfeeding, but try to maintain a balanced diet with plenty of protein, iron, and calcium, and lots of fluids, fresh fruit, and vegetables. Three good meals, with light snacks of fruit, cheese, or milky drinks in between, will keep your energy levels high and help you avoid fatigue. It is a good idea to keep taking an iron supplement daily. Taking care of an infant can be exhausting, so you should also take every opportunity to rest, or sleep, during the day. If you are diabetic, your doctor will carefully monitor your diet, and your glucose and insulin levels. When you resume lovemaking, don't use oral contraceptives until you stop breastfeeding (see p.364).

REFUSAL TO FEED

Occasionally, a baby will refuse to breastfeed. This happens most often during the early days, when he may be too sleepy to be interested in feeding. If this happens, don't give up; simply express the milk your baby would have suckled and wait for him to want food – babies feed much better when they are hungry.

However, should your baby tend to fall asleep soon after you have started to feed him, try lying on your side with him lying beside you so that he finds feeding a less tiring activity.

A refusal to feed may also be due to difficulty with latching on (see p.329). This usually happens because your breasts are engorged – the swelling this causes makes it difficult, even impossible, for your baby to latch on. If you express some milk from your swollen breasts he will be able to latch on more easily.

EXPRESSING YOUR MILK

Occasionally you may want to remove milk from your breasts without feeding – perhaps so that your baby can be fed using a bottle if you are planning to go out for the evening, or if your breasts have become engorged (see p.356). It is possible to express milk by hand, but you will find that it is quicker if you use a pump.

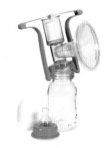

Using a manual pump
Fit the funnel of the pump over your areola to form an airtight seal, then operate the lever or plunger to express the milk.

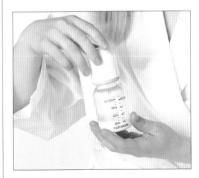

Storing your milk
When your milk has been expressed, put the cap tightly on the bottle. Refrigerate the milk until needed; it will keep for up to 48 hours in a refrigerator, or can be stored for up to six months in the freezer. Whenever you express milk, wash your hands and ensure that all equipment is sterilized beforehand.

Breastfeeding your baby

Breastfeeding your baby is a loving, nurturing experience that strengthens the bond between you. It is a continuation of the physiological relationship that began when your baby was developing in your uterus. Because your baby knows your milk will be there when he needs it and trusts it to be pure and good, it has been said that breastfeeding is the first way to tell the truth to a baby and to keep a promise.

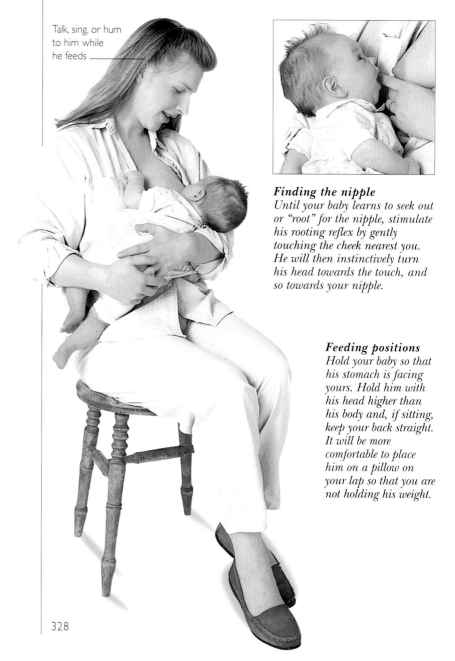

Talk, sing, or hum to him while he feeds

Finding the nipple
Until your baby learns to seek out or "root" for the nipple, stimulate his rooting reflex by gently touching the cheek nearest you. He will then instinctively turn his head towards the touch, and so towards your nipple.

Feeding positions
Hold your baby so that his stomach is facing yours. Hold him with his head higher than his body and, if sitting, keep your back straight. It will be more comfortable to place him on a pillow on your lap so that you are not holding his weight.

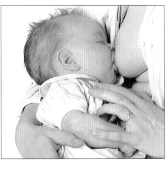

Proper feeding
When he is feeding correctly, his mouth will be wide open and, as his tongue and jaw muscles work to suck milk from your breast, you will see his ears and temples moving.

Releasing the breast
When he has finished feeding, or when all the milk has gone from the breast and you want to put him to the other, slip your little finger gently in between his jaws.

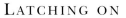

LATCHING ON

The key to happy, trouble-free breastfeeding is knowing how to get your baby's mouth correctly fixed or latched on to your breast. Proper latching on ensures that baby gets enough milk and helps you to avoid breast and lactation problems. When your baby is properly latched on, his jaws will be clamped on your breast tissue rather than your nipple, which will be completely inside his mouth.

To encourage your baby to latch on as easily as possible, give yourself plenty of time to feed and make sure you are comfortable and relaxed. Hold the baby high enough so he can reach your nipple without effort. Cradle his head in the crook of your arm, and support his back and bottom with your lower arm and hand. Express a little milk to soften the areola and ensure that his mouth contains the entire nipple.

Correct latching on is important to both you and your baby for two principal reasons. First, it prevents your baby from sucking on the nipple itself, which would cause soreness and cracking. Second, it enables him to stimulate a good flow of milk, ensuring that he gets the rich hindmilk as well as the less nourishing but thirst-quenching foremilk (see p.327). A good flow of milk also prevents your breast from becoming engorged (see p.356) because it has been inadequately emptied.

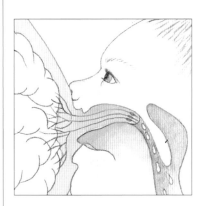

The sucking effect
A baby first stimulates milk to flow into the nipple by pressing the tip of his tongue against the areola at the base of your nipple. Then he presses the back of his tongue up towards his palate to squeeze the milk from the nipple into his throat.

BREASTFEEDING TIPS

Breastfeeding is simple – if it weren't, so many millions of infants and mothers wouldn't have managed it successfully. However, it can be challenging, so ask for help from friends, nurses, midwives, or the La Lêche League, if needed.

• Establishing breastfeeding is always easier if you put the baby to the breast within a few minutes of delivery. Once you've achieved successful suckling in the celebratory atmosphere that surrounds birth, you will feel confident about future feeding.

• If your baby has trouble locating your nipple because it is soft and small, put a cold, wet cloth on it momentarily and it will protrude and firm up.

• Milk flows in both breasts at every nursing and it is better to use both at each feed. Start with the heavier of them.

• Let your baby suck for as long as he likes on the first side so he gets both the foremilk and the hindmilk. (Foremilk is the dilute, thirst-quenching part; the hindmilk is the richer, creamier part.) Then switch to the other breast. He can stay there too as long as he likes.

PREPARING YOUR NIPPLES FOR BREASTFEEDING

In the first few days of feeding, the nipples are delicate and need time to toughen up, so increase the length of time on each breast gradually. Two minutes on each breast will give your baby sufficient colostrum at first. Build up the time on each breast to ten minutes each side by the time the milk has come in on about the third or fourth day.

All babies suck most strongly in the first five minutes, during which they take about 80 percent of the feed. When she has had enough she'll lose interest and play with your breast or fall asleep. Alternate the breast you begin feeding with each time.

BREAST CARE DURING THE EARLY DAYS

You will need to take special care of your breasts when you start breastfeeding. Buy at least two maternity bras that you can afford (see p.163) and pay strict attention to the daily hygiene of your breasts and nipples. Bathe them every day with water; don't use soap because it defats the skin and can encourage a sore or cracked nipple to develop. Always handle your breasts with care. Never rub them dry, always pat them.

After feeding, if possible, leave your nipple open to the air for a short time. Wear pads inside your bra to soak up any milk that may leak, and change these pads often. Don't leave a wet pad in contact with your breast for any length of time. To avoid cracked nipples, apply a drop of oil or cream (arachis oil or olive oil or hypercium calendula cream) to the pad.

BREAST CARE

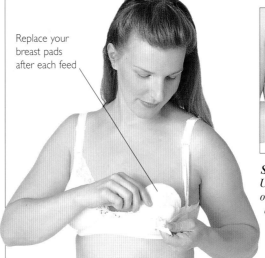

Replace your breast pads after each feed

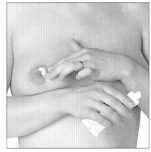

Sore nipples
Use lotion to relieve cracked or sore nipples. Apply often, especially after each feed.

Breast pads
Leaking breasts can be embarrassing and uncomfortable, can cause cracked nipples, and stain your clothes. Breast pads tucked in the cups of your bra will *soak up the leaking milk, and are easy to wear. Washable and disposable ones are available, although avoid ones backed with plastic.*

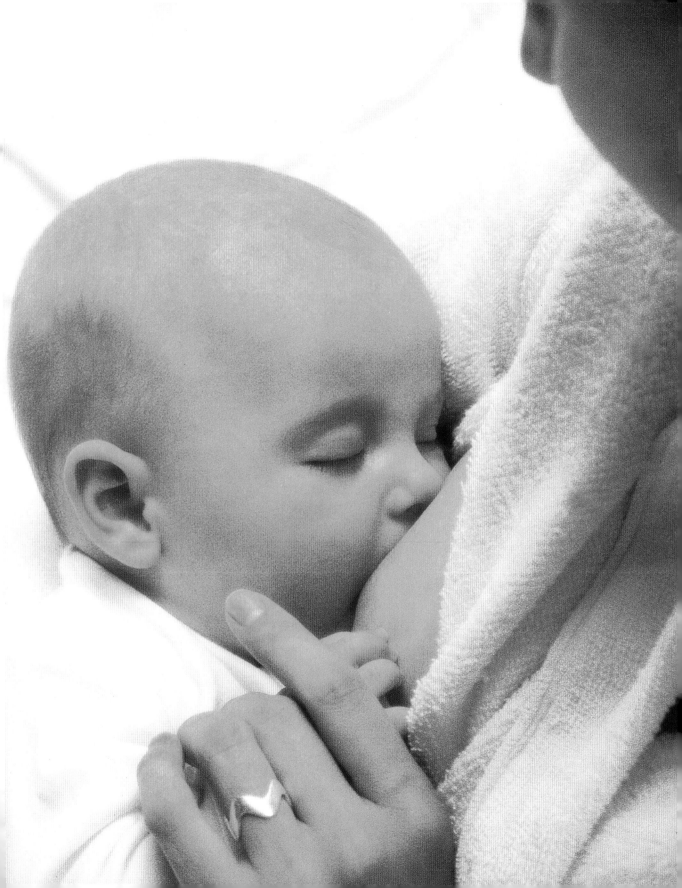

Bottlefeeding

Bottlefeeding your baby with an infant formula, instead of breastfeeding, is perfectly safe and healthy provided you follow the manufacturer's instructions carefully. Give your baby plenty of warm, loving attention and eye contact.

PREPARING FORMULAS

Infant formula products range from relatively inexpensive dried-milk-based powders to ready-to-use but expensive liquid milk products. Infant formulas are vitamin- and iron-enriched, and are carefully formulated to make them as close as possible to human milk. They are usually based on cow's milk, but soya-based formulas are available for babies who cannot digest, or who have an allergy to, ordinary milk. If you are unsure which product to choose, ask your doctor or health visitor to recommend one. Whichever formula you use, absolute cleanliness of the bottles, spoons, mixing jugs, and teats is essential, because a newborn baby is very vulnerable to infection. In addition, you must always wash your hands thoroughly before feeding.

BOTTLEFEEDING EQUIPMENT

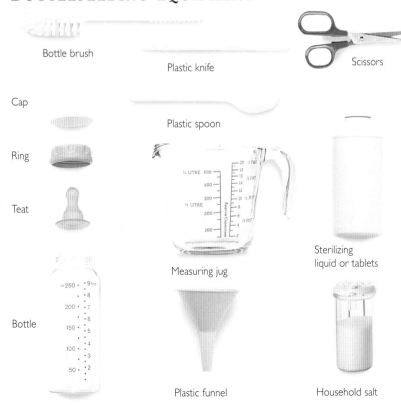

Bottle brush

Plastic knife

Scissors

Cap

Plastic spoon

Ring

Teat

Measuring jug

Sterilizing liquid or tablets

Bottle

Plastic funnel

Household salt

TAKE CARE

To reduce the risk of your baby contracting a gastro-intestinal infection, make sure that everything that comes in contact with your baby's food is thoroughly cleaned or sterilized before use. You can use a sterilizing tank, steamer, microwave sterilizer, or dishwasher (see opposite). Make sure that you wash your hands before handling any formula or equipment. Dummies and teething rings should also be thoroughly cleaned each time they are used.

Always store prepared bottles of formula in the refrigerator, and never keep it longer than 24 hours. It's best to make up formula when you need it, not in advance. If your baby does not finish a bottle or if you warm up a bottle for him but he does not want it, throw it away – reheated feeds are prime sources of infection.

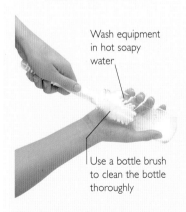

Wash equipment in hot soapy water

Use a bottle brush to clean the bottle thoroughly

Washing bottles and teats
All equipment should be washed in hot, soapy water. Scrub the insides of the bottles with a bottle brush and rub the teats thoroughly to remove any traces of milk. Rinse the bottles and teats thoroughly under warm, running water to remove any soap.

KEEPING EVERYTHING CLEAN

You will soon develop your own routine for cleaning bottles. You may use a sterilizing tank with a sterilizing chemical, or a steamer or microwave sterilizer. You can also sterilize equipment by boiling in water. You should continue to sterilize all feeding equipment until your baby is 12 months old.

Before sterilizing, wash the feeding equipment in hot, soapy water or, if you have one, in a dishwasher, and scrub inside the bottles with a bottle brush. Teats should be always be carefully cleaned, and everything thoroughly rinsed (see column, left).

To use a sterilizing tank, half-fill the tank with cold water. Add a sterilizing tablet and wait for it to dissolve. Put in the equipment, filling the bottles with water to keep them submerged. Then fill the tank with cold water, and leave for the required time.

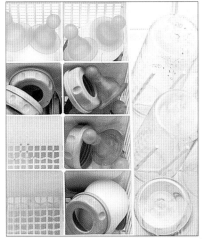

Cleaning in a dishwasher
After 12 months, if you have a dishwasher, you can put the bottles, jug, and knife straight in it. Clean teats separately before they go in (see column, left). Run the dishwasher on the normal cycle.

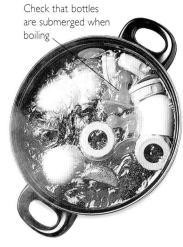

Check that bottles are submerged when boiling

Boiling
You should boil the bottles for five minutes. Then remove and allow to cool down before using.

MEASURING AND MIXING

The can or packet will give instructions on preparing formula; follow them as closely as possible. Never make the formula "more nourishing" by adding more powder than specified – your baby will get too much fat and protein and too little water. If you habitually add too little powder to the water, because you want to make the formula more thirst-quenching, you run the risk of undernourishing your baby.

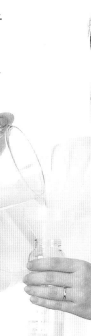

Measuring out
Using the scoop provided, measure out the quantities accurately. Use a sterilized knife blade to level off the powder in the scoop; don't heap up the powder in the scoop, or pack it down tightly.

Mixing
Use only freshly boiled water that has been allowed to cool down slightly, and measure it out after it has cooled; if you measure it out before you boil it, the made-up formula will be too strong because of the water lost by evaporation.

BREAST TO BOTTLE

If you have been breastfeeding your baby and for any reason you want to change over to bottlefeeding with formula, you should do it gradually.

Switching from breast to bottle must be done very slowly so that your baby has time to get used to bottlefeeding and to the taste of formula. Your milk supply can then slowly decline in line with the reduced demand for it.

Before beginning the change to bottlefeeding, it is important that you consult your health visitor for detailed advice on the best way to make the change.

Giving the bottle

When you feed your baby by bottle, whether with formula or with expressed breast milk be just as patient and loving as you would be if you were breastfeeding. Allow her to take a break if she feels like it and to decide when she has had enough. During feeding, cuddle her close, talk to her, and maintain eye contact. Your partner should do the same.

Warming the formula
To heat a bottle of formula, stand it in a bowl of warm water. Don't use a microwave oven as it can cause "hot spots" in the formula that might burn your baby's mouth. When it is at the right temperature, a few drops splashed onto your wrist will feel tepid. Before feeding, unscrew the teat ring a little so that air can get into the bottle when your baby sucks out the formula. This will prevent the teat from closing up.

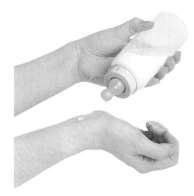

Preparing for a feed
When you feed your baby, hold her at an angle with her head slightly raised so that she can swallow easily. Until she is about ten days old, you may need to trigger her sucking reflex by gently stroking the cheek nearest you (left). When you gently insert the teat into her mouth, be careful not to push it too far back. You can make up batches of feeds and keep them in the refrigerator until needed – although you should never keep them for more than 24 hours.

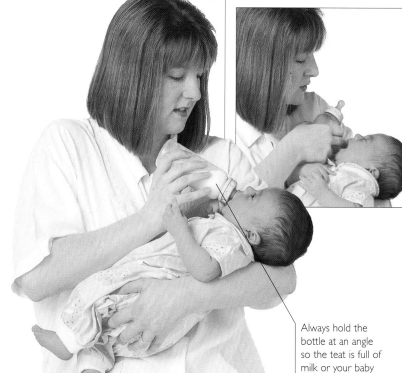

Always hold the bottle at an angle so the teat is full of milk or your baby will swallow air with the feed

Giving the bottle
Find a quiet, comfortable place in which to sit with your baby. You will probably find it most comfortable if you sit on the floor or use a chair that is low enough to support her on your lap. Rest her head in the crook of your elbow, with her back supported along your forearm. Hold her bottom securely. Make sure she isn't lying horizontally; she should be half-sitting so that she can breathe and swallow safely and there's no risk of her choking. When she begins to suck, tilt the bottle to keep the teat full of formula or milk, and free of air.

Releasing the teat
Sometimes, a baby will contentedly suck away at a bottle even though it is empty. If you want her to let go, gently slide your little finger between her gums.

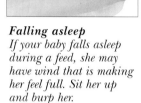

Falling asleep
If your baby falls asleep during a feed, she may have wind that is making her feel full. Sit her up and burp her.

WIND AND BURPING

The point of burping is to bring up any air swallowed during feeding or crying before feeding so as to prevent it from causing your baby discomfort. However, babies vary a great deal in their reaction to wind and, in my experience, the majority aren't noticeably more contented for having been burped.

Babies differ greatly in the amount of air that they swallow during feeding. Some swallow very little, including the vast majority of breastfed babies. Once a baby is clamped on to the breast it is virtually an airtight seal, so it's almost impossible for a baby to swallow air while on the breast.

Swallowing air is much more common in bottlefed babies, but even then it doesn't really seem to be a problem.

The one point in favour of burping is that it makes you relax, take things slowly, hold your baby gently, and stroke her in a firm and reassuring way. This is good for both of you. My attitude towards burping, therefore, is that by all means do it, but don't become fanatical.

Don't rub or pat her too hard as you may jerk her and she will bring up some of the feed. A gently upward, stroking movement is preferable to firm pats. There isn't any need to stop feeding halfway through to burp your baby; wait until she pauses naturally in the feed, and then put her on your shoulder. If she doesn't burp, don't worry; she doesn't need to.

BURPING YOUR BABY

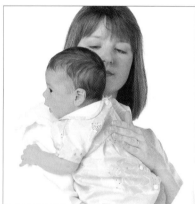

Support your baby's head with your hand so that it does not flop forward

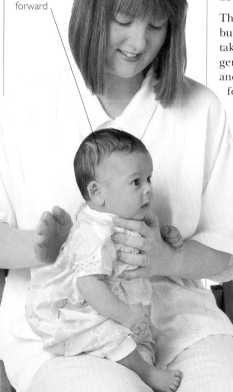

Burping positions
If your baby has wind, one of the best ways to burp her is to put her against your shoulder and gently rub her back (above). Make sure your clothing is protected by a clean towel because she might dribble or bring up a little milk (possetting).

Another way to help her to clear the wind is to lean her forwards on your lap (right), without bending her over at the waist.

YOUR BABY'S EXCRETIONS

As long as your baby's healthy you need pay little attention to the contents of her nappy.

Bowel motions vary but there are a few signs you ought to be aware of (see **Newborn health**, p.342). For example, streaks of blood in stools aren't normal. Contact your doctor right away.

Immediately after birth, your baby's urine contains urates that may stain her nappy a dark pink or red, but this is normal, so don't be alarmed. She'll urinate frequently, maybe as often as every half hour because her bladder can't hold urine for even a few minutes. You shouldn't worry unless she ceases to urinate for several hours – then consult your doctor in case there is an abnormality in her urinary tract or she is dehydrated.

Sore bottom
Nappy rash commonly occurs. Don't wash her skin with soap and water: use baby lotion, and avoid plastic pants. You can treat rashes by using special cream bought from a chemist.

Choosing nappies

Your newborn baby will need to wear nappies day and night, and for the next two to three years, until he is toilet trained, he will continue using them. It is important to choose the type of nappy that will best suit your lifestyle and budget.

TYPES OF NAPPIES

There are a variety of sizes and shapes, but the basic choice is between disposable and fabric nappies. Think which type will be comfortable for your baby, cost-effective and manageable for you.

Disposable nappies These are convenient but can be expensive in the long run. They are easy to use as the folding is straightforward and you don't need pins or plastic pants. There are two types – the two-piece is an absorbent pad that slots into specially designed plastic pants; the all-in-one has a plastic outer covering and absorbent inner layer, and is secured with adjustable adhesive tabs. Disposable nappies have elasticated legs to prevent leakage, come in boy and girl styles, and sizes that range from newborn to toddler.

Reusable nappies Reusable nappies may initially work out more expensive as you should buy at least 24 of good quality, plus fasteners (if needed), liners, and pants, although they do work out cheaper in the long term. Nevertheless, they need to be washed and dried after every use. Modern, shaped reusable nappies are softer than ordinary towelling, and are more straightforward to put on. They often come with integral velcro fastenings and you can also buy plastic fasteners so you don't have to worry about pins at all. Towelling squares are cheap and absorbent, and can fold into a variety of shapes, but they are bulky. Use reusable nappies with disposable liners that allow urine to pass through and away from the baby's skin and minimize the risk of a sore bottom. You will also need a supply of plastic pants to stop nappies soiling clothes. Choose ones with popper fasteners for a good fit, and never put them in the tumble drier.

EQUIPMENT AVAILABLE

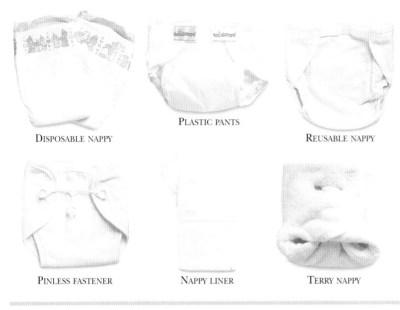

DISPOSABLE NAPPY

PLASTIC PANTS

REUSABLE NAPPY

PINLESS FASTENER

NAPPY LINER

TERRY NAPPY

DISPOSABLES

Advantages *No washing, drying, pins, or plastic pants. No risk of hurting baby with a pin. More practical when travelling as need fewer accessories and less room*

Disadvantages *Can only be used once. More expensive in the long run. Create rubbish – never flush them down the toilet*

REUSABLES

Advantages *Only require one set so don't need to keep buying a constant supply. Work out cheaper in the long run. Can be used for another child*

Disadvantages *Need adequate washing and drying facilities. Involve more labour and accessories. May prick baby with pin*

NAPPY CONTENTS

After your baby is born you'll notice changes in the colour and consistency of his stools. During the first couple of days your baby will pass meconium, a sticky, greenish black substance. This consists of bile and mucus and derives from the amniotic fluid he swallowed in your uterus. After he starts feeding, the stools will change to a greenish brown, looser consistency, and then to a yellowish brown. The colour, smell, and consistency of the stools will vary, depending on whether you are breastfeeding or bottlefeeding your baby. Breastfed babies' stools are looser and bright yellow. Bottlefed babies pass a firmer, pale brown stool, with a more pungent smell. The number of motions will also fluctuate. Some babies fill their nappies after every meal, while others are less frequent. Sometimes, a couple of days may pass without any movement – unless there are other problems (see column, left), this is normal.

NAPPY WASHING

Remove all traces of urine and faeces from fabric nappies otherwise your baby's skin will become red and sore.

Each morning fill two buckets with cold water and sterilizing solution. Put wet nappies into one bucket, and soiled nappies, after excess faeces have been flushed down the toilet, into the other bucket. Next day, rinse urine-soaked nappies in hot water before drying. Put soiled nappies through the hot programme of a washing machine, then rinse and dry. Always put nappies used during the night into a fresh batch of solution.

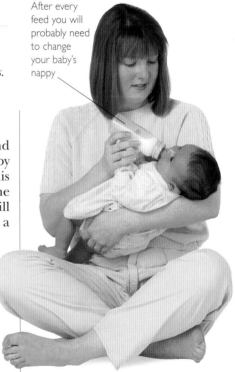

After every feed you will probably need to change your baby's nappy

NAPPY RASH

Bacteria on the skin break down urine to form ammonia, which is toxic and burns.

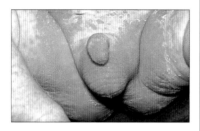

Sore bottom
Nappy rash commonly occurs. Don't wash her skin with soap and water: use baby lotion. Avoid plastic pants. You can also treat it using special cream bought from a chemist.

Changing a nappy

You will need to change your baby's nappy when it is wet or soiled which will be very often with a new baby. To prevent rashes change her nappy when she wakes up in the morning, goes to bed at night, and after feeds. Make sure you have a safe changing area with all you need close by.

CLEANING YOUR BABY

Wipe her leg creases
Remove any faeces with a tissue. Lift up her legs and fold the nappy underneath. Using one piece of cotton wool at a time, moistened with water or lotion, clean inside all the creases at the tops of her legs, wiping downwards and away from her body.

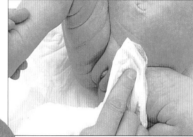

Airing her bottom helps keep it from becoming sore

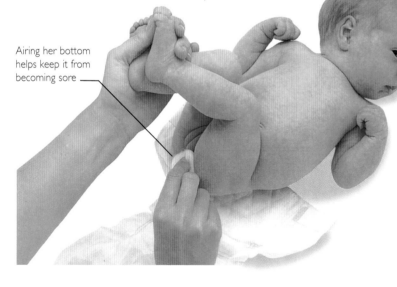

Clean her nappy area
Holding both her ankles in one hand with your finger between her heels, clean her genital area. Wipe from the vagina back towards the rectum to prevent soiling the vulva. Never pull back the labia to clean inside. Wipe her thighs and buttocks inwards towards the rectum. Remove the dirty nappy.

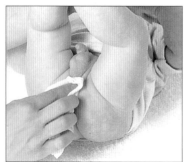

CLEANING A BOY

With baby lotion on cotton wool, clean gently under his testicles. Wipe all over his testicles and under his penis. Don't pull the foreskin back. Clean his bottom by holding and lifting his ankles with one hand; use petroleum jelly, not barrier cream, to protect his penis.

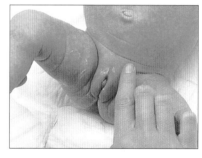

Dry her bottom
If you've used water, dry the area with a tissue, then let her kick her legs for a while, so that air reaches her bottom. Apply barrier cream gently to prevent nappy rash.

PUTTING ON A DISPOSABLE NAPPY

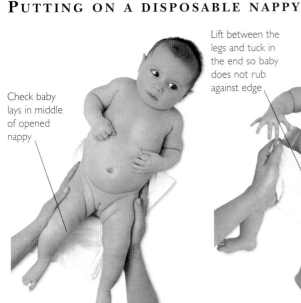

Check baby lays in middle of opened nappy

Lift between the legs and tuck in the end so baby does not rub against edge

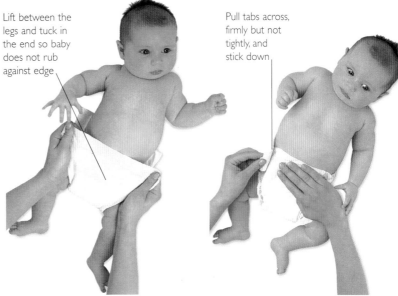

Pull tabs across, firmly but not tightly, and stick down

1 *Open out the nappy with the adhesive tabs at the top. Then lift her legs, slide the nappy underneath, and align the top with her waist.*

2 *Bring the front panel up between her legs, smoothing the sides around her tummy so they tuck neatly underneath.*

3 *Unpeel the tabs. Pull one side over and across to the front flap and stick down the tab. Repeat with the other side, keeping the nappy taut.*

PUTTING ON A FABRIC NAPPY

1 *Fold the nappy into a triangle by lifting the bottom right-hand corner to the top left, and then the bottom left to the top right.*

2 *Raise your baby's legs, and slide the nappy under, aligning the top edge with her waist.*

3 *Bring the nappy up between her legs (tuck down a boy's penis). Holding it in place, fold one side over the central panel and pull slightly to keep it firm. Then fold up the other side.*

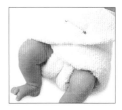

Secure the nappy
For a small baby, secure the nappy with a pin in the middle; for a bigger baby, use a pin at both sides.

Thumb on outer nappy, use fingers as a preventive measure against the saftey pin

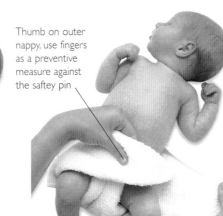

Fold over, making sure other hand has other corners secured then pin

Bathing baby

Many parents feel nervous when they first bathe their babies. Once you establish a routine, both of you can relax and enjoy the time of extra closeness.

• Warm the room to at least 20°C (68°F), and keep the time he's undressed to a minimum.

• Make sure the bath is a comfortable height for you. Wear a waterproof apron with a towel tied around your waist so you can dry your baby on your lap.

• Make sure everything you need for washing, drying, and dressing is within reach.

• Always test the water first and don't add hot water while the baby is in the bath. Add baby bath liquid to the water; this is easier to use than soap.

• Chat and smile to him constantly, and make as much body contact as possible. Most babies soon enjoy splashing around.

Your newborn baby won't need bathing very often – once a week on a regular day will be fine, although you can bathe him more often if you both enjoy it. You can bathe him in any room in your home provided it's warm enough. Always remember to test the water first to make sure it's not too hot by dipping in your elbow, or the inside of your wrist.

TOPPING AND TAILING

This is an abbreviated method of cleaning his face, neck, hands, and bottom without using a bath or removing all his clothes. Instead of a face flannel, use pieces of cotton wool dipped in cooled, boiled water and squeezed dry. Using a new piece of cotton wool each time, wipe from the inside of his eyes outwards. Clean behind his ears, over his face and chin, and around his neck. Dry him off with a soft towel.

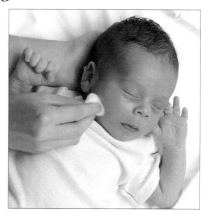

Clean his cheek and neck
Wipe his face and chin and the creases in his neck with moist cotton wool to remove any traces of milk or spittle.

Wipe inside skin creases downwards and away from his body

Clean his bottom
Undo any lower garments and remove nappy. With a new piece of cotton wool, wipe around the genital area (see p.338). If he's soiled, moisten the cotton wool with baby lotion.

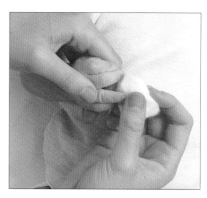

Clean his hands
Gently uncurl his fingers. Using a moistened piece of cotton wool, wipe over the fronts and backs of his hands, and in-between his fingers. With a new piece of cotton wool, wipe over his arms. Dry with a soft towel.

BATHING

Before you put him in the bath, undress him down to his vest and nappy. Wipe his eyes and face with moistened cotton wool. Then undress him completely and wrap him in a soft, clean towel.

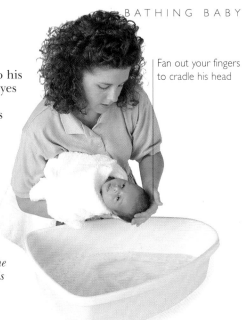

Fan out your fingers to cradle his head

Wash his head
Hold him just above the bath in a football carry, so that he lies along your arm and his head is supported by your hand. Use your other hand to carefully wash his hair with the bath water. Then gently dry his hair with a soft towel.

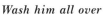

Put him into bath
Support his shoulders and neck on your forearm, hooking your hand around his far shoulder. Cradle his bottom with your other hand.

Wash him all over
Keep him semi-upright and slowly splash water over his body with your free hand. Talk and smile to him all the time. When you are finished, lift him out, with your free hand held firmly under his bottom, and wrap him gently in the towel.

Always hold him securely

CLEANING HIS CORD STUMP

Your baby's umbilical cord stump dries and drops off within a week of birth. Clean this area daily to avoid infection.

Gently wipe the skin creases around the stump with a surgical baby wipe which contains pure alcohol. Ask your midwife for a supply of these. Carry on cleaning in the same way after the stump has separated so it heals quickly. If you notice any redness, discharge or other signs of infection, ask your health visitor for advice.

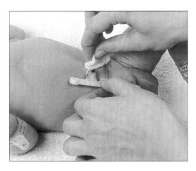

Avoid infection
Dry the area carefully after every bath. You should expose the area to the air as often as possible in order to avoid infection.

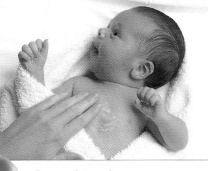

Dry and powder
Pat him dry, paying particular attention to his skin creases. If you like, apply powder, but do not apply it to his nappy area as powder will cake when wet.

As your baby gets older you will learn how to identify and cope with common minor ailments, but there are times when you must call the doctor.

Sometimes when your baby is ill you may find yourself torn between not wanting to bother the doctor unnecessarily and being increasingly worried about your baby's well-being. If this happens, you must not take chances with your baby's health – call the doctor promptly, especially if your baby is showing one or more of the symptoms set out below. Do it sooner rather than later.

• He is having convulsions.

• He is hard to rouse.

• He is having trouble breathing, is wheezing, and has a loud, dry cough.

• He has a very high temperature, or an abnormally low one.

• His stools are frequent, loose, green, and watery.

• He is vomiting a significant amount (not just the usual afterfeed possetting).

• He has refused several of his feeds in a row.

• He is showing the symptoms of dehydration (see right).

• He is listless and crying for no apparent reason.

• He seems to be bothered by his ears, head, or neck.

• He has an unusual rash.

• You have any other reason to worry about his health.

Newborn health

Newborn babies, especially those who are breastfed, are generally healthy during their first weeks of life but, because their immune systems and internal organs are not fully developed, there are a number of ailments that can affect them.

JAUNDICE OF THE NEWBORN

It is not unusual for babies to suffer jaundice – a yellowish discoloration of the skin and whites of the eyes that is a result of an excess of bilirubin in their blood. Bilirubin is a yellow pigment that is a by-product of the destruction of primitive red blood cells, which commonly occurs after birth.

Infant jaundice usually becomes apparent by the second or third day after birth, and lasts for about seven to ten days, by which time the surplus red blood cells have died off and the baby's liver has matured enough to mop up the excess bilirubin. The jaundice usually clears up without treatment, but if the bilirubin levels are particularly high, the baby may be given phototherapy. This involves exposing him to carefully controlled amounts of ultraviolet light, which breaks down the bilirubin pigment in his skin.

Haemolytic disease of the newborn This more serious condition is a result of an excessive amount of bile being present in the baby's blood. It can be caused by the breakdown of large numbers of red blood cells due to the action of antibodies from a Rhesus incompatible mother (see p.202). The chief symptoms are jaundice, pallor, enlargement of the liver and spleen, and blood abnormalities. It is usually treated by blood transfusion.

DIARRHOEA AND VOMITING

Mild cases of upset stomach or diarrhoea will soon pass but a young baby's digestive system is extremely vulnerable. Breastfed babies are less prone to these gastro-intestinal infections than are bottlefed babies, because of the protective antibodies that are present in breast milk, but all babies may suffer from them from time to time.

If your baby vomits up all his feeds over a six-hour period or is passing frequent, loose, green, watery stools, you should contact your doctor immediately.

Dehydration The major danger to babies suffering from vomiting and diarrhoea is dehydration because of the loss of fluids it causes. Its symptoms include a dry mouth, sunken eyes, abnormal depression of the fontanelle, irritability, lethargy, and refusal to feed. Never ignore these symptoms: seek medical advice at once.

CONSTIPATION

Breastfed babies do not get constipated, because the ideal composition and digestibility of breast milk keeps everything moving. Bottlefed babies can get constipated, usually because of a lack of fluid. If you are bottlefeeding your baby and he passes no stools for a day or two, then produces a hard one, give him drinks of water between feeds to increase his fluid intake. If this does not make his stools softer and more frequent, give him a little drink of diluted fruit juice twice a day, which will probably help to loosen the stools. If that fails, consult your health visitor.

Urinary problems Constipation is very easily treated and is usually nothing to worry about. However, if your baby starts to urinate infrequently it might be a sign of a fever, or of a blockage or infection in his urinary system. If he goes for a couple of hours without wetting his nappy, give him plenty of water to drink. If his nappy is still dry two hours after that, contact your doctor.

If your baby's urine becomes strong and deepens in colour, it is probable that he is not getting enough fluids. This makes the urine more concentrated, and the remedy is to increase his liquid intake by giving him several drinks of water between feeds. Should this fail to make any difference, it may be that he has a urinary infection and will need medical treatment, so contact your doctor.

FEVERS

When your baby has a fever it is a sign that his body is fighting an infection – the rise in body temperature acts to increase the activities of the defence system. If you suspect that your baby has a fever, take his temperature, then check it again in 20 minutes to see if it has varied, noting down each reading. If your baby's temperature rises slightly but he seems his usual self and shows no other symptoms of illness, the infection is probably minor and will usually pass within a day or two. You should, however, consult your doctor. Do so without delay if your baby's temperature rises by a degree or more, if he gets very hot and distressed, or shows other signs of illness such as lethargy, vomiting, or diarrhoea.

EAR INFECTIONS

Babies often get colds, and these can lead to an ear infection called otitis media. This happens when the bacteria travel along one, or both, of the Eustachian tubes (which link the middle ear to the back of the throat and which are necessary to equalize pressure in the ears) into the middle ear. Babies spend most of their time lying down, which can facilitate the passage of bacteria. Inflammation of the mucus membrane of the Eustachian tube traps the bacteria in the middle ear, where they multiply.

The symptoms include a high temperature, diarrhoea, crying for no apparent reason, and any kind of discharge from the ear. Call your doctor right away. He or she will examine your baby to confirm the diagnosis and to rule out meningitis, which has similar symptoms. Ear infections are easily cured by antibiotics.

COLICKY BABY

Colic affects male babies on the whole, and the exact causes of this exasperating blend of indigestion and inconsolable crying are not yet known.

Investigations into the cause of colic have led many researchers to suspect that it may be due to the immaturity of the baby's digestive system. Other research suggests that babies who have been subjected to maternal anxiety in the uterus are more prone to being colicky (see p.193).

In a typical colicky baby, the problem begins at about two weeks of age and disappears at about three months. The colic attacks usually happen in the evening. The baby will draw up his legs to his stomach or stick them out straight in an attempt to relieve the stomach cramps and wind, and cry loudly from distress and pain.

There is not much you can do about it except wait for him to grow out of it, but stomach massage will often ease the discomfort, as will lying him face down across your lap with a warm towel, or a hot water bottle half-filled with warm water, placed under his belly. Other measures that may work include taking the baby for a ride in a car, putting him face down across your knees and stroking his back, and giving him a dummy to suck on.

Colic is no threat to your baby's health (although it can be very frustrating for you), but when it first begins you should consult your doctor to make sure that it is nothing more serious.

HOW TO HELP YOUR BABY

In addition to all the care and attention your baby will receive from specialist staff, there are things you and your partner can do to help him thrive.

• Try to spend as much time with him as possible; he needs the same amount of love and attention as a full-term baby.

• Touch and fondle your baby, both in and out of the incubator, whenever and as soon as you can. Cuddling, stroking, and gentle caressing have positive benefits in helping him to grow and thrive.

• Express your breast milk at regular feeding times for your baby. Not only will you be giving him the best possible food, but you will be establishing your milk supply for when he is able to suck on his own.

• Research shows that the colostrum and milk of a mother whose child is preterm contain more of certain nutrients than those of mothers whose children are born at term. This makes up for a preterm baby's lack of nutrients that he would otherwise have received in the uterus, and a preterm baby fed on his mother's breast milk develops at almost exactly the same rate as he would if he were still in her uterus.

• Get involved with your baby's care. Ask the nurses to show you how to help with feeding, washing, and changing him. This will both help you bond with him and give you confidence in caring for him.

• Don't struggle with feelings of anxiety, ignorance, or worry. Seek information from the medical staff and support from your partner.

Special care baby

About one in ten of all newborn babies need to spend some time, even if only a very short time, in a special care baby unit. Most have been born too soon or have not grown as much as they should have before birth, although a small number will be ill. The aim of the special care baby unit is to protect the baby from risks to his health and to nurture him until he has outgrown them.

LOW BIRTHWEIGHT BABIES

In general, any baby weighing less than 2kg (4¼lbs) at birth is probably smaller than he should be and may need special care. About 4–8 percent of all babies have low birthweights and, of these, two-thirds are preterm and one-third small-for-dates.

Preterm babies The pace of an unborn baby's development is geared to his being born at full term (forty weeks from your LMP) so if, for any reason, he is born a few weeks or more before full term, he may not yet be ready for life in the outside world. A baby born before week 35 is said to be preterm or premature, and, depending on how premature he is, he will need the help of a special care baby unit or a neonatal intensive care unit to sustain and protect him while he catches up on his growing.

Small-for-dates babies A baby is "small-for-dates" if he weighs less than is expected for the number of weeks that have passed since he was conceived. A small-for-dates baby is usually a full-term baby who is very small at birth. A small-for-dates baby may present different problems of care after the birth from a premature baby. Babies that are only three or four weeks premature and low birthweight full-term babies who are otherwise well and feeding properly are usually cared for on the postnatal ward with their mothers, or in a so-called "transitional care" nursery where their progress will be more closely monitored than normal.

Health risks A premature baby born before 35 weeks must contend with a number of health risks that seldom affect a full-term infant, as well as more common ones such as jaundice. For example, if his internal organs are underdeveloped, he may have difficulty breathing, regulating his body temperature, and feeding; he will also be very susceptible to infection. He may also have a low blood sugar level (hypoglycaemia), which can cause brain damage if untreated, and he may need iron or calcium supplements to remedy a lack of these essential minerals.

CARING FOR BABIES WITH SPECIAL NEEDS

Today, a baby born preterm or small-for-dates, or with an illness or disability, has a far better prospect of survival than he would have 20 or even ten years ago. This is because of a tremendous growth in the knowledge of how to care for newborn babies and the application of that knowledge in special care baby units. If the baby is simply too weak or young to be able to suck, and needs tube feeding, or has jaundice and so needs phototherapy treatment, he will probably be looked after in the special care baby unit (SCBU) attached to your local maternity unit. However, if he is very premature or ill, he'll need the more specialist, "high-tech" care of a neonatal intensive care unit (NICU).

A neonatal intensive care unit is dedicated to looking after babies who need highly specialized nursing attention. In modern NICUs the tiniest premature babies – even ones born at only 24 or 25 weeks gestation and weighing barely 450g (1lb) – can be helped to thrive. Neonatal intensive care units tend to be sited in major regional rather than neighbourhood hospitals. If you go into labour very prematurely you may be taken to a hospital with an NICU even if it is not the hospital into which you were booked, or your baby may be taken there by ambulance in a special incubator immediately after the birth. This can be distressing for parents if the unit is some distance from where you live, but the unit will be designed to be as welcoming and friendly as possible. You should ask the consultant paediatrician in charge to give you a full explanation of your baby's particular needs and how you can help.

Most units encourage the parents to play an active part in the care of their baby by, for example, helping with feeding, washing, and nappy changing. Many provide rooming-in facilities so parents can stay at the hospital with their babies as much as possible. Parents are encouraged to cuddle their babies skin to skin, as this helps babies develop more quickly (see also p.348). However, it may be some time before very premature babies are strong enough to be handled outside the incubator and parents have to steel themselves for an anxious wait until their baby is strong enough.

BABIES THAT NEED SPECIAL CARE

Although every baby born prematurely or small-for-dates is assessed individually, your baby will definitely be admitted to a neonatal intensive care unit if any of the following applies:

• birth weight less than 1.5kg (3lbs)

• gestation less than 34 weeks

• severe respiratory problems (hyaline membrane disease, sometimes known as respiratory distress syndrome)

• severe birth asphyxia (lack of oxygen or fetal distress)

• severe infection

• convulsions (fits)

• jaundice that requires an exchange transfusion

• drug withdrawal, where the mother has been addicted to narcotics such as heroin.

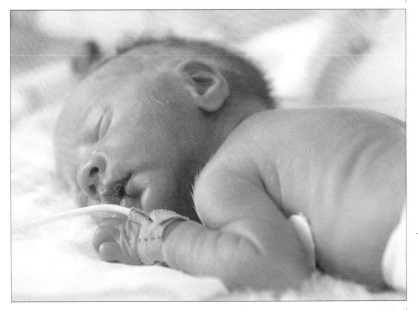

A special care baby
Most special care babies, like this one, born prematurely, spend some time in an incubator. This keeps their temperature steady and monitors their breathing.

It is common for parents of a special care baby to worry that they will miss out on the bonding process. However, be reassured that the staff will encourage you both to be as involved as possible with your baby.

• You will be encouraged to watch the nurses care for your baby and to help with the practical care and nursing.

• Don't be afraid to touch your baby as often as possible. As well as helping you to feel closer to him, this loving attention also hugely benefits your baby, helping him to thrive and grow.

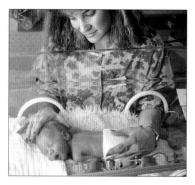

Physical contact
As well as allowing nurses to attend to your baby and attach any monitor leads, feeding tubes, or intravenous drips he might need, the circular doors in the plastic top of the incubator also allow you to reach in and touch your baby, helping you to bond with him and feel close.

Special care unit

In the special care unit your baby is cared for 24 hours a day by specially trained staff members who have a wide range of technology to help them. The main areas of concern for a special care baby are his temperature control, his breathing, his brain, his immune system, and his feeding. Be prepared for a lot of tubes, electrodes, monitors, and drips, which can be alarming when you first see them.

WHY YOUR BABY NEEDS CARE

Your baby needs special care to help him to grow and thrive independently. The following key areas are closely monitored.

Temperature control All babies are at risk of getting cold – a premature or small-for-dates baby is even more at risk, because they have little or no body fat to use as insulation. A premature baby is therefore usually placed in an incubator, an enclosed cabinet in which he can be kept warm and supplied with warmed, humidified air (or oxygen, if he needs it).

YOUR BABY'S ENVIRONMENT

A preterm or small-for-dates baby may have undeveloped internal organs and therefore needs extra assistance to help him breathe and develop. Inside the incubator (see right), the temperature, oxygen levels, and humidity are all carefully controlled to provide the optimum conditions for your baby to thrive and grow.

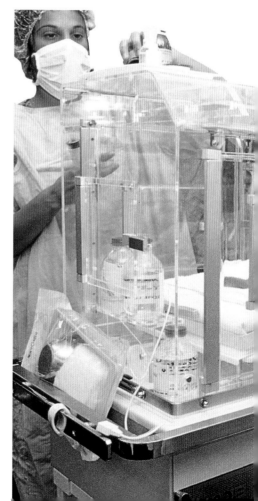

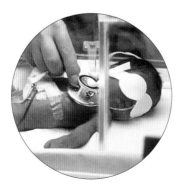

Checking heartrate
A stethoscope is placed on the baby's chest to monitor and record his heart rate.

Breathing Under 30 weeks, and certainly before 27 weeks, a baby's lungs are not sufficiently mature to allow the transfer of oxygen to the bloodstream. If you go into premature labour, you'll probably be given an injection to help mature the baby's lungs. Furthermore, because the nervous system is immature, this can have an effect on the baby's breathing mechanism, and may cause pauses in breathing, known as apnoea, sometimes accompanied by a slowing of the heart rate, known as bradycardia.

Feeding Initially, your baby will have frequent small feeds once an hour, progressing to one every three hours. A very premature or sick baby may be unable to digest milk and will have a special solution of sugar, salts, and potassium. When he is able to take milk he will be given a special infant formula or milk expressed from his mother's breasts – the ideal food for a special care baby, as for any other baby.

YOUR BABY'S NEEDS

As well as specialist medical attention, a special care baby also needs his mother and father.

Although he receives 24-hour medical care, he also needs to feel his parents' love. Physical contact with you and your partner will reassure and comfort him, and help you to develop a warm, close, and loving relationship.

He needs to hear both your voices, so talk and sing to him all the time; hold him close whenever possible so that he is familiar with your smells and can feel close to you.

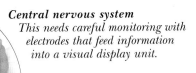

Central nervous system
This needs careful monitoring with electrodes that feed information into a visual display unit.

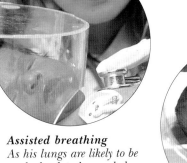

Assisted breathing
As his lungs are likely to be underdeveloped, your baby may need help with his breathing through a special ventilator.

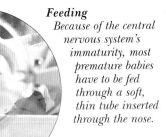

Feeding
Because of the central nervous system's immaturity, most premature babies have to be fed through a soft, thin tube inserted through the nose.

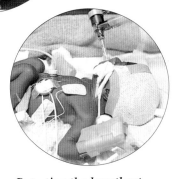

Detecting the heartbeat
Electrodes are placed on the baby's chest to monitor his heartbeat.

Premature baby

Premature babies can have a somewhat difficult start in life but the majority of them do well and grow up to be healthy, normal children thanks to the dedicated staff and advanced technology of special care units. A premature baby can look frighteningly small but most have great fighting spirit.

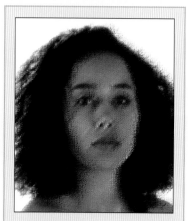

Name **Carol Scott**

Age **24 years**

Past medical history
Nothing abnormal

Obstetric history
This is Carol's first pregnancy

At 28 weeks of pregnancy, Carol noticed that her hands and feet were swollen, and that she couldn't remove her wedding ring. Two weeks later she was found to have raised blood pressure, so she was admitted to her local day centre for monitoring of her blood pressure, blood, and urine. The well-being of her baby was checked too, with regular external electronic fetal monitoring (see p.275) and ultrasound scans. Albumin was found in her urine, which is a symptom of pre-eclampsia along with high blood pressure and swelling.

BABY AT RISK

After a week of careful monitoring, Carol's blood pressure hadn't returned to normal and albumin continued to appear in her urine. At the beginning of the 32nd week there were signs of fetal distress. Her obstetrician decided that labour would have to be induced. After a straightforward induced labour, Carol delivered her baby, Alice, who weighed in at 1.4kg (3lb).

FAILING PLACENTA

Carol's obstetrician thought that the placenta had begun to fail at the beginning of the third trimester and therefore the baby's nutrition had been inadequate for some time. When this happens late in pregnancy, the baby's head is disproportionally large because of the relatively normal growth of the brain at the expense of the rest of the body.

KEEP BABY WARM

He explained that these types of low birthweight premature babies are born with insufficient energy stores and do not have enough fat to maintain their body temperature. They are more susceptible to hypothermia; hypoxia (lack of oxygen to the tissues); and hypoglycaemia (abnormally low blood-sugar)

so it's crucial that they are kept warm. Alice was put straight into an incubator and her immature lungs were helped by a ventilator. Carol was given a room next door so she could be with Alice as much as possible.

POSTNATAL REACTIONS

Carol and Mark were quite taken aback by the first sight of Alice (see box, right), even though they had had time to adjust to the idea that she would be premature. Throughout her pregnancy, Carol had dreamed of a curly-haired cherub. Instead, Alice was red and wrinkled, and her head looked very large in proportion to the rest of her body, which was very thin. Inside the incubator, attached to a ventilator and taped with wires and tubes for monitoring and feeding, Alice seemed very far away and isolated.

Seeking reassurance
Carol found herself bursting into tears at the sight of her tiny daughter, so alone and shut away. At the same time, she realized she was having considerable difficulty relating to the baby in the incubator even though she knew it was her longed-for baby. Mark encouraged Carol to explain her difficulties to the counsellor on the ward who reassured Carol that

her feelings were common and normal. The staff of the special care unit were understanding; they encouraged Carol and Mark to make contact with Alice by touching and stroking her through the portholes of the incubator. Recent studies show that this helps a premature baby to establish breathing more readily. The staff explained to Carol that her love was more important for the baby's survival than all the technology they could offer. I encouraged Carol and Mark to express all their feelings and to forget their perfect dream-baby. It was important for them to be honest about their feelings and to know that many parents of premature babies feel the same.

GETTING INVOLVED

As Carol became involved in caring for Alice, she realized that she loved her and desperately wanted her to survive. The nurses showed her how to express her colostrum (see p.327) so that it could be fed to Alice via the tube. The colostrum of the mothers of premature babies is extra rich in trace minerals – those minerals the baby would be getting if she were still in the uterus – and their milk contains extra protein to help their babies grow.

Meanwhile, Mark became very interested in the machines in the special care unit. He wanted to know what each one was doing for his daughter. Busy though they were, the staff found time to answer his questions.

Skin-to-skin contact

Once Alice had gained weight and her breathing had improved, she was taken off the ventilator and feeding tube. The staff of the postnatal unit then encouraged Carol to tuck Alice under her blouse and hold her in an upright position between her breasts. Alice was naked except for a nappy and this meant that mother and baby were in skin-to-skin contact for long periods of time. Premature babies thrive on this treatment. A mother's body is better than an incubator for keeping a baby warm because her temperature rises automatically if her baby is cold, then falls again once the baby has warmed up. The nurses called it kangaroo care, because it is similar to the way in which kangaroos keep their infants in a warm, protective pouch. This skin-to-skin contact also strengthens the mother-and-baby bond that is so important for survival. Alice began to suckle spontaneously. The unit staff were delighted with her progress and Carol and Mark were now eager to take Alice home. The obstetrician explained that it wasn't a question of Alice reaching any target weight; each baby was considered as an individual case and allowed home when her weight and general health were satisfactory given her circumstances. Generally, babies are usually kept in hospital until they reach 2.5kg (5lb).

BACK AT HOME

Once Carol and Mark were able to take Alice home, they found themselves confronting a new set of problems. Most normal newborn babyclothes were too big for Alice. Carol's mother found a specialist mail order catalogue and Mark found one or two large department stores had a stock of tiny clothes (see **Addresses**, p.370).

Ordinary nappies came almost to Alice's armpits, so Carol made smaller ones by cutting disposable nappies down to fit Alice and fastening them with tape. Alice thrived at home and soon began to catch up with full-term babies of the same age.

CAROL'S BABY

Born eight weeks early, Alice had none of the fat that a baby normally accumulates in the last few weeks, so she looked much too small for her skin, which was wrinkled and red. She made a pathetic picture.

• Her head looked very large in comparison to her body, which was thin and tiny.

• Her skin was loose-fitting and rather dry.

• She had lanugo (fine downy hair) on her back and the sides of her face.

• Her chest looked small with prominent ribs.

• As she breathed her chest rose and fell dramatically.

• Her bottom looked bony and pointed due to lack of fat.

• Her movements tended to be jerky because of her immature nervous system.

• She seemed to have to make a huge effort to take every breath. Sometimes her breathing would stop for a few seconds, but this is not abnormal in a preterm baby.

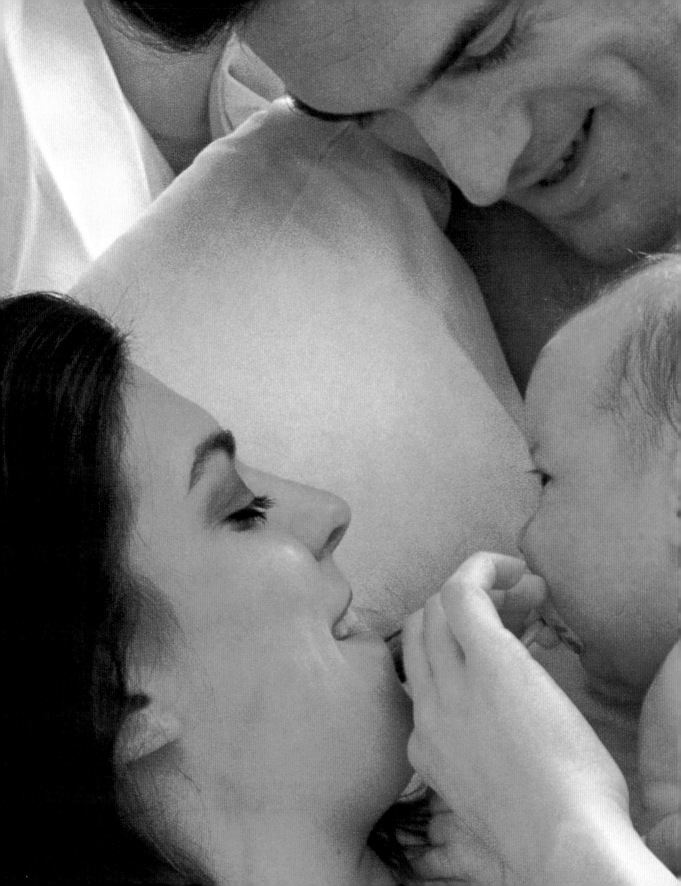

CHAPTER 16

Adjusting to
PARENTHOOD

*The responsibilities of parenthood
may weigh heavily upon you, particularly
if they mean dramatic changes to your lifestyles.
However, watching your baby grow and
develop will bring you great joy as you
start to experience the closeness that
only a family can bring.*

Plan to take some time out immediately following the birth of your baby. Don't feel you have to get back to normal straight away – if you try, you'll become overtired and miss out enjoying your new baby.

Provisions Make sure you are well stocked-up before the birth with everything you will need – favourite nutritious foods, drinks (you'll need a lot of fluid if you're breastfeeding), clothes, sanitary towels, cotton wool, nappies.

Nurturing You and your partner will nurture your newborn baby and your partner will nurture you. Spoil yourselves!

Bonding Give yourselves both time and space to get to know and bond with your baby.

Nesting Make your bed the centre of the household – talk, entertain, cuddle, and picnic there.

Visitors Restrict visiting hours. Don't feel obliged to play hostess, and do put a card on the front door saying you are resting if you don't feel like seeing anyone just then – they can always come back another time.

Callers If you have an answerphone you could alter the message to include the birth announcement, and perhaps explain that you are resting at present, but that you would love to talk to them in a few days.

The first weeks

Traditionally, women were not expected to reappear in society until some while after their babies' births. They spent this time regaining their strength. Nowadays we see a period of peace and relaxation in the days immediately following the birth of a baby as vital. It gives both partners a chance to celebrate the birth, welcome and bond with the new baby, and adjust to their new roles as parents.

BECOMING PARENTS

It usually takes new parents some time to adjust to becoming parents. Many report a degree of panic at the overwhelming responsibility they suddenly have to take on for this tiny, dependent human being. As with all major changes, it can take time for you to accept and feel comfortable in your new roles and, at the beginning, you may catch yourself hoping that someone else is going to come and take over.

The answer is to give yourselves time and space to get to know and feel comfortable with your baby. The initial few weeks are important too in establishing breastfeeding. Successful breastfeeding requires that you are as rested and relaxed as possible, and that you continue to eat well.

Welcoming your baby Every mother will daydream about her unborn child. Fitting the image of this "dream child" to the reality of the newborn baby in your arms may be difficult – especially if it is the opposite sex to the one you wanted, or isn't quite "perfect", or is simply different from what you expected.

It takes time to fall in love with your baby and to learn how to be a mother – or a father. Time spent together will give you the space you need to become adjusted, and to enable you both to make a smooth transition into parenthood.

You may find it preferable to keep your baby with you in your bedroom just at first, even if you have already prepared a room for her. Feeding will be easier and you may have more restful nights.

RESTING AND RELAXING

The first few weeks can seem like a never-ending round of feeding and changing, with snatches of catching up or resting for you when your baby is asleep. If you are exhausted all the time this can take most of the pleasure out of looking after your baby and end up making you feel resentful and irritable.

Earmarking the time straight after your baby's birth for you and your family to be together, nurturing each other, marvelling at the new life with which you have been entrusted, and nesting and picnicking in your bed, will ease you into parenthood and help you regain your strength before you get back to real life.

Friends and family A close friend or relative could make this an extra-special period for you by taking on the household chores, food preparations, etc. You may also find this person an invaluable source of support, particularly if he or she is knowledgeable about aspects of baby care and behaviour. On the other hand, you may find that, as new parents, you are offered advice that may be confusing or contrary to your own ideas. In such cases, do not hesitate to discuss things with your midwife or health visitor, who will be able to clear up any confusion.

You are bound to receive a lot of friendly enquiries, either personally or by phone. Discuss this with your partner and decide together how you will deal with it. Don't feel that you have to entertain. You need to conserve your strength, and being a good hostess every afternoon for the first week or so really will wear you out, so please don't feel guilty about restricting visiting hours. Do put a note on the front door saying "Mother and baby resting. Please do not disturb" if you want to rest. You could also add an announcement, such as "Matthew born at 11.35 p.m., July 20th, 7lb 2oz. Mother and baby doing well." If you own an answerphone, you could include the birth message here as well.

Other children

If you already have a child or children, then this period can be structured to include them. If you've had the baby in hospital and have been away from home, your other children will want their share of your attention. They will enjoy cuddling up with you, talking or reading to the baby, and playing on the bed, and it will help to offset any feelings of jealousy. However, they probably won't want to sit still for long and you may be grateful for someone they like and trust to give them some extra individual attention.

Your baby's experience

He has arrived in a brand-new world and in a warm, intimate, and loving environment.

Daily routine At first he won't have a recognizable baseline of behaviour. It will be 3–6 weeks before he will begin to settle down into an established routine of feeding and sleeping.

Sensations He will prefer looking at your face than at unfamiliar people and things; he will be reassured by the smell of your skin and his father's; he will look towards new sounds, and will be startled if they are loud or unexpected; he will enjoy the taste of your milk; he will love being cuddled, touched, and massaged.

Communicating His main means of communicating is by crying. He will cry if he is hungry, tired, upset, bored, or feels lonely. He will also cry if he senses that you or his father are tense or tired.

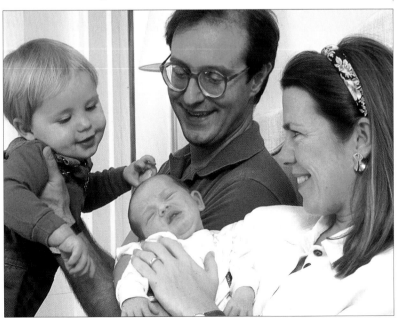

Family togetherness
Time spent cuddling, talking, and just being together without everyday demands will enable you to adjust to the changes within your family.

LOCHIA

While your uterus contracts and returns to its normal size and condition after delivery, you will have a vaginal discharge known as lochia.

Lochia is the normal vaginal discharge from a healing uterus. The duration of lochia loss varies widely from woman to woman, its average length being about 21 days, although it may be as short as 14 days or continue for up to six weeks. Breastfeeding helps to reduce the duration of lochia production, because the oxytocin that triggers the let-down reflex (see p.326) also causes uterine contractions, and these help the uterus to shrink back to its normal size, cutting down on bleeding.

However long it continues, lochia secretion goes through three distinct stages as the placental site heals. For the first three or four days, the lochia is bright red, then it gradually reduces in quantity and changes to pink or brown as the uterine lining is shed, and by about the tenth day it becomes yellowish-white or colourless.

Lochia should have a fresh, blood-like odour; if it becomes at all foul-smelling you should tell your doctor immediately because such a change indicates an infection. You should also tell your doctor if the flow suddenly becomes bright red again. This usually means that the placental site is not healing properly, perhaps because you are over-exerting yourself. Your doctor will probably recommend that you rest for a couple of days and generally take things easier.

Because there is a risk of infection, you should not use tampons until about six weeks after delivery, so you will need to use sanitary towels until the lochia flow ceases.

Postnatal health

After your baby has been born, your body begins to reverse the changes it underwent during pregnancy and labour. The withdrawal of the huge amounts of pregnancy hormones is like the withdrawal of a lifeforce, and the period immediately following labour and delivery – known as the postnatal or postpartum period – can be a very tiring one for you. Try to get as much rest and relaxation as you can, and also make sure that your diet is healthy and includes an adequate amount of fluids (at least a pint of milk a day and four pints of other liquids such as water or fruit juice). If you are breastfeeding, you will need to take good care of your breasts and nipples.

PELVIC AREA

After delivery, your uterus, cervix, vagina, and abdomen begin to shrink back to approximately their pre-pregnant and pre-labour sizes. The shrinkage of your uterus is accompanied by a vaginal discharge known as lochia (see column, left) and by contractions or spasms called afterpains or afterbirth cramps.

Afterpains All women feel uterine contractions throughout their fertile lives. During menstruation they are known as menstrual cramps, during pregnancy as Braxton Hicks' contractions, and following delivery as afterpains. After delivery, the uterine contractions are stronger and more painful than usual because they are the means by which the uterus contracts down to its former non-pregnant size; the faster and harder it contracts down, the less likelihood there is of any postpartum bleeding. Afterpains are usually more noticeable if you have had a child before, because the muscles of your uterus will have been stretched by your previous pregnancy and so will have to work harder to help get your uterus down to its non-pregnant size. You may also feel these muscular spasms when you breastfeed, as the hormone oxytocin involved in the milk let-down reflex (see p.326) also causes uterine contractions. They usually disappear after three or four days.

Bowels and bladder You should get out of bed to use the toilet as soon as you possibly can after delivery. However, the bowels have often been cleared out prior to delivery so you may not want to move them for 24 hours or more, and this is quite normal. When you move your bowels you may feel the urge to bear down. Any pressure in the perineal region will stretch your tissues and cause pain if you have a episiotomy wound (see column, right). To prevent stretching, hold a clean pad firmly against the stitches and press upwards while you bear down. Do everything you can to prevent constipation and the need to strain. Eat lots of roughage, vegetables, and fruit, especially prunes and figs, and drink lots of water (see column, p.357).

Drinking plenty of water, in addition to getting up and walking about, will help to get both your bowels and your bladder working normally. There may be some hesitancy before the urine starts to flow for the first time. This is nothing to worry about and is usually the result of swelling of the perineum and tissues that surround the bladder and urethral opening. A good way to start to pass urine is to sit in some water and try out the pelvic floor exercises (see p.148), passing urine into the water. This is not as unhygienic as you may think, if you wash yourself down afterwards, because urine is sterile. Urine flow is often triggered off by turning on the bath taps and letting them run while you stand over the lavatory pan.

Cervix and vagina These will have been stretched considerably during labour and will be soft and slack for a while. It takes about a week for your cervix to narrow and firm up again, which it will do unaided, but you can help the recovery of your vagina by contracting and relaxing its muscles (pelvic floor exercises). You ought to begin these exercises within about 24 hours of giving birth, beginning with five contractions three times a day and gradually working up to five contractions ten times a day. You can also use exercises to tone up your abdominal muscles (see p.358), but do not begin these until the flow of lochia has stopped.

Caesarean wound If you have had a Caesarean section, you should avoid beginning any abdominal exercises until the wound has completely healed. It is better to avoid lifting heavy weights; try not to climb stairs more than once a day; be careful how you move when you are getting up from a lying or sitting position; and generally try not to put too much strain or pressure on your abdominal muscles.

Piles Haemorrhoids (piles) are quite common after childbirth; they are caused by the great strain imposed on the veins in the pelvic floor during labour and delivery. They appear as lumpy swellings just inside your anus, and with proper care (consult your doctor or midwife) they will eventually shrink away.

MENSTRUATION AND OVULATION
The dramatic fall in the exceptionally high levels of pregnancy hormones following delivery brings the eventual resumption of menstruation and ovulation, as well as sometimes causing cold and hot flushes (sometimes occurring both at once, which can be disconcerting). Menstruation will usually restart some time between the eighth and the sixteenth week following the delivery, but both it and ovulation may be significantly delayed if you are breastfeeding your baby. However, if you want to resume making love (see p.364) before your periods have started, you must use birth control because ovulation will precede menstruation.

EPISIOTOMY WOUND

The pain from an episiotomy wound gets worse before it gets better. The wound is positioned where fluid can accumulate in the cut edges. The skin then swells, with the result that the stitches become tighter and tighter and bite into the tender skin surrounding the wound.

If you are bruised or if the stitches are really painful, it will help to sit on an inflatable rubber ring, so try to keep one with you at all times. Good hygiene is vitally important while the wound is healing, so make sure that it is kept clean. Most stitches dissolve after five or six days.

Warm baths and showers, and special perineal pads that fit between your sanitary towel and the wound, are soothing and encourage the healing process, as do pelvic floor exercises. You may also find that ice packs or local anaesthetic creams are helpful. Your doctor or midwife will advise you on their use.

Don't use antiseptics in your bath as they can cause irritation. After bathing, dry the area thoroughly with a hairdryer instead of using a towel, which will cause pain.

If you sit down when you use the lavatory, urine, which is strongly acid, will run over the episiotomy wound and make the raw skin sting. Standing up will probably help. You could also try pouring warm water over yourself as you're passing urine, in order to dilute the acid and reduce the sting.

FATIGUE

Getting enough rest and sleep is essential if you are to combat the inevitable fatigue of the first weeks of caring for your newborn baby.

Try to rest whenever you can, especially during the first week or so when you will still be recovering from the exhaustion of labour. Avoid climbing stairs and heavy lifting as much as possible, and get your partner or someone else to help you with the baby and the housework. Take advantage of your baby's daytime naps – rest or nap yourself then, and try not to waste these valuable opportunities for rest by using them to catch up on the housework.

Ensure that you get enough sleep. At night, go to bed half an hour or so before you plan on going to sleep, and unwind by sipping a warm, milky drink and listening to the radio, watching television, or doing a little light reading to relax you physically and mentally before you sleep. If you are breastfeeding, express milk into bottles (see p.327) so that your partner can share the night-time feeding duties just as he should if you are bottlefeeding.

A healthy diet is an essential part of combating fatigue, but don't eat too much late at night because digesting it might interfere with your sleep pattern.

BREASTS AND NIPPLES

Because of the increased size and weight of your breasts, a good quality, well-fitting cotton maternity bra will be both convenient and comfortable. Change to a clean one every day and, if you are using breast pads to prevent leaking milk from staining your clothes, avoid those that are lined or backed with plastic. Change pads after each feeding and whenever they become wet.

Cleaning and washing Clean your breasts and nipples daily with cotton wool and baby lotion or water, but avoid using soap because it strips away the natural oils that protect the skin from drying and cracking, and it can aggravate a sore or cracked nipple. Always treat your breasts with care – don't rub them dry for example, very gently pat them dry instead.

There is no need to wash your nipples before or after each feed but, before you fasten or put on your bra after feeding, let your nipples dry in the air, and always wash your hands before handling your breasts in order to prevent infection.

Engorgement About three or four days after you have given birth, your breasts will fill with milk. They will become larger and heavier, and feel tender and warm when you touch them. If they overfill it is known as engorgement. Engorgement usually only lasts a day or two, but it can be uncomfortable and may recur.

To ease engorged breasts, take off milk either by manual expression or by feeding your baby (although you may have to express a small amount of milk so that he can latch on, see also pp.328 & 330). In addition, you may find that it helps to bathe them with warm water or cover them with warm towels, or to stroke them gently but firmly towards the nipple.

Engorgement can recur at any time during the period of breastfeeding, particularly if your breasts are never properly emptied or if your baby misses a feed.

Blocked ducts A blocked milk duct may occur in the early weeks of breastfeeding. It may result from engorgement, from a bra that is too tight, or from dried secretions on the nipple tip blocking a nipple opening. If you get a blockage, your breast will feel tender and lumpy and there may be a reddening of the skin.

To clear a blocked duct, start feeds with the affected breast and gently massage it just above the sore area while feeding to ease the milk gently towards the nipple. If the blockage will not clear, don't offer the breast to your baby and consult your doctor immediately as it could become infected and result in a breast abscess, which is painful, although not a catastrophe.

Sore nipples When you begin breastfeeding, your nipples may feel slightly tender for the first minute or so of suckling. This tenderness is quite normal, and it usually disappears after a few days. Sore nipples, however, are a common problem in the early weeks and can turn what should be a pleasure into something of an ordeal. Incorrect latching on and carelessness when taking your baby off your breast (see p.328) are the principal causes of sore and cracked nipples, but taking care to start and finish feeding properly can prevent these problems arising, and is essential if they are to heal after they have become sore or cracked.

Sore nipples heal quickly when they are exposed to the air so, if possible, go topless or bra-less occasionally, especially when resting, in order to let the air circulate over them.

Cracked nipples If a sore nipple becomes cracked, you may need to keep the baby off that breast for up to 72 hours and express milk from the breast to avoid engorgement. Cracked nipples can be very painful, and they can lead to breast infection. To help avoid cracked nipples, apply a drop of baby lotion to your breast pad.

Mastitis The first signs of mastitis (breast infection) are swelling, tenderness, and reddening of the affected area, accompanied by flu-like symptoms, which can include a high temperature, chills, aches, headaches, and perhaps nausea and vomiting. If you think you have developed an infection, contact your doctor; if treated promptly with antibiotics, mastitis usually subsides within a day or so. You cannot pass the infection on to your baby, because it only affects your breast tissue, not your milk.

PROTECTING SORE NIPPLES

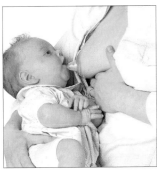

Your baby will adjust quickly to the feel and taste of the shield

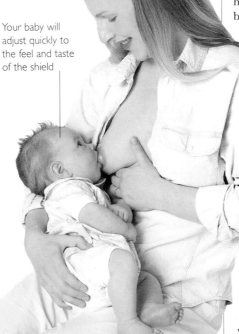

Using a breast shield
If your nipples get sore, use breast shields to protect them during feeding. The shield fits over the nipple and the baby sucks through it. To ease your nipple into the shield, slip your hand between breast and ribcage and push gently upwards; this is also useful without a shield, as it helps your baby get the nipple fully into his mouth – and that helps prevent sore nipples in the first place.

CONSTIPATION

Many women suffer from constipation after giving birth. If you find you are affected, exercise, a sensible diet, and lots to drink will help you to deal with it.

After delivery, the passage of faeces through your bowels tends to slow down, and this can lead to constipation. The slowing down occurs mainly because your abdominal muscles are relaxed and stretched and so the pressure within your abdomen is lower than normal. Relaxation of the bowel muscles themselves, because of the high levels of progesterone during pregnancy, may also slow down bowel movements. If you have had an episiotomy you might, consciously or unconsciously, hold back from passing stools for fear of causing pain.

Medication, such as laxatives, stool softeners, or suppositories, can help to get things moving again, but if you are breastfeeding it is best to avoid taking anything by mouth because it can be passed on to your baby via your milk, and can cause you stomach cramps and watery stools.

The best remedy for constipation (and a good way to prevent it) is to eat dried prunes or figs. It helps to drink plenty of fluids; eat plenty of fibre-rich foods; avoid inactivity by getting out of bed and walking around; and, after the lochia discharge has ceased, exercise your abdominal muscles to restore their tone (see p.358). Practising your pelvic floor muscles exercises will return tone to your anal muscle and the anal sphincter.

FIRST DAYS

You can do a few gentle exercises just days after giving birth. Whether lying in bed, or sitting in a chair, try to get into the habit of doing something to tone your muscles.

Remember the importance of your pelvic floor muscles (see p.148). Strengthening these will help to prevent incontinence.

Tone up your stomach muscles by pulling them in as you breathe out, then holding for a few seconds. Relax, and then repeat as often as possible.

You can prevent, or reduce, swollen ankles and feet simply by moving your feet up and down as though you were pedalling.

TAKE CARE

If you've had a Caesarean, wait for 4–6 weeks before starting to exercise, and check with your doctor first. If you have had a tear or an episiotomy, don't practise stretching exercises until it has healed.

Postnatal exercises

A few weeks after giving birth, try to establish a daily exercise routine. This may not seem like a top priority when you're faced with the new demands of being a mother. However, exercising will tone muscles that were stretched during pregnancy and delivery, and increase your energy supply. Exercise twice or several times a day rather than for one long period. It's also good for morale.

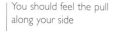
You should feel the pull along your side

Side bends
Stand with your feet about 1m (3ft) apart. With your left hand on your thigh, slowly bend over to the left. Run your left hand down your leg as far as you can without straining, raise your right hand over your head, and breathe deeply. Hold your breath for a short while, then straighten up as you breathe out. Repeat the exercise, bending over to the right.

Gently slide your hand down your thigh so that you can feel when it's time to stop

Try to keep your pelvis level; this will improve the stretch

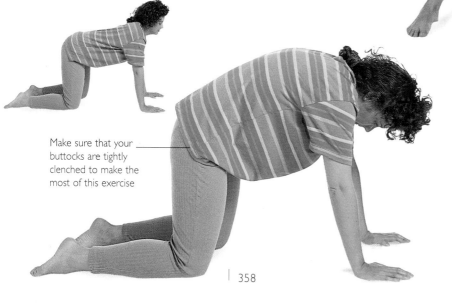

Make sure that your buttocks are tightly clenched to make the most of this exercise

Pelvic tuck-in
You may have practised this exercise before giving birth as it helps to correct the tilt of your pelvis. Kneel down on all fours with your knees about 30cm (12in) apart, then tighten your buttock muscles, tucking in your pelvis and arching your back upwards into a hump. Hold for a few seconds, then release. Don't let your back sink downward. Repeat several times.

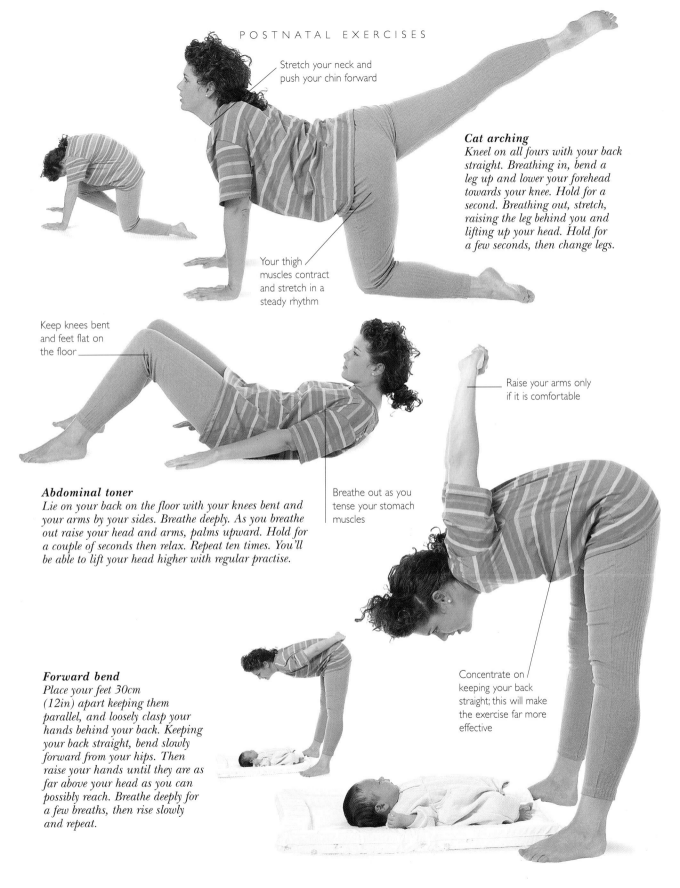

Stretch your neck and push your chin forward

Cat arching
Kneel on all fours with your back straight. Breathing in, bend a leg up and lower your forehead towards your knee. Hold for a second. Breathing out, stretch, raising the leg behind you and lifting up your head. Hold for a few seconds, then change legs.

Your thigh muscles contract and stretch in a steady rhythm

Keep knees bent and feet flat on the floor

Raise your arms only if it is comfortable

Abdominal toner
Lie on your back on the floor with your knees bent and your arms by your sides. Breathe deeply. As you breathe out raise your head and arms, palms upward. Hold for a couple of seconds then relax. Repeat ten times. You'll be able to lift your head higher with regular practise.

Breathe out as you tense your stomach muscles

Concentrate on keeping your back straight; this will make the exercise far more effective

Forward bend
Place your feet 30cm (12in) apart keeping them parallel, and loosely clasp your hands behind your back. Keeping your back straight, bend slowly forward from your hips. Then raise your hands until they are as far above your head as you can possibly reach. Breathe deeply for a few breaths, then rise slowly and repeat.

POSTNATAL CHANGES

The sudden change in hormone levels following childbirth is thought to be a principal cause of the baby blues and postnatal depression.

Very soon after you conceive, the levels of certain hormones in your body, especially progesterone and oestrogen, rise steeply and stay high throughout the months of pregnancy. Then, during the first 72 hours after giving birth, the levels of these hormones crash.

The amount of progesterone in your blood falls from about 150 nanograms (thousand millionths of a gram) per millilitre to less than 7ng/ml, and the amount of oestrogen falls from around 2,000ng/ml to 20ng/ml. After that, the amount of progesterone dwindles to zero and the oestrogen settles down at about 10ng/ml.

When the levels of oestrogen and progeserone drop, your body finds it very difficult to adjust. This can have a marked effect on your emotions and mental processes, and, along with other factors such as personal or relationship problems, may lead to the baby blues or even postnatal depression.

Severe exhaustion, another possible postnatal problem, may be made worse by a lack of potassium in your body. Low potassium levels are easily corrected by eating plenty of potassium-rich foods such as bananas or tomatoes.

Your changing emotions

During the days and weeks following the birth, you will be in an emotionally labile state because of the abrupt cessation of your pregnancy hormones (see column, left). And, because it is such a major event in your life, giving birth is liable to accentuate any underlying personal or emotional problems you may have, and to resurrect any unresolved issues. It is, however, difficult to predict just how you will react to the birth of your baby – sometimes an elated, trouble-free pregnancy can be followed by a low-key postnatal period.

If there are postnatal emotional problems, their nature, severity, and duration can vary greatly from one woman to another, and from one pregnancy to another. A woman can have a trouble-free postnatal period after the birth of one child, then have a rough time following the birth of a subsequent one.

THE "BABY BLUES"

Because the most important single cause of postnatal emotional problems is the abrupt and unavoidable drop in hormone levels, you should not be surprised if, like most women after giving birth, you suffer from the baby blues to some extent. As many as 80 percent of mothers do, so it really is the norm rather than the exception, and women who escape it entirely are in a fortunate minority. For the nine months of pregnancy, you have been experiencing very high levels of hormones and suddenly they are plunged back to the comparatively low levels of normality. This drastic but normal swing renders the majority of women weepy, prone to sudden mood swings, irritable, indecisive, and anxious.

The baby blues usually set in about three to five days after the birth and last for about a week to ten days. The onset often coincides with the beginning of your milk production (which itself is governed by your changing hormones) and for this reason the baby blues were known, in the nineteenth century, as "milk fever".

Becoming a mother If you get the baby blues, you usually find that the reality of motherhood seems difficult to cope with once the initial euphoria of having your new baby wears off. In addition to the symptoms mentioned above, you might feel confused, anxious about your ability to look after your baby, and frustrated because it seems to be taking you so long to learn to be a good mother. Be easy on yourself; no woman has the expertise for instant motherhood – it is something that can be acquired only with time.

You might also find that you are beginning to feel differently about your partner. This does not mean that you are feeling less for him, you are just feeling different, and it is not a sign that your relationship is deteriorating. It is more likely that eventually it will mature and become richer. Talking things through openly with your partner is important, because this is one of the best ways to keep the stresses and strains of motherhood in perspective, and prevent them from escalating into a serious emotional disturbance.

It is also important not to overdo things. Tiredness is inevitable in the early days, but it should never be ignored. If you feel tired, stop whatever you are doing if it's not essential, and lie down with your feet raised slightly above your head. You don't have to go to sleep to conserve your strength; a good rest may be all you need.

POSTNATAL DEPRESSION

About ten percent of all mothers develop postnatal depression (PND). This is, in many respects, different and separate from the baby blues. PND is longer-lasting, more serious, and needs rapid medical attention. It is a psychiatric disorder that can get out of hand if left untreated, and it is vital that you get medical help early. With treatment, your depression should resolve in a few weeks; the longer PND is untreated, the longer it will take to resolve.

Symptoms There are many symptoms associated with PND, and these are experienced by different women in varying combinations. In addition to depressive symptoms, such as hopelessness and despondency, sufferers can experience lethargy, anxiety, tension, panic, sleep difficulties, loss of interest in sex, obsessional thoughts, feelings of guilt, and lack of self-esteem and concentration.

Treatment Drugs will help postnatal depression, but support from family and friends is also vital. There are also some things you can do for yourself (see column, right). Your doctor will normally prescribe antidepressant drugs, taking into account whether you are breastfeeding. Over a period of time, these will bring about a gentle and gradual improvement, so it's important to keep taking your medication even after you start feeling better. Some drugs may involve side effects such as a dry mouth, drowsiness, and confused thoughts. If these side effects interfere with your daily life, consult your doctor about changing your medication.

If the feelings of depression worsen premenstrually, tell your doctor. He or she may be able to prescribe further medication, such as progesterone pessaries or injections, in order to prevent this severe form of premenstrual tension.

PUERPERAL PSYCHOSIS

In this rare psychotic form of postnatal depression, affecting about one in 1,000 mothers, the sufferer loses contact with reality, may experience delusions or hallucinations, and always has to be hospitalized. Intensive treatment with drugs, psychotherapy, and/or electro-convulsive therapy will be offered.

SELF-HELP FOR DEPRESSION

If you are feeling low, there are a number of things you can do to help yourself. The most important thing is to convince yourself that you will get better, no matter how much time that takes.

Rest as much as possible Being tired definitely makes depression worse and harder to cope with. Catnap during the day and, if possible, get someone to help with night feeds.

Maintain a proper diet Eat plenty of fruit or raw vegetables; don't snack or binge on chocolates and sweet biscuits. Eat little and often. Do not go on a strict diet.

Take gentle exercise Give yourself a rest from being indoors or taking care of the baby. A brisk walk about in the fresh air can help to lift the spirits.

Avoid major upheavals Don't move house or redecorate.

Try not to worry unduly Aches and pains are common after childbirth, and more so if you are depressed. Try to take them in your stride; they will almost certainly fade away as soon as you can relax.

Be kind to yourself Don't force yourself to do things you don't want to do or that might upset you. Don't worry about not keeping the house spotless or letting household tasks lapse. Concern yourself with smaller, undemanding tasks and reward yourself when you finish them.

Talk about your feelings Don't bottle up your concerns; this can make matters worse. Talk to others, particularly your partner.

The depressed mother

While mild feelings of depression are not uncommon for a few days after a birth, depressive feelings that deepen and last longer than about two weeks may signal a serious condition requiring medical treatment. Women with postnatal depression (PND) become increasingly withdrawn and lose touch with reality and their baby.

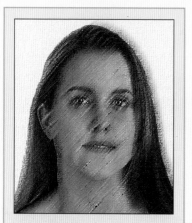

Name **Christine Rance**

Age **33 years**

Past medical history
Nothing abnormal

Obstetric history **Three children, a boy aged four, a girl aged two and a half and a boy of four months. All pregnancies and deliveries normal**

Christine sailed through all her pregnancies, although afterwards she came down with rather a bump. After the birth of her first baby, she went through a short spell of "baby blues", although she recovered in a few days. After her second baby was born she felt tired and dejected for about two weeks. She also put on a lot of weight which she can't lose. Three weeks after the birth of this baby she's depressed and unable to cope. Her GP has diagnosed postnatal depression.

SOME PREDISPOSING FACTORS

Christine has never been very good at handling change within her life; she prefers a stable permanent situation. She has always felt a little inferior and unsure of herself, doesn't have a particularly clear sense of her own identity, and is rather lacking in self-respect. Obesity has become a problem, particularly as she overeats when she is depressed. She has gained weight with each pregnancy, which she has found increasingly difficult to lose. After her first pregnancy, she was almost a stone overweight and it took a year to slim down. She then became pregnant with her second child, Laura, and the weight piled on again. After Laura's birth, she found it impossible to lose weight and in fact gained more in the first months of Laura's life than she had when she was pregnant.

Christine's husband, Stephen, often complains that she no longer looks like the woman that he married and Christine has been on countless diets in order to try to get herself into shape, without success. She feels extremely self-conscious about her size, and tends to wear shapeless clothes in order to disguise it. Sometimes she thinks that she

hasn't been too good a mother and she often feels inadequate about her maternal instincts.

FEELING HELPLESS

Christine is used to the feeling of baby blues and was expecting to be sad after her third child. When depression set in it was almost a self-fulfilling prophecy. By the third day postpartum she was extremely weepy and the smallest obstacle seemed insurmountable and molehills became mountains. She started behaving in rather a helpless way, and refused to get out of bed.

Stephen's mother came to live at the family home in order to take care of Thomas and Laura and to help with running the house. Even though she tried to be helpful, Christine repaid her with criticism. The atmosphere became tense and her mother-in-law tended to leave her alone rather than risk upsetting her.

Christine and Stephen then began to have arguments. Christine felt that Stephen didn't really understand her situation. She wanted him to take time off work in order to support and comfort her. Stephen, not understanding completely what was going on, started to become depressed himself and his work began to suffer.

Christine was so drowned in her own misery – at feeling so exhausted, hopeless, and guilty, at having three children to look after (especially as the two eldest had started to be difficult and misbehave), having to coordinate the household, and the tense relationships between herself and Stephen, and herself and her mother-in-law – that she could think of nothing else. She stopped communicating with her family and only talked to the baby. Then, after a week of this, she found herself unable to even relate to baby Oliver, and she started thinking of the awful things she could do in order to stop him from crying. She didn't care about feeding him. She left him to scream.

PARTNER'S ROLE IN PND

There is quite a lot of research which shows that a decisive factor in determining whether a woman succumbs to PND is having a supportive and helpful partner; second is an understanding family. So I suggested to Christine that she and Stephen should think of ways that he could take the pressure off her. There are many ways in which he could be really constructive such as:
• hold Christine close a lot and tell her he's proud
• stay with Christine and Oliver whenever possible, hold them both, or nurse Oliver for Christine
• get used to having Oliver in a sling and carry him around all the time he's at home
• do the shopping, the chores, and the cooking when he can
• carry Oliver around in the sling when he goes out to give Christine a real break

• take the children to his mother's for a day or the best part of a day so that Christine can have time on her own or with the girls, have her hair done, or see a film, etc.

HELP IS OFFERED

After about two weeks of this behaviour, during which her midwife reassured her that everything would get better soon, she was visited by her social worker, who realized that Christine's reactions were far from normal. She contacted Christine's doctor, who visited her three weeks after delivery. He diagnosed early postnatal depression, and called in a psychiatrist, who visited Christine in her own home.

About two weeks after the psychiatrist's visit, Christine started to improve, mainly as a result of the advice that he had given her. First he advised her to forget what was happening in the rest of the house. She should think only about the baby and herself and let everything else take care of itself. Second, he advised her to let someone else see to the baby overnight so she

could get a full night's sleep. Third, he advised Christine to attend the Well Baby Clinic twice a week where she could talk to women in a similar situation. He also advised her to contact MAMA (the Meet-A-Mum-Association – see **Addresses**, p.370), which offers good advice and support.

In addition to the above advice, Christine's doctor prescribed a mild antidepressant and mild sleeping pill to tide her over the first difficult few weeks only. He said that he would continue the antidepressants after this, and it was agreed that he would reduce its dosage gradually as soon as Christine felt able to take charge of herself and her life.

FUTURE LOOKS BRIGHT

After six weeks, Christine was sleeping so much better that she asked to stop the sleeping pills. She is now continuing on the antidepressant medication and is determined to halve the dose over the next four weeks and be free of it in another six. Stephen feels much happier now that she is almost back to normal, and the children, too, are more relaxed.

CHRISTINE'S CHILDREN

No permanent harm will have been done to Christine's ability to bond with her baby, and once she started to feel better, she was able to rebuild her relationships with her older children.

• However, while she was feeling depressed and was unable to give them much attention, her children became very anxious, difficult, and rather naughty.

They rebelled against their grandmother's care, and demanded more of their parents' attention and affection.

• In cases of postnatal depression, children need support, either before or after their mother has improved. Various groups exist (see **Addresses**, p.370) to help with the effects of postnatal illness on families.

BIRTH CONTROL

You need to consider some form of contraception when you resume intercourse after birth because ovulation could occur at any time.

If you start having intercourse before your periods have come back, don't assume that the absence of menstruation means that you won't get pregnant. You will ovulate two weeks before your first period, so if you have put off using contraception until after that, you may have waited too long. Even when you are breastfeeding your baby, and your periods are absent until you wean her, ovulation may still occur – so intercourse without contraception can result in pregnancy.

Contraception Pills containing oestrogen are not prescribed for women who are breastfeeding, because oestrogen reduces milk production. Progestogen-only "mini-pills" may be prescribed instead; these do not inhibit milk production, but their long-term effects on babies are not yet known. They are also thought by some to worsen any postnatal depression by inhibiting the natural production of progesterone.

Because of this, if you are breast-feeding you might prefer to use a different form of contraception, such as condoms with contraceptive gel or cream. If you want to use a diaphragm or an IUCD (coil) you will have to wait until your six-week check-up before you can get one; if you previously used a diaphragm, you will need to be fitted for a new one because your cervix may have enlarged and your old diaphragm may no longer fit. Until you get your new diaphragm or IUCD, use condoms and spermicidal cream.

Resuming sex

You probably won't be in the mood for making love in the first days, or even weeks, after giving birth, because the sheer physical exhaustion of labour and the drastic changes in your hormone levels after delivery combine to inhibit sexual desire. An initial lack of interest in sex is both natural and desirable, because your body needs time to recover from the changes and stresses of pregnancy and childbirth, and you need time to adjust to your new baby. Talk to your partner – he will probably feel totally sympathetic and understanding.

YOUR PARTNER

The arrival of the baby can also have a dampening effect on your partner's libido; it is not uncommon for a father to feel a lack of desire and even to lose his ability to maintain an erection, and he might find it difficult to adjust to his and your dual, sometimes contradictory, roles as parents and lovers.

Both of you must be prepared for such problems and should not take them personally. If you are philosophical and open about problems, and discuss them lovingly and sympathetically, you will prevent them developing into long-term difficulties.

WHEN TO RESUME

The point at which sexual desire returns varies greatly from one couple to another, and even from one pregnancy to another. For instance, a woman might have desired sex three weeks after one pregnancy, but have had no interest in it for three months or more after the next one.

There is also the question of just when it is physically safe for intercourse to take place; couples were once advised to give up sex six weeks before the expected date of delivery and to abstain from it for six weeks afterwards (until after the six-week check-up). This well-meaning advice is now thought to be unnecessarily cautious, and the general opinion today is that penetrative sex can continue as late in pregnancy as you wish – provided there are no medical reasons to avoid it (see p.234) – and that it can begin again as soon as you like. You can also restart non-penetrative sex as soon as you like after giving birth. If you or your partner are at all unsure about whether it is safe to make love again, discuss things with your doctor or obstetrician.

If both of you are feeling happy about it, and there is no medical objection to it, you can resume sexual activity as soon as you feel the desire to. In addition, making love can have a beneficial effect for a number of reasons. For example, it reaffirms your affection and desire for one another, and the hormones released during sexual activity cause contractions of your uterus, which will help it to return to its pre-pregnant state.

LACK OF DESIRE

Don't worry about loss of libido – it's natural. There are, however, many factors that can conspire against both your desire for and enjoyment of postnatal sex. Apart from any lingering discomfort you might feel, it is quite common for women to see themselves as unattractive at first, and this can make them shy away from sex or think negatively. Your still-bulging tummy may make you feel unsexy, so starting exercises to get back into shape (see p.358) is important for your self-esteem, and pelvic floor exercises will help to reduce the slackness of your vagina.

Anxieties and distractions may also diminish your sexual desire or enjoyment. Fear of getting pregnant again may bother you, and resuming birth control can be worrying or annoying. Even your baby can have a considerable influence on your enjoyment of lovemaking, because it is often hard to adjust to this new presence in the house. You may not feel as free as before or as able to abandon yourself, and you may not be able to relax and enjoy lovemaking because you half expect your baby to cry for attention at any time. It is also possible for you to get so absorbed with your baby that you find you have little need for other emotional ties or physical contact, to the exclusion of your partner. Even your sexual responses may become focused on your baby. This is because oxytocin, the hormone that is produced during breastfeeding, is sexually stimulating, and sometimes during a feed a woman can be stimulated up to and even including orgasm.

MAKING INTERCOURSE MORE ENJOYABLE

You might find that it takes a long time for you both to regain your previous level of sexual interest. You may both need extra fondling, kissing, and other foreplay before you become sexually aroused. For the first few times you make love, you should avoid penile penetration and stick to gentle oral or manual sex. And because an episiotomy site can be surprisingly painful during intercourse and may take months to become totally pain-free, please be honest with your partner and tell him if sex causes you discomfort or pain. Getting him to feel your scar will help him to be sympathetic, and a warm bath before lovemaking and using a water-soluble vaginal lubricant or saliva, can be a great help.

Whether or not you have had an episiotomy, extra lubrication is usually necessary because, until your hormone levels are back to normal, your vagina will not lubricate itself as quickly as in pre-birth days, no matter how much foreplay you have. Avoid non-water-soluble lubricants such as petroleum jelly because they can prevent air from reaching the lining of your vagina and this can encourage the growth of harmful bacteria.

After you have resumed intercourse, you may well find that man-on-top positions are uncomfortable. Experiment with other positions (see p.234) – side-by-side positions are especially good ones to try if you are suffering from a sore episiotomy site. Whichever positions you use, be patient, do not do too much at first, and build up your sexual activity levels gradually.

POSTNATAL CHECK-UPS

Your last visit to your obstetrician will be at about six weeks after delivery, when you will be thoroughly checked.

Your check-up At your visit, you will be weighed, your blood pressure will be checked, and your breasts examined for lumps (although this is not always done if you are breastfeeding, because lumps are not easy to distinguish from milk glands). You will have a pelvic examination to check that, among other things, an episiotomy has healed well, your cervix is closed, and your uterus is back to normal. The doctor will usually ask you how you are feeling emotionally and how you are coping. She or he will also discuss your future method of contraception with you and provide you with a diaphragm or an IUD should you need one.

Your baby's first check-up This will usually be a separate visit. The GP or paediatrician will check his ears, eyes, limbs, and muscle tone, listen to his heartbeat, check his control over his head movements, measure the circumference of his head, check for hip displacements, and weigh him. His weight will be recorded on his weight chart every time he subsequently attends the clinic, and the chart will be an important record of progress.

TIME FOR YOURSELVES

Find time in your daily routine when you and your partner can be alone together. This is an important part of keeping your relationship alive and well.

At home Continue small rituals as part of your daily life together. If you always had a sundown drink together at the end of the working day, shared a bath in the evenings, did the crossword together, or read your own books and papers while chatting or reading bits out to one another, continue to do so. Not only is it precious time together, it will also help you maintain normality in your everyday lives.

Going out Your new baby will be surprisingly portable in the first few months of her life, but you will also need to go out together alone. Turn to someone you trust for a babysitter. If you're breastfeeding, express your milk so that your baby can be fed with it while you're out. It may be difficult or seem too much hassle, but persevere. It is important for you and your partner to have time together away from your baby.

As a couple If you want to learn a new sport or skill, or resume an old one, why not plan to do it together now? Putting aside two or three hours every week when you are booked to do something as a couple will ensure that you have time together as individuals rather than just as parents.

Changes to your lifestyle

Many people underestimate just what is involved in caring for a new baby. It is a demanding and exhausting job that can turn your lives upside down. You may find yourself wondering whether you and your partner will ever be able to spend time together. Fitting in all the demands on your time and energy can be difficult, but if you approach the situation sensibly and discuss it together before the birth, you should be able to minimize the disruption and manage to spend some time alone. It does require planning, but it is possible.

KEEPING ON TOP OF IT ALL

Taking care of your newborn baby will probably be much harder than you expected. In the first place, labour and birth are physically and emotionally draining; in the second you'll find that during the day, one job or activity succeeds another almost without respite.

Getting enough rest is most important – it is rare for a new baby to allow you more than four hours' sleep at a time during the night, so you should learn to catnap. Your diet is also important, especially if you are breastfeeding. Continue to eat as well as you did throughout your pregnancy, and drink plenty of fluid.

Taking short cuts, such as occasionally buying prepared meals, at least for the first few months, will help you cope, as will getting your priorities right – ensuring enough rest, for example, is far more important than cleaning the house, and your partner can always dust and vacuum when he gets home, or perhaps you could do it together at weekends.

Avoid guilt Feeling guilty seems to be a burden carried by most new mums, and quite a few well-established mums. Remember that you can only do your best, and that it is important that you put yourself and your health high on your list of priorities. Bear in mind too that it takes about a year for your body to regain its pre-pregnancy state, so make sure that your family does not demand too much of you at first – and that you do not demand too much of yourself, because just after delivery you will find that you have very little stamina and will become easily exhausted.

Find a routine This does not mean training your baby to eat, sleep, and play according to your timetable but rather following his lead and fitting your life around his daily routine. It won't necessarily mean rearranging your entire lives to accommodate him; much of your routine and lifestyle will continue as before.

APPRECIATE YOUR NEW ROLES

At first, it may be more difficult than you had hoped to embrace your new roles as parents. You may resent the loss of your own income and the satisfaction of doing a demanding job well, and you may envy your partner his relatively free and independent lifestyle.

Your partner, on the other hand, may find it difficult to cope with the stress and demands of being the only wage earner, and may feel shut out from your intimate relationship with your baby. He may also feel envious of your home-based lifestyle, especially if he doesn't appreciate how demanding a baby can be.

These different experiences can result in your wondering where the closeness and intimacy of pregnancy went, and also whether you will ever get back to the easy understanding you had before you became pregnant. You will, but you need to keep talking to each other, explaining your thoughts and feelings, and trying not to let misunderstandings alienate you from each other.

MAKING TIME FOR YOURSELVES

One of the most difficult changes to manage is lack of time. Most of your waking and sleeping hours must be devoted to the care of your new baby; this can be frustrating and might make you feel resentful. Maintaining outside contacts, continuing with your usual lifestyle, and keeping the lines of communication open between you and your partner will go a long way to helping you cope with the various conflicting demands on your time and energy.

Sharing Doing things together is especially important once you have a baby. Young babies are very portable so don't hesitate to include him in your plans. He can come with you when you visit friends, and you may be surprised at how little effect he has on your social life in the first few months of his life.

However, you also need time together alone and, although it may seem odd having to make a formal appointment to spend time with your partner, it really can help you to maintain your relationship. One of the problems you will find following the birth of your first child is that the spontaneity you had as a free and easy couple does tend to get rather lost, so planning to spend time together becomes vitally important. It needn't be elaborate – it could be something as minor as always having a ritual drink together at the end of the day, or it could be planning to go swimming together for two hours every Sunday while a friend looks after your baby.

Time alone We all need time and space to recharge our batteries. When you have a baby it is very easy to get so caught up in the never-ending round of babycare that you lose sight of this need.

It is very important that you arrange to have at least a few hours every week when you can just please yourself, whether that be planning a special outing, seeing a friend, or following a particular interest. Make an arrangement with someone you trust to babysit for you – your partner, a close friend, or relative. Not only will you benefit, your baby will also benefit from the social contact.

SHARING YOUR BABY'S CARE

You'll get many offers from friends and relatives to babysit. Take advantage of other people who are willing to share the care of your baby.

Father As far as your baby is concerned, her father is the second most important person in her life after you. Daddy can do anything that Mummy can – he can even give breast milk in a bottle, so encourage your partner to take equal responsibility for the care of your baby.

Grandparents Perhaps itching to help and thoroughly experienced in childrearing, her grandparents can be the ideal people to help with babysitting and general babycare. She and they will relish the contact, and this will help them to form strong bonds of affection from the very beginning.

Relatives and friends Your family will probably enjoy helping you look after the new addition to the family. Friends may also be enthusiastic about babycare – and the ones who have already had children can be invaluable. Always make sure that childless or young assistants know how to handle a baby properly, but try not to watch so closely or anxiously that you make them feel uncomfortable – young babies are more resilient than they look.

New parents

During Sue's pregnancy, Tiberio and Sue wanted to find out all they could about pregnancy, childbirth, and parenthood. They read books, attended antenatal classes, and got hands-on experience with friend's children. However, they realized that nothing totally prepares you for parenthood and that you have to be adaptable and flexible.

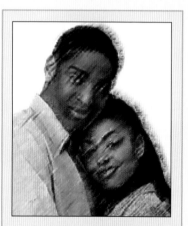

Names **Tiberio and Sue Benton**

Age **33 and 29 respectively**

Past medical history
Nothing abnormal

Obstetric history **Sue recently gave birth to a baby girl weighing 7lb 5oz**

Tiberio works in an engineering firm; Sue is a secretary in a large pharmaceutical company. Tiberio and Sue had been waiting for the right time to have a baby – until they realized that there was no such thing as a right time. After moving to a larger house, Sue talked to her personnel manager about maternity rights. Sue then gave up alcohol, examined her diet, and came off the pill. Tiberio cut down his smoking to under five a day, and moderated his alcohol intake. Sue became pregnant a few months later.

MAKING PLANS

Tiberio and Sue agreed from the start that parenthood should be a shared responsibility. Sue was determined not to stay at home playing the role of a traditional mother and, as her company operates flexitime, she planned to go back to work three months after the baby had been born. Tiberio was concerned about how much their lifestyle would have to change but Sue assured him newborn babies are very portable so wherever they went, the baby could go too. Having discussed the different issues and thought about how they would manage, they felt reassured about being able to cope with parenthood.

THE BIRTH EXPERIENCE

I had advised Sue and Tiberio to acquire some basic facts about birth and the types of birth that were available in their area so that they could make a birth plan and discuss their choices from an informed standpoint. They visited their local hospital, talked to the staff, read books, and made a birth plan for a hospital birth with a request for no drugs and no episiotomy if at all possible.

When Sue went into labour, however, she found that she was finding it increasingly difficult to cope with the intensity of the labour pains. Tiberio found it hard to see her in such pain, although he managed to remain calm, supportive, and encouraging. Towards the end of the first stage, when her contractions were coming very close together, Sue was becoming tense and distressed, and eventually she asked for pain relief. Tiberio encouraged and praised her, and helped her to change position. However, she still found the contractions difficult to cope with, so the midwife gave her a small dose (50mg) of pethidine, which took effect quite quickly. This helped Sue to relax and stay calm.

About an hour later, Sue was found to be fully dilated and she started to push. The baby's head didn't take long to crown. At this point the midwife urged Sue to stop pushing so that the perineum had time to stretch fully. Sue allowed her contractions to push her baby out and moments later Emma was born.

Postnatal feelings

Sue and Tiberio fell in love with Emma as soon as she was born. Tiberio couldn't get over how tiny and perfect she was, while Sue's maternal feelings were very strong from the start. However, Sue also felt a touch guilty that she hadn't managed to have Emma without painkillers, although she was sensible and tried not to let this detract from the pleasure and pride she took in Emma's birth. I told Sue that it's impossible to know your own pain threshold in advance, and that she shouldn't feel guilty about requesting pain relief that was essential. Sue and Tiberio have a normal, healthy baby girl and Sue has every reason to be proud of herself and all that she has achieved.

BECOMING NEW PARENTS

In the first few days after the birth, Tiberio and Sue found that friends and relations were keen to offer advice. Although they occasionally found this irritating, they also appreciated that much of this advice reflected other parents' own experience and was often illuminating and reassuring.

Everyday care

When Sue and Tiberio had to deal with the day-to-day care of their newborn baby, they were quite shocked at just how much was demanded of them. For the first ten days Tiberio was at home, but even with two of them, the round of feeding and changing, with short periods of sleep in between, seemed endless.

Sue wondered how she would ever be able to manage on her own and wished that she was going back to work while Tiberio stayed at home to look after the baby. She told me that on her first day alone she had felt abandoned, like a new girl at primary school. However, she coped – despite feeling that she had never been so exhausted in her life – and, as

Emma started to respond to her and then to smile properly, she confessed that she was rather surprised to find that she really enjoyed being with her and looking after her. She also made friends with other new mothers in her area, which gave her an opportunity to compare notes with friends who understood exactly how she felt and what she was experiencing.

Sue and Tiberio managed to socialize with their friends more than they'd ever thought they would be able to because, just as Sue had said, Emma proved to be very portable. They even managed to take Emma abroad on a short holiday.

A new perspective

Work felt as if it was in the very distant past for Sue and she found she wasn't looking forward to going back as much as she had expected. Tiberio enjoyed being back at work, despite finding the disturbed nights a bit of a strain.

He found himself really looking forward to coming home in the evening, seeing and cuddling Emma, and chatting to Sue about what had happened during her day. He was pleased that Sue was enjoying being at home, but he soon realized that they couldn't afford to keep up with their mortgage payments unless Sue returned to her job.

Consequently, Sue returned to work as she had arranged with her employers and Emma was cared for during the day by Sue's mother until Sue came to pick her up at 4.30p.m.

Although things were exactly as Sue had planned them before Emma's birth, she no longer had quite the same feelings about motherhood being restrictive as she had earlier. She confessed that if Tiberio had been earning enough for them to manage, she would have changed her mind about returning to work so soon and become a full-time mum, at least until Emma went to nursery.

TIBERIO AND SUE'S BABY

Sue breastfed Emma until she returned to work, which gave Emma a flying start. In addition, Sue expressed milk for Emma for an extra two months after she returned to work.

• She enjoyed the close contact that she had with her mother during her first three months of her life.

• While on maternity leave Sue made the effort to make friends with other new mothers who were at home with their babies so Emma has had the chance to mix

with other babies. As a result Emma is outgoing and sociable and has a ready-made circle of friends with whom she can play whenever Sue wants.

• She loves being with her father and mother during the evenings and at weekends.

• She has formed a close and loving bond with her grandparents, especially her grandmother who looks after her during the day now that Sue has returned to work.

369

USEFUL ADDRESSES

The Active Birth Centre
25 Bickerton Road,
London N19 5JT
Tel: 0171 482 5554
*Information and classes on
non-mechanized childbirth*

**AIMS (Association for
Improvements in Maternity
Services)**
2 Bacon Lane, Hayling Island,
Hampshire P011 ODN
Tel: 01753 652781

APEC (Action on Pre-eclampsia)
31–33 College Road,
Harrow, Middlesex HA1 IEJ
Tel: 01923 266778

**Association of Breastfeeding
Mothers**
PO Box 441, St Albans,
Hertfordshire AL4 OAS
Tel: 0171 813 1481
*24-hour telephone service for
breastfeeding mothers*

Association for Postnatal Illness
25 Jerdan Place,
London SW6 1BE
Tel: 0171 386 0868
*Advice for women with postnatal
illness, including depression*

Birthworks
Unit 4E, Brent Mill Trading
Estate, South Brent, Devon
TQ10 9YT
Tel: 01364 72802
*Advice on water births, videos for
sale, and birth pools for hire*

**BLISS (Baby Life Support
Systems)**
17–21 Emerald Street,
London WC1N 3QL
Tel: 0171 831 9393
*Helpline for parents of special needs
babies*

British Diabetic Association
10 Queen Anne Street,
London W1M 0BD
Tel: 0171 323 1531
Advice for pregnant diabetic women

Down's Syndrome Association
155 Mitcham Road,
London SW17 9PG
Tel: 0181 682 4001
*Advice on the care of children with
Down's syndrome*

**FRES (Federation of
Recruitment and Employment
Services)**
36–38 Mortimer Street,
London W1N 7RB
Tel: 0171 323 4300
*Send SAE for a list of nanny and
au pair agencies*

The National Fertility Association
114 Lichfield Street,
Walsall WS1 1SZ
Tel: 01922 722888
*Information and support for people
experiencing infertility*

**Independent Midwives'
Association**
1 The Great Quarry,
Guildford, Surrey, GU1 3XN
Tel: 01483 821104
*Send SAE for register of midwives
offering private care*

**MAMA (Meet-a-Mum
Association)**
Cornerstone House
14 Willis Road,
Croydon CRO 2XX
Tel: 0181 771 5595
*Help for new parents, especially
mothers with postnatal depression*

Maternity Alliance
15 Britannia Street,
London WC1X 9JP
Tel: 0171 837 1265
*Advice and information about
maternity rights and benefits*

Miscarriage Association
c/o Clayton Hospital,
Northgate, Wakefield,
West Yorkshire WF1 3JS
Tel: 01924 200799
*Advice and information on a
national network of miscarriage
support groups*

National Childbirth Trust
Alexandra House,
Oldham Terrace,
Acton, London W3 6NH
Tel: 0181 992 8637
Antenatal classes and postnatal help

**National Council for
One Parent Families**
255 Kentish Town Road,
London NW5 2LX
Tel: 0171 428 5400
Advice and referral service

**PAL (Parents Anonymous
[London])**
6 Manor Gardens,
London N7 6LA
Tel: 0171 263 8918
24-hour helpline for stressed parents

Rowe & Maw (public law group)
20 Blackfriars Lane,
London EC4V 6HD
Tel: 0171 248 4282
Legal advice on fertility and surrogacy

Royal College of Midwives
15 Mansfield Street,
London W1M 0BE
Tel: 0171 312 3535

**SANDS (Stillbirth and
Neonatal Death Society)**
28 Portland Place,
London W1N 4DE
Tel: 0171 436 5881
*National support network for
bereaved parents*

**TAMBA (Twins and Multiple
Birth Association)**
Harnott House,
309 Chester Road, Little Sutton,
Ellesmere Port CH66 1QQ
Tel: 0151 348 0020
*Provides encouragement and support
for parents of multiple birth babies*

Women's Health
52 Featherstone Street
London EC1Y 8RT
Tel: 0171 251 6580
*Telephone service or send SAE for
advice on reproductive health*

INDEX

emotions 360–3
exercises 358–9
health 354–7
Postpartum haemorrhage 223, 291
Posture, in pregnancy 69, 88, 160
Pre-eclampsia 70, 224, 226–7
Pre-labour 270–1
Pregnancy
antenatal care 174–89
body care 158–61
complaints 206–13
emergencies 218–27
exercise 144–51
food 128–39
late stages 258–9
preparation for 8, 16–27
signs of 60–1, 72
tests 61–2
trimesters 66–89
Premature babies 80, 84, 348–9
breathing problems 299, 347, 349
special care units 344, 345, 346–7
Premature labour 298–9
Preserved food 139
Processed foods 138–9
Progesterone
and contraception 364
and infertility 42, 44
ovarian cycle 28, 29
postnatal emotions 360
in pregnancy 60, 72
sensual pregnancy 230
Projectile vomiting 199
Prolactin 43, 47, 326–7
Prolonged labour 296–7
Prostaglandins, induction of labour 300, 301
Proteins 131, 132, 134, 136, 137
Pudendal block 281
Puerperal psychosis 361
Pushing, in labour 284–5, 286, 289
Pyloric stenosis 199

QR

Quickening 78, 80, 194
Rashes
nappy rash 336, 338
in pregnancy 161
Reflex actions, newborn baby 320–1
Registering birth 323
Relaxation
in labour 289
massage 152–3
pain relief 125
in pregnancy 151, 258–9
Reproductive tract
female 28
male 31
Respiratory distress syndrome 198-9, 344–5
Rhesus incompatibility 54, 177, 185, 187, 200, 202–3, 342
Rib pain 212–13
Rights and benefits 64–5, 164
Rooting reflex 321, 328
Rubella *see* **German measles**

S

Safety
babies 243
food hazards 139
nurseries 241
in pregnancy 168–71
working mothers 164, 165, 169–70
Salmonella 139
Screening tests 184–5, 188–9
Seminal fluid (semen) 30
donor insemination 55
ejaculation 31
infertility tests 8, 39, 40–1
Sensual pregnancy 12, 230–7
Serum screening 184–5
Sex, of baby 31, 33, 81
Sex chromosomes, abnormalities 25
Sexual intercourse
after childbirth 100
after delivery 364–5
in pregnancy 69, 230–1, 234–7
Sexually transmitted diseases 19
Shivering 291
Shoes 162–3
Show 237, 267, 271
Shunt, urinary tract problems 201
Siblings *see* **Children**
Sickle-cell anaemia 25, 26, 178, 186
Sight
newborn baby 320
in unborn child 192, 193
Single parenthood 166–7
Sit-ups 145
Skin
birthmarks 318
care of 158
newborn baby 316, 318
pigmentation 68, 69, 78, 158–9, 161, 231
in pregnancy 74, 158–9
problems 161
stretch marks 80, 159
Sleep
after delivery 356
baby 102
in pregnancy 71, 84, 88, 210–11, 258
Slings 242
Small-for-dates babies 344
Smell, sense of 61
Smoking 16
Sneezing, newborn baby 321
Socks 163
Sonicaid 178, 265
Special care babies 344–9
Sperm
donor insemination 49, 54, 55
ejaculation 30, 31
fertilization 32–3
genes 22, 23
infertility 34, 38–41
infertility treatments 49, 52
production of 30
and sex of baby 31
Spider veins 80, 159
Spina bifida 17, 20–1, 197, 293
Sports 144–5

Squatting 151
Squint 318
Step reflex 320
Sterilization, bottlefeeding equipment 332, 333
Sterilization, reversal of 47
"Sticky eye" 317–18
Stillbirth 261, 312
Stitches
Caesarean section 309, 311, 322–3
episiotomy 110, 293, 355
Stockings 163
Stork bites 318
Strawberry birthmarks 318
Stretch marks 80, 159
Stretching exercises 146–7
Sucking reflex 321
Superstitions 156
Surgery
Caesarean section 308–11
fetal 200–1
infertility treatment 46, 47
Surrogate mothers 54, 55
SUZI (sub-zonal insemination) 49
Swimming 145, 182
Syntocinon 291, 297
Syntometrine 116, 265, 291, 311

T

Tailor sitting 150
Tay-Sachs disease 25, 26
Tears, perineum 109–10, 285, 291
Teats, bottlefeeding 333, 334
Teeth, in pregnancy 159
Teething rings 332
Television, safety 169
Temperature
after delivery 291
baby's 343
TENS 283
Tense-and-relax technique 258–9
Termination of pregnancy 189
TESE (testicular sperm extraction) 49, 52
Testes (testicles) 30, 38, 39
Testosterone 30
Thalassaemia 25, 178, 186
Thrush 18, 212–13
Tights 163
Tiredness
after delivery 356, 361
in labour 98, 277
loss of libido 236
in pregnancy 60, 71, 74, 164
Topping and tailing 340
Toxoplasmosis 139, 169, 178
Toys 241
Trains 171
Transition stage 273, 279
Travel
to hospital 267
in pregnancy 171
with baby 242
Trial of labour 298, 308
Trimesters 66–89
first 66–7, 72–5
second 68–9, 76–85

ACKNOWLEDGMENTS

PHOTOGRAPHY Ranald Mackechnie
ILLUSTRATIONS Annabel Milne: 23, 28, 29, 31, 33, 45, 109, 183, 186, 203, 219–221, 224, 271, 273, 275, 281, 298, 301, 329 Howard Pemberton: 45, 73, 75, 77, 79, 81, 83, 85, 87, 89, 286, 287, 309
MEDICAL CONSULTANTS Dr. Sarah Reynolds; Dr Sarah Temple Gwen Atwood; Leonora Branski; Dr. Nigel Brown; Dr. Felicity Challoner; Prof. Geoffrey Chamberlain; The Hallam Medical Centre; Dr. Kypros Nicolaides; Prof. Cheryl Tickle; Dr. Robert Whittle
FILM OUTPUTTING Brightside
ADDITIONAL EDITORIAL ASSISTANCE Jane Cooke; Kathy Fahey
ADDITIONAL DESIGN ASSISTANCE Johnny Pau; Chris Walker
MODELS: Deanne Barnes; Joe and Jack; Sharon Caines; Nagihan Tunali Caykara and Nyazi; Charlotte Chance; Lyndel Donaldson; Hilary and David Goodman, and Alexander; Jashu Halat; Amy Lewis; Susan Lipman and Stephanie; David Todd
EQUIPMENT Mothercare UK Ltd – maternity and baby clothes; equipment and toys
ADDITIONAL PHOTOGRAPHY Dave King;

David Murray; Ray Moller; Stephen Oliver; Susanna Price; Jules Selmes
INDEX Hilary Bird
PICTURE CREDITS The publisher would like to thank the following for their kind permission to reproduce their photographs: (Abbreviations key: t=top, b=below, r=right, l=left, c=centre, a=above).
Ace Photo Agency: 350-351; **Attard:** 14-15; **CARE: Centres for Assisted Reproduction, Nottingham:** 52cr; **Collections:** Anthea Sieveking 126-127, 125r, 281br, 307; **Family Life Picture Library/Angela Hampton:** 172-173; **Genesis:** 81b; 81tl; 83b; **Sally & Richard Greenhill:** 106b; 115bl; 117bl; 121bl; 284b; 286b; 287t c b; 290cl; 318bc; 318bl; 318br; 347br; **Howard Sochurek/Hillelson:** 75t; 77b; 85br; 87br; 87tl; 89cl; 181b; **Hutchison:** 293br; 316bl; **Image Bank:** Marc Romanelli 58-59; Tosca Radigonda 2-3, 90-91; **Images Colour Library:** 228-229; **Marcia May:** 262-263; **Mother & Baby Picture Library:** 204-205; **University of Nottingham:** 39b; **Parthenon Publishing Group:** Dr John Yovich 41t; **Science

Photo Library: 23tr; 29br; 30l; 32bl; 32br; 32cl; 32tl; 33c; 39cr; 39tr; 45c; 45tr; 73br; 73tl; 75b; 77t; 79b; 79t; 85tl; 137t; 193bl; 338tr; Andy Walker 338tl; Antonia Reeve 45b; Bsip Bajande 346-347; David Leah 42cl; Hank Morgan 48bl; 50b, 139br; Hattie Young 24bl; James Stevenson 30br; 347cb; John Greim 347ca; John Walsh 40bl; Manfred Kage 345bl; Moredun Animal Health Ltd 309l; P M Motta & S Makabe 42bl; Peter Ryan 364bc; Petit Format/CSI 50cr, 353br; Secchi 199bl; Stevie Grand 40bl, 89br, 346cl; **Dr I D Sullivan:** 196cl; **Telegraph Colour Library:** 252bl; Antonio Mo 111, 235; Genna Naccache 104-105; Ian McKinnell 319; J Cummins 238-239; John Slater 331; Mel Yates 294-295; Sana: Martine Loornis 190-191; V.C.L 251; **Tony Stone Images:** 33b; 292b; Chris Harvey 1, 179; David Joel 347cl; Dennis O'Clair 103, 314-315; Lori Adamski Peek 142-143; Philip & Karen Smith 216-217; **The Wellcome Trust:** 52tl; 309br; **Zefa Picture Library:** Howard Sochurek 183cr.